GRAINGER & ALLISON'S DIAGNOSTIC RADIOLOGY

Interventional Radiology

SIXTH EDITION

GRAINGER & ALLISON'S DIAGNOSTIC RADIOLOGY

Interventional Radiology

SIXTH EDITION

EDITED BY

Anna-Maria Belli, FRCR, EBIR

Michael J. Lee, MSc, FRCPI, FRCR, FFR (RCSI), FSIR, EBIR

Andreas Adam, CBE, MB, BS(Hons), PhD, FRCP, FRCR, FRCS, FFRRCSI(Hon), FRANZCR(Hon), FACR(Hon), FMedSci

ELSEVIER

London   New York   Oxford   Philadelphia   St Louis   Sydney   Toronto

ELSEVIER

ISBN: 978-0-7020-6933-8

Executive Content Strategist: Michael Houston
Content Development Specialist: Louise Cook
Project Manager: Andrew Riley
Design: Christian Bilbow
Marketing Manager: Rachael Pignotti

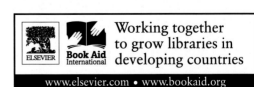

Working together to grow libraries in developing countries

www.elsevier.com • www.bookaid.org

Contents

PREFACE

The 11 chapters in this book have been selected from the contents of the Interventional Radiology section in *Grainger & Allison's Diagnostic Radiology, Sixth Edition*. These chapters provide a succinct up-to-date overview of current imaging techniques and their clinical applications in daily practice and it is hoped that with this concise format the user will quickly grasp the fundamentals they need to know. Throughout these chapters, the relative merits of different procedures and techniques are described, variations are discussed and recent imaging advances are detailed.

Grainger & Allison's Diagnostic Radiology has long been recognized as the standard general reference work in the field, and it is hoped that this book, utilizing the content from the latest sixth edition of this classic reference work, will provide radiology trainees and practitioners with ready access to the most current information, written by internationally recognized experts, on what is new and important in the subspecialty field of interventional radiology.

LIST OF CONTRIBUTORS

Anna-Maria Belli, FRCR, EBIR
Professor of Interventional Radiology; Consultant
  Radiologist, Radiology Department, St George's
  Healthcare NHS Trust, London, UK

David J. Breen, MRCP, FRCR
Consultant Abdominal Radiologist; Honorary
  Senior Lecturer in Radiology, Department of
  Radiology, Southampton University Hospitals,
  Southampton, UK

Joo-Young Chun, MBBS, MSc, MRCS, FRCR
Consultant Interventional Radiologist, Royal London
  Hospital, Barts Health NHS Trust, London, UK

**Bhaskar Ganai, BSc(MedSci) Hons, MBChB, MRCS,
FRCR, EBIR**
Lecturer in Interventional Radiology, Royal College
  of Surgeons in Ireland, Department of Radiology,
  Beaumont Hospital, Dublin, Ireland

Christopher J. Hammond, BMBCh, MA, MRCS, FRCR
Consultant Vascular Radiologist, Department of
  Radiology, Leeds General Infirmary, Leeds, UK

James E. Jackson, FRCP, FRCR
Consultant Radiologist, Department of Imaging,
  Hammersmith Hospital, London, UK

Konstantinos Katsanos, MSc, MD, PhD, EBIR
Consultant Vascular and Interventional Radiologist,
  Endovascular, Spine and Interventional Oncology,
  Department of Interventional Radiology, Guy's and
  St Thomas' Hospitals, London, UK

Aoife N. Keeling, FFRRCSI, MRCPI, MSc
Consultant Interventional Radiologist, Beaumont
  Hospital, Dublin, Ireland

**Michael J. Lee, MSc, FRCPI, FRCR, FFRRCSI,
FSIR, EBIR**
Professor of Radiology, Royal College of Surgeons in
  Ireland; Consultant Interventional Radiologist,
  Beaumont Hospital, Dublin, Ireland

Michael M. Maher, MD, FRCSI, FRCR, FFRRCSI
Professor of Radiology, University College Cork;
  Consultant Radiologist, Cork University Hospital
  and Mercy University Hospital, Cork, Ireland

James F.M. Meaney, FRCR
Consultant Radiologist; Director, Centre for Advanced
  Medical Imaging, St James's Hospital, Dublin,
  Ireland

Robert A. Morgan, MB ChB, MRCP, FRCR, EBIR
Consultant Vascular and Interventional Radiologist,
  Radiology Department, St George's NHS Trust,
  London, UK

Richard J. Morse, MBBS, MRCP, FRCR
Consultant Radiologist, Royal Cornwall Hospital,
  Truro, Cornwall, UK

Jonathan G. Moss, MB ChB, FRCS(Ed), FRCR
Professor of Interventional Radiology, Department of
  Radiology, North Glasgow University Hospitals,
  Gartnavel General Hospital, Glasgow, UK

**Anthony A. Nicholson, BSc, MSc, MB, ChB, FRCR,
FFRRCSI(Hon), FCIRSE, EBIR**
Consultant Vascular and Interventional Radiologist,
  Leeds Teaching Hospitals, Leeds, UK

**Owen J. O'Connor, MD, FFRRCSI, MB, BCh,
BAO, BMedSci**
Inerventional Radiology Fellow, Radiology,
  Massachusetts General Hospital, Boston, MA, USA

Uday Patel, MB ChB, MRCP, FRCR
Consultant Radiologist, Department of Radiology,
  St George's Hospital, London, UK

Lakshmi Ratnam, MBChB, MRCP, FRCR
Consultant Interventional Radiologist, Radiology,
  St George's Hospital, London, UK

Jim Reekers, MD, PhD, EBIR
Professor of Radiology, Department of Radiology,
  Academic Medical Centre Amsterdam, University of
  Amsterdam, The Netherlands

**Elizabeth E. Rutherford, BMedSci, MBBS,
MRCS, FRCR**
Consultant Radiologist, University Hospitals
  Southampton NHS Trust, Southampton, UK

Tarun Sabharwal, FRCR, FRCRI, EBIR, FRSIR, FCIRSE
Consultant Interventional Radiologist, Clinical Lead
  Interventional Radiology, Guy's and St Thomas'
  Hospitals, London, UK

Beth Shepherd, MBBS, MA(Cantab), MRCS, FRCR
Radiology Registrar, University Hospital Southampton NHS Foundation Trust, Southampton, Hampshire, UK

Anthony Watkinson, BSc, MSc, MBBS, FRCS, FRCR, EBIR
Consultant Radiologist, The Royal Devon and Exeter Hospital; Honorary Professor of Interventional Radiology, The Peninsula Medical School, Exeter, UK

Reddi Prasad Yadavali, MBBS, MRCS, FRCR, EBIR
Consultant Interventional Radiologist, Department of Radiology, Aberdeen Royal Infirmary; Honorary Senior Clinical Lecturer, School of Medicine and Dentistry, University of Aberdeen, Aberdeen, UK

CHAPTER 1

Basic Clinical Requirements of Interventional Radiology

Jim Reekers

IR

Interventional radiology (IR) is a recognised subspecialty of radiology both within the Union of European Medical Specialties (UEMS) and the European Society of Radiology (ESR). IR is unique and distinct from all other surgical, radiological and medical subspecialties and specialties.

IR is performed by trained IR specialists who have expertise in interpreting diagnostic imaging as well as expertise in image-guided minimally invasive procedures and techniques as applied to various diseases and organs. There are a huge variety of therapeutic procedures performed by IR. They can be divided into broad categories of vascular, non-vascular and oncological interventions. For a more detailed description of IR and what interventional radiologists do, please read the Global Statement on IR.[1]

TRAINING

Training in IR should be under an accredited training programme and the minimum length of training is 2 years. In several countries there are special training curricula for IR and there is also a European IR training curriculum which can be viewed at <http://www.cirse.org>.

There is a European IR examination which can be taken by every interventional radiologist after the completion of training. This examination is called the European Board of Interventional Radiology (EBIR) and is held under the auspices of an independent European Board. Maintenance of IR skills by performing an adequate number and range of procedures and demonstration of continuous medical education by CME certification is an essential requirement.

CLINICAL INVOLVEMENT

Interventional radiology involves interaction with patients and their families, taking decisions and judging outcome and risks. Most important is the clinical evaluation and management of patients with diseases or conditions amenable to image-guided interventions. The IR as a clinician should keep the following questions in mind when entering into a patient consultation: Is the proposed procedure necessary? Is the patient suitable or fit for the procedure? What is the potential for harm? Are there better alternatives for the patient?

For these reasons an IR should be clinically trained. Clinical involvement may include seeing patients in consultation particularly for complex treatments (see the next section), but this is not always feasible and for more routine work it is often not necessary. It is becoming more common for IRs to have their own clinics and beds. Access to day case and inpatient beds is necessary to optimise provision of an IR service. An on-call service should also be provided on a 24/7 basis, which means having an adequate number of IRs available or providing an on-call service through formation of a network of IRs from adjacent hospitals.

INFORMED CONSENT

Informed consent is an essential requirement in contemporary medicine, especially in cases where there is clinical equipoise, as is sometimes the case in IR treatments. Informed consent should be based on an ethical assessment of the clinical situation, including the invasiveness of the procedure, the clinical indications and not simply on practical issues. Focusing on the whole decision-making process, effective communication and an individualised approach to consent is essential, also because it will reduce much of the patient's anxiety for the procedure to follow. A combination of information both written and verbal is often the best approach. Informed consent should ideally be obtained by the operator performing the procedure or, if this is not possible, the task can be delegated to a suitably trained doctor. Informed consent should also be obtained at least 24 h before any procedure so that the patient has time to digest the information and make an informed decision. The risks, intended benefits and alternatives should be discussed with the patient and any follow-up care that is planned should be itemised. Informed consent is a prerequisite for good clinical IR practice as IR is increasingly the first line of treatment and the interventional radiologist the primary clinician.[1]

IR CHECKLIST

In 2009, Haynes et al. published the results of a study which implemented a 19-item surgical safety checklist to determine whether this checklist could reduce complications and deaths associated with surgery.[2] A significant reduction in the rate of death and complications occurred after the introduction of the surgical safety checklist. The death rate fell from 1.5% before the introduction of the checklist to 0.8% afterwards. The complication rate fell from 11 to 7%. Although complications in IR are significantly fewer than with surgery, patient contact before IR procedures is often quite short, and sometimes it is difficult for the interventionalist to gather all the necessary clinical information in a timely manner. This increases the risk of complications. A standarised checklist has the advantage of ensuring that human error, in terms of forgetting key steps in patient preparation,

intraprocedural care and postoperative care are not overlooked.[3] This checklist can be downloaded and modified through <http://www.cirse.org/files/files/Profession/IR_Checklist_new.pdf>.

However, the patient safety checklist is only one part of a comprehensive patient safety strategy. Regular morbidity and mortality meetings, reporting of errors, participation in hospital risk management committees and a culture of patient safety are all important items in the overall strategy for patient safety. In an ideal world, competence should match performance but this is not always the case. Performance may be hindered by both system and individual influences. Individual influences on performance can be aided by a lifelong commitment to learning, while system influences may be difficult to deal with and may involve not peforming some procedures if the necessary support is not available locally.

COAGULATION

Management of coagulation status and haemostasis risk in percutaneous image-guided interventions is very important. Haemorrhage is a major complication of IR procedures and guidelines for the management of coagulation status and haemostasis risk are available.[4] IR procedures can be divided into two categories: those with low and those with moderate risk of bleeding. For each category special attention should be given to the clotting status of the patient. In elective treatments, the coagulation status should be optimised unless there are other important contraindications to stopping anticoagulation. General rules for haemostasis management are given in Table 1-1.

TABLE 1-1   IR Procedure Categories: Haemorrhagic Risk

Low Risk of Haemorrhage		
Vascular	• INR: Routinely recommended for patients receiving warfarin anticoagulation or with known or suspected liver disease	• INR > 2.0: Threshold for treatment (i.e., FFP, vitamin K)
• Dialysis access interventions		• PTT: No consensus
• Venography		• Platelets: Transfusion recommended for counts < 50,000/µL
• Central line removal	• Activated PTT: Routinely recommended for patients receiving intravenous unfractionated heparin	
• IVC filter placement		
• PICC line placement		
Non-Vascular		
• Drainage catheter exchange		
• Superficial abscess drainage		
Moderate Risk of Haemorrhage		
Vascular	• INR: Routinely recommended for patients receiving warfarin anticoagulation or with known or suspected liver disease	• INR: Correct above 1.5.
• Angiography, arterial and venous intervention with access size up to 7Fr		• Activated PTT: No consensus (trend toward correcting for values _1.5 times control, 73%)
Non-Vascular	• Activated PTT: Routinely recommended for patients receiving intravenous unfractionated heparin	• Platelets: Transfusion recommended for counts > 50,000/µL
• Intra-abdominal, chest wall or retroperitoneal abscess drainage or biopsy		• Hematocrit: No recommended threshold for transfusion
• Lung biopsy		• Plavix (clopidogrel): Withhold for 5 days before procedure
• Transabdominal liver biopsy (core needle)		• Aspirin: Do not withhold
• Percutaneous cholecystostomy		• Low-molecular-weight heparin (therapeutic dose): Withhold one dose before procedure
• Gastrostomy tube: initial placement		
• Radiofrequency ablation: straightforward		
• Spine procedures (vertebroplasty, kyphoplasty, lumbar puncture, epidural injection, facet block)		

CONTRAST MEDIUM ALLERGY

Contrast medium carries a risk for allergic reactions, but this has been reduced to a very low level since the advent of low-osmolar contrast media. A treatment protocol for anaphylaxis and allergy should be available in the interventional suite. Patients with known previous allergic reactions to contrast media should be pretreated with steroids. An oral regimen often used is dose 1, prednisone 50 mg 13 h prior; dose 2, prednisone 50 mg 7 h prior; and dose 3 (final dose), prednisone 50 mg 1 h prior to the intervention. If oral prednisone is not an option for the patient one of the following equivalent alternatives should be considered: 8 mg Decadron (dexamethasone) IV × 3 doses starting 13 h prior to intervention or 200 mg Solu-Cortef (hydrocortisone) × 3 doses starting 13 h prior to the procedure.

KIDNEY FUNCTION

Low-osmolar contrast medium has a small but definite benefit over high-osmolar contrast media for patients with pre-existing renal impairment.[5] Pre-procedural hydration may have a protective effect in high-risk patients and some newer drugs may also have a role in protection from contrast medium-induced nephrotoxicity (CIN). For the purposes of this standard, CIN as a major complication is clinically defined as an elevation of serum creatinine requiring care which delays discharge or results in unexpected admission, readmission or permanent impairment of renal function. This definition focuses on the outcome of renal impairment, which is the central issue in any monitoring programme. The threshold chosen is 0.2% and is based on consensus and a review of the pertinent literature. Three factors have been associated with an increased risk of contrast-induced nephropathy: pre-existing renal insufficiency (such as creatinine clearance <60 mL/min (1.00 mL/s)), pre-existing diabetes and reduced intravascular volume.

Adenosine antagonists such as the methylxanthines theophylline and aminophylline may help, although studies have produced conflicting results. Administration of sodium bicarbonate 3 mL/kg/h for 1 h before, followed by 1 mL/kg/h for 6 h after administration of contrast medium was found superior to plain saline in one randomised controlled trial of patients with a creatinine level of at least 1.1 mg/dL (97.2 μmol/L).[6]

A randomised controlled trial involving patients with a creatinine over 1.6 mg/dL (140 μmol/L) or creatinine clearance below 60 mL/min studied the use of 1 mL/kg of 0.45% saline per hour for 6–12 h before and after the administration of contrast medium[7] and suggested that N-acetylcysteine (NAC) 600 mg orally twice a day, on the day before the procedure, *may* reduce nephropathy, but the results are inconclusive.

SEDATION AND PAIN MANAGEMENT

Sedation and pain management during IR procedures are becoming more important as many complex

TABLE 1-2   **Common Side Effects of Conscious Sedation**

Hypotension	• Volume replacement therapy by crystalloids or colloids • Sympathomimetic agents such as ephedrine (5–10 mg boluses) or phenylephrine (100 μg boluses)
Respiratory depression	• Reversal of narcotics by naloxone (0.1–0.3 mg IV every 30–60 s, with no specific maximum dose) • Reversal of benzodiazepines by flumazenil (0.2 mg IV every 60 s, usually up to 1 mg) • Respiratory support
Nausea	• Reversal with antiemetic agents
Prolonged sedation	• Reversal with naloxone or flumazenil

percutaneous procedures are performed without general anaesthesia. Sedation should, however, only be performed in those circumstances when adequate resuscitative equipment and organisational support are available. For more complex cases in ill patients and in instances where deep sedation is desired, the assistance of a dedicated anaesthetist is mandatory. Conscious sedation is often used in interventional procedures to minimise discomfort. There are three main categories: benzodiazepines, opioids and intravenous anaesthetics. The most common side effects of conscious sedation are described in Table 1-2.

Benzodiazepines

These drugs are reasonably safe to use during IR procedures, as their cardiorespiratory suppressive effects are minimal. However, even commonly used doses of benzodiazepines can cause apnoea. Therefore, it is important to adequately monitor patients receiving benzodiazepines. The most commonly used benzodiazepines include midazolam and lorazepam. Midazolam has a rapid onset and short duration of action, which makes it an ideal drug for most interventional procedures.

In patients where a benzodiazepine overdose occurs, **flumazenil** (0.2 mg IV every 60 s, usually up to 1 mg) should be administered.

Opioids

For most interventional radiological procedures, and especially for elderly patients, shorter-acting narcotics like fentanyl and alfentanil are preferred. The regular dose for fentanyl is 25–50 μg IV. Duration of effect becomes longer with higher doses/infusions

In case of opioid overdose, **naloxone** (0.1–0.3 mg IV every 30–60 s, with no specific maximum dose) should be administered.

Intravenous Anaesthetics

Ketamine and propofol can be used for conscious sedation in IR procedures. These drugs should, however, only be reserved for situations in which all necessary provisions for administration of general anaesthesia are available, which includes the participation of an anaesthetist.

COMPLICATIONS REGISTER

The periprocedural management of patients undergoing image-guided interventional procedures is continually evolving. Local factors such as procedure types and patient selection will influence management. In addition, advances in technology and image guidance may have a significant effect on periprocedural management. The use of arterial closure devices, smaller-gauge catheters and biopsy devices, adjunctive haemostatic measures such as postbiopsy tract plugging/embolisation and colour flow ultrasonography or computed tomographic fluoroscopy can affect the incidence of periprocedural haemorrhagic complications. One of the most effective methods of improving the safety of IR procedures is to maintain a local complication register and to hold a regular complication meeting. This should lead to improved local procedural guidelines, protocols for interventional radiological procedures and training.

THE INTERVENTIONAL RADIOLOGY SUITE

Common medications used during arterial interventions and their doses are indicated in Table 1-3.

INVENTORY

An inventory of interventional radiological devices, catheters and guidewires should be available. Also the essential materials to deal with complications, such as covered stents, in case of an arterial rupture after angioplasty, should be part of the inventory. In general it is recommended to keep the stock small, as technology changes rapidly and most devices have a limited period

TABLE 1-3   Doses of Common Medications Used during Arterial Interventions

Glyceryl trinitrate (nitroglycerin)	0.1 mg/mL/dose IA, repeated up to 3 times	Treatment of vasospasm
Heparin	75–100 IU/kg IV	Prevent arterial thrombosis
Protamine	10 mg IV per 1000 IU heparin	Heparin reversal
Papaverine	1 mg/kg IA	Treatment of vasospasm
Lidocaine	0.5 mL/kg (5 mg/kg) 1% (without adrenaline)	Local anaesthesia

of sterility. No specific recommendations can be given here and local practice will dictate how sufficient stock and stock control is achieved. In many European countries separate storage of interventional equipment outside the interventional room is required by hospital infection committees.[8]

REFERENCES

1. Kaufman JA, Reekers JA, Burnes JP, et al. Global statement defining interventional radiology. Cardiovasc Intervent Radiol 2010;33:672–4.
2. Haynes AB, Weiser TG, Berry WR, et al. A surgical safety checklist to reduce morbidity and mortality in a global population. N Engl J Med 2009;360:491–9.
3. Lee MJ, Fanelli F, Haage P, et al. Patient safety in interventional radiology: a CIRSE IR checklist. Cardiov Intervent Radiol 2012;35:244–6.
4. Malloy PC, Grassi CJ, Kundu S, et al. Consensus guidelines for periprocedural management of coagulation status and hemostasis risk in percutaneous image-guided interventions. J Vasc Interv Radiol 2009;20:S240–9.
5. Sigstedt B, Lunderquist A. Complications of angiographic examinations. Am J Roentgenol 1978;130:455–60.
6. Merten G, Burgess W, Gray L, et al. Prevention of contrast-induced nephropathy with sodium bicarbonate: a randomized controlled trial. JAMA 2004;291:2328–34.
7. Solomon R, Werner C, Mann D, et al. Effects of saline, mannitol, and furosemide to prevent acute decreases in renal function induced by radiocontrast agents. N Engl J Med 1994;331:1416–20.
8. Humphreys H, Coia JE, Stacey A, et al. Guidelines on the facilities required for minor surgical procedures and minimal access interventions. J Hosp Infect 2012;80:103–9.

CHAPTER 2

ANGIOGRAPHY: PRINCIPLES, TECHNIQUES AND COMPLICATIONS

James E. Jackson • James F.M. Meaney

INTRODUCTION

The non-invasive imaging of blood vessels continues to evolve and there have been significant new developments in cross-sectional imaging techniques since the 5th edition. As discussed in the previous edition of this textbook these have made many diagnostic catheter angiographic techniques almost obsolete; this is a welcome change as they are clearly less invasive and, therefore, safer and will in many instances give more diagnostic information than could be obtained by conventional catheter arteriography because of the concurrent visualisation of surrounding tissues and the ability to reconstruct the data in any plane.[1] A good understanding of the basic principles and techniques of catheter angiography remains essential, however, for those intending to become interventional radiologists and this information is still included in this chapter. The newer cross-sectional techniques for imaging blood vessels will, however, be discussed first as these will, quite rightly, be requested before (and often instead of) conventional catheter angiography.

Ultrasound plays a key role in a few areas, notably evaluation of the carotid bifurcation and follow-up of peripheral bypass grafts for patency, but it falls to CT and MR to provide detailed information of the vasculature for most other territories. The major advance in CT has been the introduction of multiple rows of detectors, which, in combination with a continuously rotating X-ray source and continuous table movement, allows rapid imaging of a large region of interest during first pass of an intravenously injected bolus. For MR, the key development has been the progressive increase in gradient speed, which, when coupled with parallel imaging that greatly increases acquisition speed, also allows rapid imaging of a large region of interest during first pass of an intravenously injected bolus. MR has the additional advantage that for some indications intravenous contrast injection is not necessary.

MULTIDETECTOR CT ANGIOGRAPHY (MDCTA) TECHNIQUES

The development of CT equipment combining a fan-shaped X-ray source, multiple detector rows and continuous table movement has led to the ability to acquire image data from a large tissue volume in a short time period.[1] Two major advantages result from rapid CTA acquisition times: firstly, blood vessels of the thorax and abdomen can be imaged during breath-holding; and secondly, it is possible to capture the relatively short 'arterial' phase following injection of contrast medium intravenously. Optimal imaging of the vessels during the first arterial passage of contrast material requires both a relatively rapid IV injection of iodinated contrast medium (usually 3–5 mL/s) to ensure adequate arterial opacification, and data acquisition at the appropriate time of vascular enhancement. The latter can be estimated based upon the 'expected' time of arrival of the contrast medium within the organ being imaged, but as this varies between patients it can be inaccurate and may result in poor-quality studies. These have been replaced by automated contrast bolus detection techniques in which the 'arrival' of contrast medium within a large vessel is measured on images obtained at a single level and data acquisition is initiated when a certain increase in density within the region of interest has been reached. 'Tight' boluses of contrast medium using a chaser of normal saline may be useful not only to improve vascular opacification but also to reduce the total volume of contrast medium required.

Rapid acquisition of images results in large data sets; for example, comprehensive evaluation of the peripheral vasculature from the level of the renal arteries to the feet with an acquired slice thickness of 0.8 mm will generate approximately 1500 images. Whilst all the diagnostic information is available in this data set, evaluation of the source images is not only extremely time-consuming but also confusing and is helped considerably by reconstruction of the data in axial, coronal and oblique planes without loss of resolution, so-called multiplanar reconstruction (MPR). Tortuous vessels can be 'straightened' by curved MPR to aid in the assessment of luminal narrowing caused by, for example, atheromatous disease or encasement by tumour. Maximum intensity projection (MIP) and volume rendering (VR) techniques are additional tools that help greatly in the assessment of blood vessels.[2] Each of these reconstruction techniques has its advantages and disadvantages:

1. *MPR* is very useful for the rapid review of blood vessels in any plane, including the relationship to surrounding bone and soft tissues. It also allows the assessment of vessel walls that might be obscured in MIP and VR techniques by, for example, calcification or endoluminal stents. Each image, however, gives only one 'slice' of information and multiple separate images are often required to demonstrate the vessel in its entirety.

2. *MIP techniques* produce a planar image from a volume of data within which the pixel values are determined by the highest voxel value in a ray projected along the data set in a specified direction. The images format mimics a conventional arteriogram but a disadvantage of this technique is that any tissue of high density (such as bone, fresh haematoma or vascular calcification) will be reprojected in the final image and may misrepresent the blood vessel. This is a common cause of overestimation of vascular stenoses.

3. *Volume-rendering techniques* assess the entire volume of data with an attenuation threshold for display and produce a three-dimensional image. Typically, tissues are assigned a colour that is dependent upon their attenuation values, facilitating the differentiation of structures of differing density. The final images can be rotated in real time to find the best projection to display anatomy and pathology and this is the most important feature of this technique. Vascular stenoses can be overestimated, however, and small vessels may not be clearly visualised.

It should be remembered that, whilst these postprocessing techniques are very helpful for diagnostic assessment and for display in multidisciplinary team meetings, the axial source images are essential and allow the operator to distinguish between artefact and disease when an abnormality is suggested on reformatted views.

MAGNETIC RESONANCE ANGIOGRAPHY (MRA) TECHNIQUES

Magnetic resonance angiography is a method for generating images of blood vessels with magnetic resonance imaging (MRI). With improved understanding of the nature of the signals emanating from blood vessels on MR images, it became evident that rather than simply contributing a source of artefacts on MR images, flow phenomena could be harnessed to generate diagnostic 'angiograms'.[3] Although MR angiograms can be generated without use of contrast medium, non-contrast techniques suffer from frequent artefacts and are time inefficient. Contrast-enhanced techniques, which can be completed within seconds rather than the several minutes of earlier methods, have revolutionised clinical practice over the last decade and extended the reach of MRA into all vascular territories with the exception of the coronary arteries.[3]

Contrast Mechanisms

Unenhanced Time-of-Flight (TOF) MRA

TOF angiography relies on the fact that the blood enters the volume under consideration with relatively high velocity and traverses it rapidly, so that it receives very few radio frequency (RF) pulses.[3] In order to maximise inflow effect, protons within the imaging volume must be replenished between successive repetition times (TRs), although maximal inflow may not be necessary in clinical practice and some trade-offs can be accepted. Oblique course of the blood vessel being imaged in relation to the slice orientation and short TRs adversely affect signal-to-noise ratios (SNR) as a result of protons under these circumstances experiencing more RF pulses whilst in the imaging slice. The severity and length of stenoses also tend to be overestimated on TOF MRA images because of intravoxel dephasing secondary to turbulent, slow or pulsatile flow.[3]

As a result of these limitations, TOF MRA has failed to offer a viable non-invasive screening alternative to conventional arteriography, and has not had a major impact on clinical practice outside the brain, where it remains the primary approach for evaluation of the intracranial arteries.

Phase-Contrast MRA

Phase-contrast angiography (PCA) is now seldom used in clinical MRA. The methodology underpinning the technique is somewhat complex and, like TOF MRA, images are prone to artefacts and data acquisition is lengthy.[4]

Contrast-Enhanced MRA (CEMRA)

Because of their unmatched high contrast-to-noise ratios, high spatial resolution, rapid speed of acquisition and relative freedom from artefacts, contrast-enhanced techniques have almost universally replaced non-contrast techniques in clinical practice.[5-9] Unlike TOF and PCA techniques, where the intravascular signal is dependent on inherent properties of flow and is, therefore, at the mercy of alterations in flow rate secondary to vascular disease, intravascular signal for contrast-enhanced MRA (CEMRA) depends on a T1 shortening effect induced by the injection of a paramagnetic contrast agent (usually gadolinium based). Images can, therefore, be acquired in any plane, including coronal, which affords the best anatomical coverage for virtually all vascular territories outside the brain.[5] In addition, the ability to exploit ultrafast 3D acquisitions (by using the shortest TRs possible and parallel imaging), allows rapid image acquisition that can easily be accommodated within a single breath-hold, an important factor when imaging in the chest and abdomen. In order to generate 'selective' arteriograms, images are acquired during the first arterial passage of the contrast agent before its arrival within the veins. The synchronisation of data acquisition with the peak arterial bolus is one of the major challenges of CEMRA, as the rate of transit of contrast medium from the peripheral vein injection site to the vessel of interest is affected by a number of factors, including heart rate, stroke volume and the presence or absence of proximal steno-occlusive lesions. Although the circulation time can be measured using a test bolus, or can be inferred by making some assumptions about the patient's cardiovascular status, the process is now automated by employing an MR fluoroscopic approach—a technique that demonstrates contrast medium arrival in real time on the display monitor, thus signalling the appropriate time for data acquisition.[7,8]

The unique nature of k-space (the array of data from which the final image is generated), whereby the central lines determine image contrast and the peripheral lines determine image resolution, can be uniquely exploited to generate CEMRA images with unrivalled signal-to-noise ratios. In situations where breath-holding is not required (e.g. vascular territories which do not move with respiration such as the peripheral arteries and carotid arteries), assuming acquisition of the contrast-defining central lines of k-space is completed during the arterial peak, the continued collection of resolution-defining peripheral lines of k-space during venous enhancement does not result in venous contamination of the images. CEMRA is now the standard of reference for MRA against which all new techniques must be measured.

New Non-Contrast Techniques

Because of concerns regarding nephrogenic systemic fibrosis,[10] there has been renewed interest in non-contrast techniques for body (extracranial) imaging where TOF and PCA techniques are limited.[11,12] A new family of 'balanced' techniques, where image contrast reflects the ratio of T1/T2, have been developed which portray the vessels as high signal structures. Background tissues are suppressed and either arteries or veins can be highlighted. In many instances the information provided allows contrast injection to be avoided.[11,12]

CLINICAL APPLICATIONS OF CTA AND MRA

Although CT and MR generate broadly similar angiographic images, the former is still favoured in many instances for a number of reasons: MR remains less widely available than CT especially out-of-hours and requires more expertise and operator input; although the

time required for acquisition of first pass contrast-enhanced MRA and CTA is similar, the set-up time for MRA is greater; and it is more difficult to monitor unstable patients in the MR environment.[1]

It is clear, however, that the role of MRA has markedly increased since the last edition of this book, particularly in elective studies of thoracic and abdominal vessels, and it remains important in patients in whom contrast medium is contraindicated.

Thorax
Thoracic Aorta and Great Arteries

Because of the relatively large size of these vessels, conditions such as aneurysms, stenoses, aberrant anatomy and the relationship between blood vessels and adjacent tumours are equally well demonstrated with both CTA or MRA (Figs. 2-1 and 2-2).[13,14] With improvements in spatial resolution, the blood supply to the thoracic cord can be delineated with either technique, information that is useful to the surgeon and helps prevent spinal cord infarction in patients undergoing repair of thoracic aortic aneurysms.

Pulmonary Arteries

CTA (CTPA – CT pulmonary angiography) has been the technique of choice for detection of pulmonary embolism for at least the last decade (Fig. 2-3).[15,16] Advantages include high accuracy compared to catheter angiography in a wide range of reported studies, wide availability (including out of hours), short total examination time, ease of patient monitoring during the study and a high degree of clinician confidence in the test. Although several studies have established high accuracy for MRA compared with pulmonary angiography for the evaluation of suspected pulmonary embolism, it is not widely used clinically[17,18] (Fig. 2-4). Reasons for this include a reluctance to refer potentially unstable patients to MRI and the availability of CT pulmonary angiography.

Improvements in spatial resolution for MRA and additional techniques, such as MR perfusion and ventilation (mirroring the ventilation and perfusion components of nuclear medicine studies albeit at much higher resolution), offer additional functionality to determine the location and distribution of small emboli and may improve the acceptability of MR for PE.[17,18]

Abdomen
Abdominal Aorta and Abdominal Veins

Assessment of the abdomen in virtually all patients with suspected acute vascular emergencies such as abdominal aortic aneurysm rupture and acute mesenteric ischaemia is performed with CTA but the elective assessment of vascular pathology within the abdomen can be performed with either CTA or MRA.[5 7,19,20] Abdominal aortic aneurysm morphology can be equally well assessed by CTA and MRA (external dimensions, tortuosity and relationship to visceral arteries) but calcium within the wall is

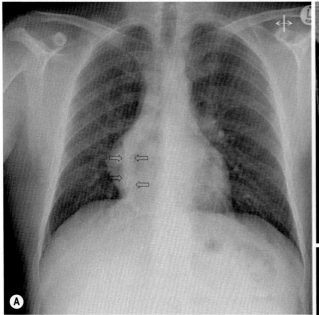

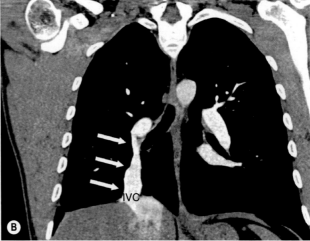

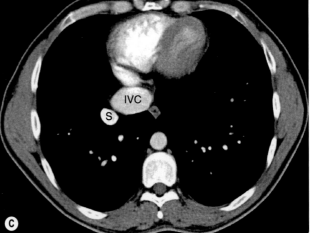

FIGURE 2-1 ■ **Asymptomatic patient undergoing pre-operative assessment.** CXR (A) shows an unusual tubular structure (arrows) projected behind the right heart border. Coronal reformat (B) from CTA demonstrates an abnormal vein (arrows) draining from the right lung into the IVC. The axial source image (C) demonstrates the vein (S) just before it joins the IVC. The appearance is that of a Scimitar syndrome, a variant or anomalous pulmonary venous drainage in which part or all of the right lower lobe drains into the inferior vena cava.

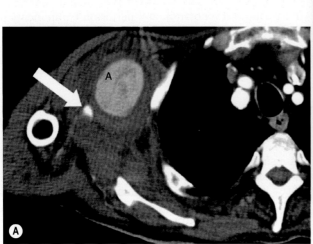

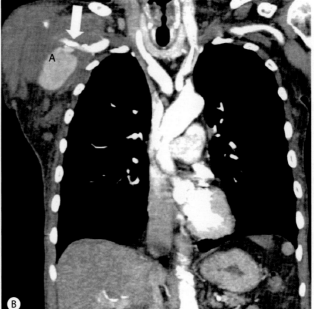

FIGURE 2-2 ■ **Patient with embolic episode to right arm.** CTA in axial (A), coronal (B), sagittal (C) reformat demonstrates a large pseudoaneurysm arising from the subclavian artery (denoted by the arrow). The arrow denotes the subclavian artery and A, the aneurysm sac in all 3 parts.

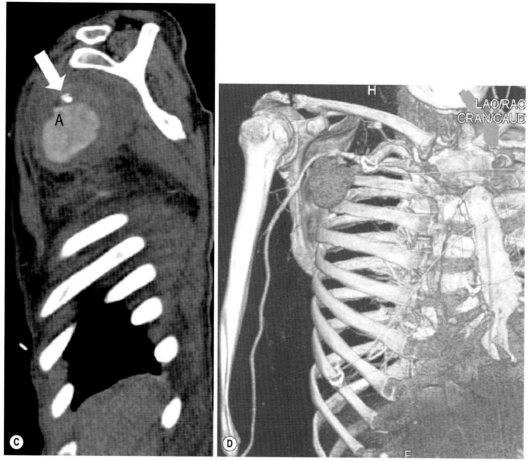

FIGURE 2-2, Continued ■ Surface shaded display (D) shows the relationship of the aneurysm to the parent artery and the status of the distal run-off arteries.

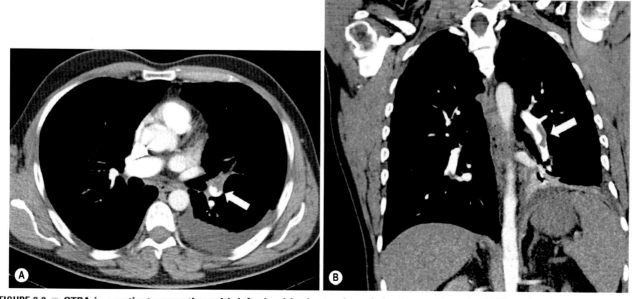

FIGURE 2-3 ■ **CTPA in a patient presenting with left pleuritic chest pain and shortness of breath.** (A) There is a large filling defect within the left lower lobe pulmonary artery (arrow) consistent with acute pulmonary embolism. Coronal reformat (B) confirms the extensive clot (arrow).
Continued on following page

better demonstrated by CTA; for this reason aneurysm assessment before and after endovascular stenting is usually performed with CTA.[19]

Thrombosis of the spleno-portal system or IVC is usually detected by performing delayed imaging after acquisition of the arterial phase for CTA or MRA (Fig. 2-5). An advantage of MRA is that venographic images can also be acquired using a non-contrast technique.

Renal, Mesenteric and Hepatic Arteries

The assessment of native and transplant renal arteries and the staging of hepatopancreaticobiliary neoplasm is well

performed with both CTA and MRA, supplemented by additional standard imaging of the parenchyma as indicated.[19,20] CEMRA, however, has many advantages for imaging the renal arteries and proximal mesenteric arteries.[10] (Fig. 2-6). Numerous studies and meta-analyses attest to the accuracy of MRA in the assessment of significant visceral artery stenotic disease.[8] An additional significant benefit of MRA lies in its ability to measure

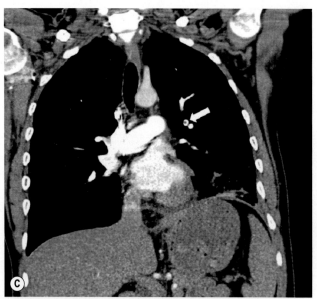

FIGURE 2-3, Continued ■ (C) A more anterior image confirms further embolism to the upper lobe pulmonary artery (Arrow points to filling defect of embolus within the artery).

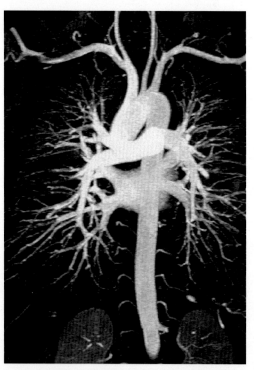

FIGURE 2-4 ■ Normal pulmonary MRA.

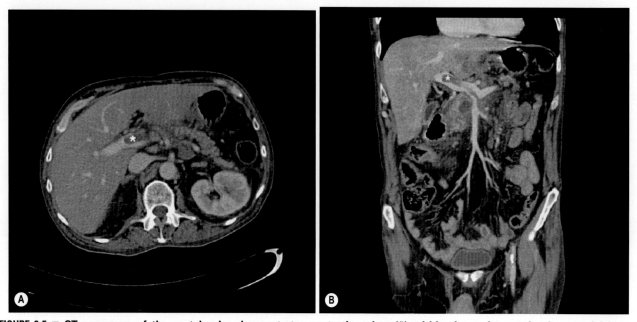

FIGURE 2-5 ■ CT venogram of the portal veins demonstrates acute thrombus (*) within the main portal vein on axial image (A) and coronal reformat (B).

directly the flow rate to each kidney using a two-dimensional (2D) cardiac-triggered, phase-contrast approach, which facilitates both the assessment of end-organ damage and the likelihood of success of transluminal angioplasty.[1]

As mentioned above, renewed interest in non-contrast techniques has led to the development of reasonably robust techniques which benefit the patient in avoiding the risks of contrast agents in patients with renal impairment or other contraindication to gadolinium contrast agents.[11,12]

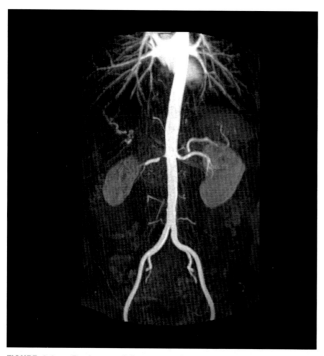

FIGURE 2-6 ■ **Patient with severe hypertension refractory to treatment.** CEMRA demonstrates severe proximal right renal artery stenosis with reduced size of the right kidney.

Carotid and Vertebral Arteries and Intracranial Arteries

TOF MRA remains the technique of choice for depiction of the intracranial arteries (Figs. 2-7 to 2-10).[1,3] Because of the requirement accurately to differentiate stenoses at a 70% cut-off within a relatively small (internal carotid) artery, there are stringent spatial resolution requirements for carotid evaluation[9] (Fig. 2-9). For CTA, excellent quality is achieved but the presence of intramural calcification (calcified plaque) at the bifurcation may interfere with accurate stenosis grading, whereas the signal void of calcium on MR does not interfere with image interpretation.[1]

A further advantage of MRA lies in the assessment of patients with suspected subclavian steal syndrome. Although both CTA and MRA are equal in their ability to detect subclavian stenosis, the reversed flow within the vertebral artery that confirms the diagnosis can only be made with MRA.[1]

A particular situation exists in the imaging of carotid and vertebral artery dissections where imaging of the lumen alone with CTA or MRA simply demonstrates narrowing indistinguishable from other causes.[1,9] In all cases of suspected carotid or vertebral dissection, therefore, pre-contrast T1- and T2-weighted fat-saturation MR images should be performed, as these will demonstrate the bright appearance of an intramural haematoma, which is typically crescent-shaped. Failure to do so results in the identification of a focal stenosis only, and robs the patient of the opportunity to receive anticoagulation therapy, the treatment of choice for dissection.

Peripheral Arteries

For assessment of the peripheral arteries, both CTA and MRA are well validated.[7,21,22] In the peripheral arteries, as in most other areas, TOF MRA has been superseded by CEMRA.[7,23] Although the spatial coverage offered by single-field-of-view imaging is insufficient to address all of the relevant anatomy, the introduction of moving-table

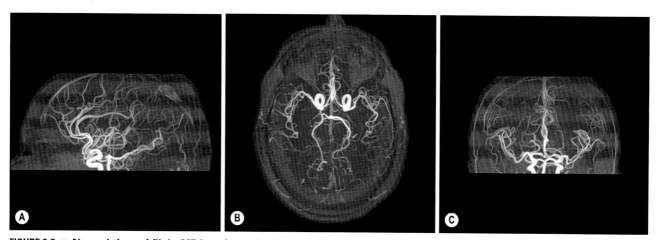

FIGURE 2-7 ■ **Normal time-of-flight MRA performed at 3.0 tesla.** Note excellent detail of the intracranial arteries on lateral (A), basal (B) and anteroposterior (C) MIPs.

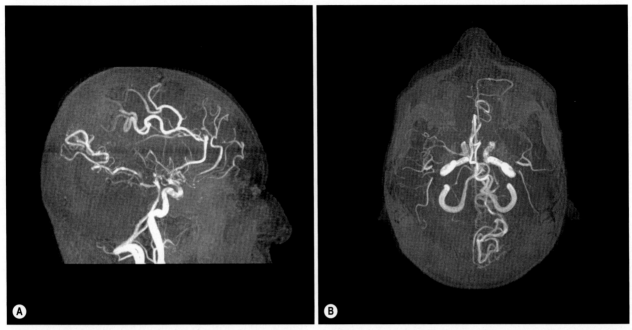

FIGURE 2-8 ■ **Patient with left cortical blindness.** Lateral (A) and basal (B) projections from TOF MRA demonstrate a large left occipital arteriovenous malformation.

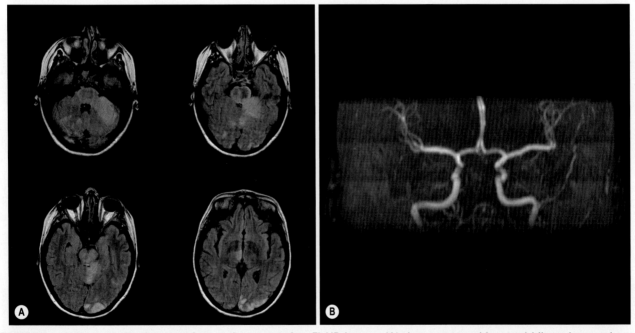

FIGURE 2-9 ■ **Patient admitted unconscious and unresponsive.** FLAIR images (A) demonstrate widespread bilateral parenchymal abnormality affecting both cerebellar hemispheres, pons, midbrain, right thalamus and left occipital lobes. TOF MRA in anteroposterior (B) and basal (C) projections demonstrates absence of the basilar artery, indicating thrombosis.

MRA has opened the way for routine non-invasive MRA of the entire run-off arteries in a short timeframe (<20-min examination)[23] (Figs. 2-11 and Fig. 2-12). The major limitation of moving-table MRA is venous contamination in the legs. Methods to eliminate this include the use of tourniquets inflated to subsystolic pressures to delay onset of venous enhancement, careful attention to detail in setting up the examination (to avoid any redundancy in anatomical coverage), the use of high

parallel-imaging factors and the exploitation of ultra-short TR imaging.[23]

FUTURE DIRECTIONS

Following the breathtaking developments in both CT and MR technology over the last two decades, clinicians now have at their fingertips readily available, reproducible

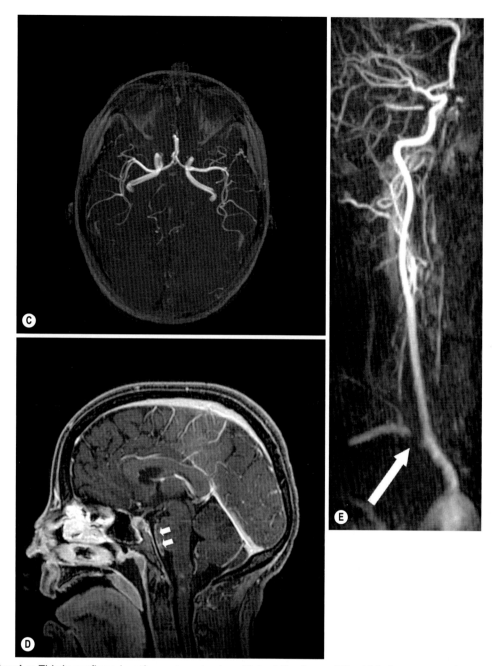

FIGURE 2-9, Continued ▪ This is confirmed on the post-contrast sagittal midline image (D), which demonstrates intravascular thrombus within the basilar artery (arrows). Contrast-enhanced MRA of the neck vessels (E) demonstrates a tight stenosis at the origin of the right subclavian artery (arrow), thought to be the source of embolism. Note also irregularity of the right vertebral artery consistent with atheroma.

and accurate modalities in both CTA and MRA for non-invasive assessment of virtually all vascular territories. CTA offers ease of use, rapid performance, wide availability and ease of interpretation. MRA offers virtually identical, or, in some cases, improved 'road-mapping' potential and, in addition to the widely implemented contrast-enhanced techniques, a number of non-contrast techniques that offer truly non-invasive vascular imaging. Additionally, it allows assessment of functional aspects of flow and the ability to perform follow-up studies without risk to the patient. Further improvements in spatial resolution can be expected in CTA but this is likely to result in only modest diagnostic benefit given the excellent image quality already achievable. Improvements in spatial resolution are also likely in MRA, together with greatly improved temporal resolution facilitated by better coil efficiency and new parallel imaging methods that increase acquisition speed and/or spatial resolution by a factor of 2–16. 3-Tesla imaging (3T imaging),[24] new targeted contrast agents and the potential for routine functional imaging of end-organ damage offer exciting prospects for the future.

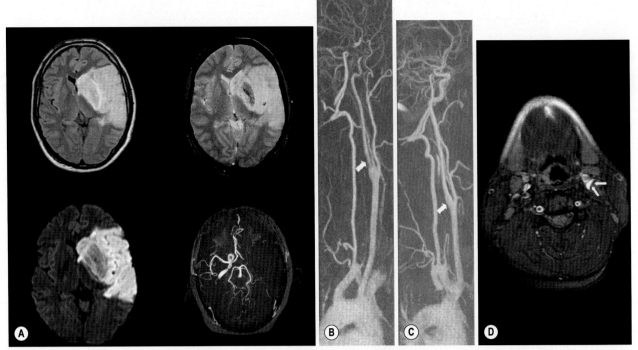

FIGURE 2-10 ■ **Patient admitted with sudden-onset dense right hemiplegia.** (A) Panel of 4 images (top left FLAIR, top left GRE T2, bottom left DWI, bottom right TOF MRA) demonstrates widespread acute left middle cerebral artery infarction with some haemorrhage and mass effect secondary to left middle cerebral artery occlusion. CEMRA (B) demonstrates diffuse narrowing of the internal carotid artery at the bulb (arrow). The normal right side is shown for comparison (arrow denotes normal carotid bulb) (C). Axial fat-saturation image (D) through the area of narrowing shown on (B) demonstrates crescentic high signal intensity (arrows), confirming the presence of acute carotid artery dissection.

CATHETER ARTERIOGRAPHY

Technique

The risks associated with modern arteriography are extremely small. Arteriography is still, nevertheless, an 'invasive' procedure and it should never be undertaken unless the radiologist is satisfied that the likely benefits justify the potential risks. An arteriogram should never be carried out simply because it has been scheduled or 'routinely requested' by a clinical team; mistakes inevitably occur and the radiologist responsible for the procedure should be satisfied in every case that proper indications exist for the particular study requested.

Preparation of the Patient

Informed consent should be obtained for arteriography. A doctor, preferably the responsible radiologist or a member of the radiology department, should see the patient before the procedure to explain what is to be done, check that no contraindications to the study exist, check the appropriate pulses and ensure that adequate premedication is arranged. The groin should be shaved if a femoral approach is to be used. It is generally recommended to ask the patient to stop solid foods for a few hours before the procedure but to permit free oral fluids unless general anaesthesia or heavy premedication is being used. Dehydration should be avoided and adequate measures should be taken to avoid this during the procedure and the recovery period.

Contraindications

There are very few absolute contraindications to arteriography but there are many factors that considerably increase the hazards of the technique. Always check that a patient is not pregnant before arteriography, as the radiation dose may be considerable. If arteriography is essential in a pregnant patient, the dose to the fetus should be minimised by protection, field collimation and careful choice of filming sequences. Caution should be exercised in patients on anticoagulant therapy or with other bleeding diatheses. Arteriography should be avoided if possible in such cases; if it is essential, then all possible steps should be taken to correct or improve the coagulation defect before and during the procedure if this is clinically acceptable. Other factors that increase the risk of bleeding from an arterial puncture site include systemic hypertension and disorders predisposing to increased fragility of the vessel wall such as Cushing's syndrome, prolonged steroid treatment and rare connective tissue disorders such as certain Ehlers–Danlos subtypes (especially type IV).

Arteriography may be necessary in a patient with a suspected or known previous adverse reaction to contrast medium. Arteriography can require larger doses of contrast medium than any other radiological procedure and particular care must be exercised in infants and in dehydrated or shocked patients, patients with serious cardiac or respiratory disease, patients in hepatic or renal failure, and other patients with serious metabolic abnormalities.

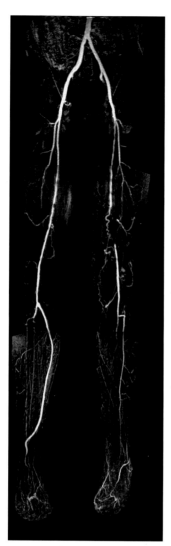

FIGURE 2-11 ■ **Peripheral MRA performed using a three-station, moving-table approach.** The study demonstrates excellent visualisation of the entire run-off arteries from the mid-abdominal aorta to the level of the pedal arch. Note extensive vascular stenoses and occlusions and a bypass graft from the right popliteal artery to the right anterior tibial artery.

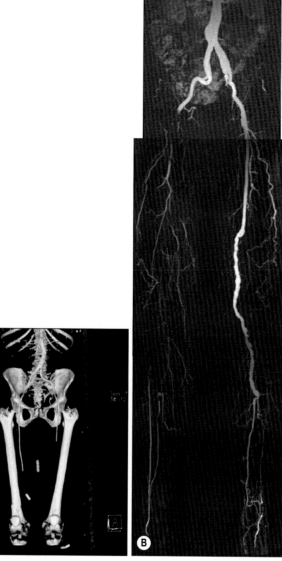

FIGURE 2-12 ■ (A) Patient with acute onset of rest pain in both lower legs. Peripheral CTA using a surface-rendered reformat demonstrates acute cut-off of the superficial femoral arteries on both sides consistent with bilateral acute embolism. (B) Patient with long-standing claudication right leg: peripheral MRA demonstrates occlusion of the right common femoral, superficial femoral and popliteal arteries with reconstitution of flow via collaterals.

Anaesthesia

Most arteriography is performed under local anaesthesia, though general anaesthesia is necessary for babies and young children, for confused, difficult or very nervous patients, and in some complex procedures. Although general anaesthesia can be more pleasant for the patient than local anaesthesia and reduces motion artefact on the radiographs, it nevertheless adds to the risks of arteriography. This is not only because of the (small) risks inherent in general anaesthesia but also because it masks the patient's subjective symptoms and reactions. These may provide the radiologist with immediate warning of a mishap such as the subintimal injection of contrast medium or the inadvertent wedging of the catheter tip in a small artery: a warning that may well prevent more serious injury.

Arterial Puncture

It is often said that the most important part of an angiographic procedure is the initial vessel puncture and there is no doubt that a good technique is likely to make the subsequent angiogram not only more comfortable for the patient but also easier for the angiographer. It should go without saying that the most suitable route of access in order to achieve the aims of the study should have been chosen before the patient enters the angiographic suite; this decision will often depend upon a number of factors, including previous imaging studies, operation notes and clinical examination.

The most common vessel punctured for diagnostic and therapeutic angiography is the common femoral artery. Axillary, brachial or radial approaches can be used, but these routes are usually reserved for those patients in whom a femoral approach is not possible due to iliac occlusive disease. A popliteal artery puncture may be useful in certain instances such as angioplasty of the superficial femoral artery when it is not possible to catheterise this vessel via an antegrade approach.

The technique of arterial puncture and catheterisation of the common femoral artery will be described. Access via other less commonly used vessels such as the brachial, radial and popliteal arteries will not be discussed further in this chapter. Interested readers are referred to previous editions of this textbook or specialist interventional radiology texts.

Retrograde Femoral Artery Puncture
(Fig. 2-13)

The artery is palpated to select the site of puncture before local anaesthetic is injected. Various anatomical descriptions are given regarding the site at which to puncture, but the aim should be to enter the common femoral

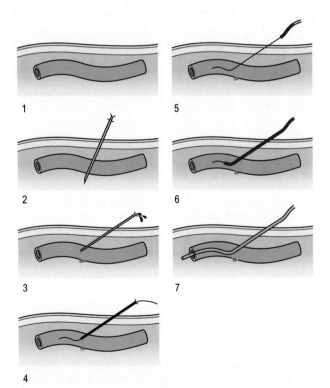

FIGURE 2-13 ■ **Percutaneous catheterisation.** One of the commonly used techniques of percutaneous arterial catheterisation. The artery (1) is transfixed (2). The needle is partially withdrawn and re-angled (3). A guidewire is passed into the needle during free backflow of blood (3, 4), the needle is removed and a catheter or introducer is inserted over the wire (5, 6). When the catheter is safely within the arterial lumen, the wire is withdrawn (7).

artery a short distance below the inguinal ligament. This is best achieved by puncturing the vessel where it can be most easily palpated, irrespective of the relationship of this point to the inguinal skin crease. Since this is the point where the artery crosses the femoral head, it is also the easiest point at which to achieve haemostasis afterwards. Ultrasound is also recommended to help select the most appropriate site of puncture, avoiding atherosclerotic plaques, and is also used to guide needle entry.

It is important that the arterial puncture site should be adequately anaesthetised. After cleansing the skin with a suitable preparation, 5–10 mL of 0.5–1% lidocaine is infiltrated around the artery. It is important to inject the local anaesthetic agent posterior to the artery as well as anterior to it, even if a single-wall puncture of the vessel is subsequently made, as it makes the arterial puncture and subsequent catheter manipulation much more comfortable for the patient. In addition, if the puncture site is inadequately anaesthetised arterial spasm is more likely, which may make selective catheterisation very difficult because of the lack of free catheter movement.

After local anaesthesia, a small scalpel incision is made in the skin (large enough to accommodate the anticipated catheter), the skin being temporarily drawn laterally during the incision to avert the risk of a scalpel injury to the arterial wall. A pair of fine artery forceps is inserted into the incision and used to create a tunnel through the subcutaneous tissues down to the artery. This manoeuvre is particularly important in large or obese patients, for it not only facilitates catheterisation but also reduces the risk of a postoperative haematoma: any escaping blood emerges through the incision and is immediately apparent, instead of collecting subcutaneously.

The technique employed for puncturing the artery is a matter of personal preference. A reliable way is to feel the artery with the middle and index fingers of the left hand and insert the needle (held in the right hand) between the two palpating fingers. The needle is held angled forwards and passed through the anterior wall alone or right through the artery, depending upon the angiographer's preference. A single-wall puncture technique is most commonly performed with a one-part needle, in which case free pulsatile blood flow will occur as soon as the needle enters the vessel lumen. When a double-wall puncture technique is performed a two-part needle is used; after passing through the vessel, the central stylet is removed, the needle angled slightly more towards the horizontal and then withdrawn at an even rate, assisted by gentle rotatory movements to avoid any sudden jerking. When the tip of the needle is safely in the arterial lumen there will be a free, spurting backflow of blood from the hub. While the needle is held steady with one hand, the soft tip of a guidewire is threaded through the needle into the artery. When a sufficient length of wire is inside, the needle is removed and firm manual pressure maintained on the puncture site until the needle has been exchanged for a catheter or dilator. The guidewire is removed when the tip of the catheter is in a satisfactory position and the catheter is then flushed free of blood with heparinised saline. At the end of a correctly conducted insertion procedure there should be no bleeding around the catheter, which will move freely and painlessly through the puncture site when manipulated.

There are arguments in favour of both single- and double-wall arterial punctures; some radiologists prefer to puncture only the anterior wall of the artery to minimise the trauma to the vessel, although puncture to both vessel walls does not increase the risk of complications as these are usually caused by the subsequent manipulations with guidewires and catheters. Proponents of a double-wall puncture technique maintain that this method is safer, particularly when first learning angiography, with a lesser risk of intimal dissection when introducing the guidewire through the needle when compared with a single-wall technique. Whichever method is employed, if a guidewire does not pass freely into the arterial lumen it should not be forced; this technique is never successful and usually causes an intimal dissection. If there is good backflow of blood the reason for failure of the wire to pass freely may be either that the needle is angled sharply towards one wall of the blood vessel or that the wire is passing into a small branch vessel such as the deep circumflex iliac artery. A number of manoeuvres may help, including fluoroscopy, cautious repositioning of the angle of the needle or changing to a J-wire. A gentle injection of contrast medium is possible to help ascertain the nature of the problem but only if good backflow is present. If there is poor backflow then the needle may be positioned near an atheromatous plaque or a stenosis, may be only partially in the lumen, or may have caused an intimal dissection. In these circumstances discretion is advised and it is wise to start again with a fresh puncture. In difficult cases remember that there is usually a patent femoral artery in the opposite leg! Better two groin punctures than a dissection or a large haematoma.

The catheter is flushed with a heparinised saline solution throughout the procedure to prevent clotting. It is almost always preferable to give a firm hand flush intermittently, rather than maintain a continuous slow flush infusion. This technique not only leaves the proximal end of the catheter free for manipulation but also is more effective, since a slow infusion may only clear the proximal holes of a catheter with multiple side-ports; clot forms in the end-port and the more distal side-ports, and is then blown out into the vascular system when a pressure contrast injection is performed.

Antegrade Femoral Artery Puncture

The most common indication for an antegrade puncture of the femoral artery is when performing ipsilateral superficial femoral, popliteal or infragenicular artery angioplasty. Once again, the aim should be to puncture the common femoral artery just below the inguinal ligament. The most common problem associated with this procedure is catheterisation of the profunda femoris and many methods have been described in order to manipulate the catheter out of this vessel into the superficial femoral artery when this has happened. With a good technique and ultrasound guidance, however, this complication should rarely occur.

Preparation of the patient is important; obese patients may have an abdominal 'apron' that hangs over the groin

and this should be lifted superiorly and strapped out of the way with heavy-duty tape. It is well worthwhile when performing an antegrade femoral puncture to screen over the femoral head to determine the correct site for vessel puncture, as this is often considerably higher than anticipated when using palpation alone. The fovea of the femoral head is a useful landmark for the correct site of arterial access and this can be marked on the skin before local anaesthetic is infiltrated in the same way as for a retrograde puncture. A skin incision is made with a scalpel blade and blunt dissection is again performed of the soft tissues over the femoral artery. The vessel is then punctured with the needle angled slightly towards the feet. The best wire to use is a wide-angled J-wire with a curvature of radius 7.5 mm. This should be introduced through the needle with the tip of the curve directed anteriorly, so that, as it exits the needle tip within the vessel lumen, it is directed into the superficial femoral artery rather than the profunda femoris. A straight guidewire is much more likely to pass directly into the latter vessel because of the posterolateral orientation of this artery.

Selective Catheterisation

By manipulating a catheter under fluoroscopic control it is possible to insert the catheter selectively into various branches of the vascular system such as the renal artery, coeliac axis, axillary artery, etc. Different catheter shapes are available, each of which is suitable for a particular manoeuvre or for catheterising certain arterial branches. Superselective catheterisation (also known as subselective embolisation) is the term used for the catheterisation of small subsidiary arteries that themselves arise from named branch arteries and is most frequently performed during embolisation procedures. A coaxial catheter (one that passes through the lumen of a diagnostic or guiding catheter) is often used for the catheterisation of these small vessels.

DIGITAL SUBTRACTION ANGIOGRAPHY

With any DSA examination, particular attention must be paid to the elimination of movement artefact. Respiratory motion needs to be controlled (a nose-clip is often helpful) and in the case of abdominal and pelvic examinations the effects of bowel movement can be minimised by the use of paralytic agents. Multiple mask acquisition is a simple and much neglected technique for counteracting the effect of inevitable movement such as, say, the artefacts produced in pulmonary arteriograms by cardiac motion. If several pre-contrast images are taken so as to embrace all the different phases of the cardiac cycle, then appropriate mask selection will subsequently permit virtually any contrast-filled image to be presented free of artefact. The same technique can be used in those individuals who are unable to hold their breath for any length of time. Such patients should be asked to breathe normally throughout the run and multiple images are obtained *before* the injection of contrast medium so that a suitable mask for subtraction is available for every phase

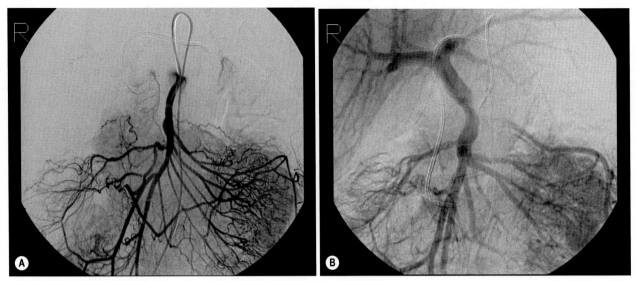

FIGURE 2-14 ■ **Example of use of breathing technique during visceral angiography.** Arterial (A) and venous (B) images from a superior mesenteric arteriogram acquired during patient respiration. Intestinal peristalsis has been obliterated with hyoscine butylbromide. The arterial and venous images were acquired at different phases of respiration but the use of different masks (mask 2 for the arterial image and mask 10 for the venous image), acquired before the injection of contrast medium, has resulted in excellent-quality images.

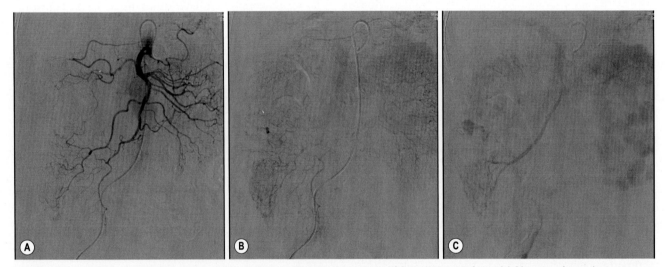

FIGURE 2-15 ■ **Superior mesenteric artery angiogram in a 79-year-old patient with acute gastrointestinal haemorrhage.** Images were obtained with the patient breathing throughout the acquisition using the technique described in the text. (A) Arterial phase image demonstrates normal arterial anatomy. (B) Late arterial/early capillary phase image demonstrates an area of active contrast medium extravasation into a proximal ascending colon diverticulum. (C) Delayed image demonstrates that extravasated contrast medium has spilled into the colonic lumen. Normal venous drainage is seen from the caecum.

of respiration. This technique is particularly suited to visceral angiography (Fig. 2-14) and allows the acquisition of images during arterial and late venous phases that are often of much better quality than those obtained in patients who are asked to hold their breath (Fig. 2-15).

AFTERCARE

When an arteriographic study is completed, the catheter is withdrawn and firm manual pressure applied to the puncture site for 5–10 minutes. The radiologist should be absolutely satisfied that bleeding has stopped before the patient leaves the angiography suite. The wound site is then checked at regular intervals by the nursing staff, who should also record pulse and blood pressure observations for a reasonable period following the procedure and check that distal pulses remain palpable. Pressure pads, sand bags and other accoutrements are generally a waste of time. It is much better to be able to see the puncture site than to cover it up. If bleeding does not stop from a puncture site, press for longer! Almost all post-catheterisation bleeding can ultimately be controlled by local pressure unless the artery has been torn or there is a coagulation abnormality. Several devices are now available that are used to seal the puncture point in the vessel wall at the time of catheter withdrawal in order to allow rapid mobilisation and discharge of the patient, often within 1–2 h.[25-27] These have become popular in many centres following cardiac catheterisation and are being utilised more commonly in peripheral angiography. A description of the various devices that are currently available and a discussion of the arguments for and against their use lie outside the scope of this chapter and the interested reader is referred to specialist texts.

An adequate record of the procedure should be entered in the patient's case notes. This should include:
- date
- name of the operator
- puncture site
- catheter size
- studies performed
- names and doses of anaesthetic agents
- volumes and concentrations of contrast medium and other drugs administered
- preliminary findings
- any complications during the procedure
- integrity or otherwise of the pulses peripheral to the puncture site at the end of the procedure
- post-procedural nursing instructions.

These notes are important not only for patient care but also as a medico-legal record and they should be comprehensive and accurate.

COMPLICATIONS

Puncture Site Complications

Haemorrhage

Haemorrhage may occur from the puncture site and may cause external blood loss or a subcutaneous haematoma, which can result in extensive bruising. Retroperitoneal bleeding is uncommon but may occur if the arterial puncture is performed above the inguinal ligament. Perhaps the commonest reason for this is the introduction of the needle during retrograde femoral artery catheterisation at too acute an angle so that it passes through the back wall of the external iliac artery above the inguinal ligament. It is less well recognised, however, that this complication may also occur when the femoral artery is correctly punctured; this is probably due to a downward extension of the pelvic and abdominal wall fascial layers around the femoral artery and vein, the so-called femoral sheath. If this sheath is transgressed at the time of vessel puncture, and bleeding subsequently occurs from the puncture site after catheter or sheath removal for any reason, then blood may spread along the fascial planes continuous with the femoral sheath into the retroperitoneum or, indeed, into the anterior abdominal wall.

Four types of haematoma may occur after femoral artery puncture: (A) abdominal wall, (B) retroperitoneal, (C) groin and thigh and (D) intraperitoneal. The first three may all result from puncture of the common femoral artery (i.e. below the inguinal ligament), with (A) and (B) resulting when there is bleeding into the femoral sheath and (C), the commonest, when there is spread into the femoral triangle. Intraperitoneal haemorrhage is even less frequent than retroperitoneal bleeding and generally requires transgression of the peritoneum itself, which is more likely to occur if vessel puncture is performed above the level of the inguinal ligament. Some intraperitoneal bleeding has also been described, however, when the arterial puncture is below the inguinal ligament; it has been postulated that this may be due to the presence of defects in the parietal peritoneum.

Excessive bleeding is usually the result of bad technique. Particular caution is necessary in patients with a bleeding diathesis or hypertension and following the use of balloon catheters in transluminal angioplasty. If inexplicable bleeding continues, check that inadvertent over-heparinisation has not occurred. This can be corrected if necessary by the administration of protamine sulphate (10 mg of which counteracts the effects of approximately 1000 IU heparin).

Intramural and Perivascular Contrast Medium Injection

Contrast medium may be inadvertently injected into the wall of a vessel or outside the vessel (perivascular). In most cases little harm (apart from pain) results from a perivascular injection but it is possible to dissect and occlude an artery with a subintimal injection of contrast medium. Never inject into a needle or catheter that does not exhibit free backflow.

Vascular thrombosis can result from severe trauma to the vessel at the puncture site or from a subintimal contrast injection. It is also possible that thrombus wiped off the outside of the arterial catheter during its extraction forms a nidus for thrombus at the puncture site. Vascular trauma at the puncture site can be minimised by good technique. Never use force to introduce a wire into a vessel; if it does not pass easily something is wrong! It is often better for the inexperienced operator to start again with a fresh needle puncture and/or call for help than to persist with one that is causing problems. A 10-minute delay with a successful outcome is always preferable to a dissection and/or a groin haematoma.

Peripheral embolisation from the puncture site probably occurs to a minor degree in many cases but clinically obvious embolisation is rare.

Local vascular complications such as false aneurysm (pseudoaneurysm) or AV fistula formation and late stenosis or occlusion can all result from arterial procedures. Good technique is the best preventative measure. Femoral artery pseudoaneurysms are usually caused by a combination of a low puncture—the superficial femoral or profunda femoris arteries have often been cannulated instead of the common femoral artery when this complication occurs—and inadequate compression of the vessel at the end of the procedure.

Local sepsis may occur following an arterial puncture (although it is extremely rare) and this factor is particularly important if early surgery is contemplated. The utmost care should be taken to observe sterile precautions and when a study is performed in a patient with local skin contamination (e.g. open wound, ileostomy, etc.) a protective adhesive sheet helps to keep the operative field uncontaminated.

Injury to local structures such as nerves, joints and bones is rarely of clinical significance. Occasionally damage to branches of the femoral nerve gives rise to areas of cutaneous anaesthesia or paraesthesia in the thigh.[28] These normally recover completely, although this may take several months in some instances.

Catheter-Related and General Complications

1. *Thrombi* can form in or on a catheter and be ejected into the vascular system. This is always undesirable and in areas such as the cerebral or coronary circulation is extremely dangerous. Catheters should be flushed assiduously during all arteriographic procedures to prevent thrombus formation. Other types of embolism that may occur are air embolism (sometimes from incorrectly loaded pressure injectors) and thread embolism from fragments of gauze swab.

2. *Vascular injuries* distant from the puncture site may be produced by the catheter or guidewire, or by the intramural injection of contrast medium or saline. If there is ever any doubt about whether a needle or catheter tip is in a satisfactory position, contrast medium should always be injected in preference to saline. Under fluoroscopic control, it is then possible to stop the injection immediately if any extravasation or other mishap is apparent. The most common injury is dissection of the tunica intima from the tunica media and this complication is far more likely to occur in previously diseased vessels than in normal vessels. The intima forms a raised flap that may completely occlude the vessel. It is also possible to perforate vessels with a guidewire or to rupture them when a forced injection is made through a catheter wedged into a vessel of the same calibre.

3. *Injuries to organs* are normally caused by ischaemia during arteriographic procedures (other than those related to the effects of contrast medium). This may occur through wedging of the catheter so that the normal flow to an organ is obstructed; dissection of the feeding artery; spasm, thrombosis or rupture of the feeding artery; or embolism. The ischaemia resulting from one or more of the earlier mentioned events may have no observable clinical sequelae, may result in temporary or permanent functional abnormalities in the affected organ or system, or may cause infarction of the organ. The clinical importance of these accidents depends very much on the vascular territory in which they occur; complete occlusion of a carotid, coronary or renal artery is likely to have disastrous consequences whereas occlusion of, say, a hepatic artery may not necessarily produce any adverse effects.

4. *Guidewire fracture.* Occasionally fragments of guidewire or catheter may become detached within the vascular system. Catheters may also become

knotted during overenthusiastic manipulation procedures. With good technique these complications should not occur.

5. *Injection accidents.* Tragedies have occurred when toxic substances have been inadvertently injected into blood vessels. Skin-cleansing fluids should always be removed from the instrument trolley immediately after the puncture site has been prepared. Drugs should always be double-checked before injection through a catheter.

6. *Vasovagal reactions.* Vagally mediated reactions may occur during arteriography in response either to the injection of contrast medium or to the discomfort and psychological effects of the procedure. Bradycardia is a prominent feature of such reactions, which must be distinguished from acute allergic responses to the contrast medium or local anaesthetic. The incidence of vasovagal reactions is considerably reduced if proper premedication is employed.

REFERENCES

1. Cowell GW, Reid AW, Roditi GH. Changing trends in a decade of vascular radiology—the impact of technical developments of non-invasive techniques on vascular imaging. Insights Imaging 2012;3(5):495–504.
2. Lell M, Fellner C, Baum U, et al. Evaluation of carotid artery stenosis with multisection CT and MR imaging: influence of imaging modality and postprocessing. Am J Neuroradiol 2007; 28(1):104–10.
3. Ozsarlak O, Van Goethem JW, Maes M, Parizel PM. MR angiography of the intracranial vessels: technical aspects and clinical applications. Neuroradiology 2004;46(12):955–72.
4. Dumoulin CL, Souza SP, Walker MF, Wagle W. Three-dimensional phase contrast angiography. Magn Reson Med 1989;9: 139–49.
5. Prince MR, Narasimham DL, Stanley JC, et al. Breath-hold gadolinium-enhanced MR angiography of the abdominal aorta and its major branches. Radiology 1995;197(3):785–92.
6. Zhang HL, Schoenberg SO, Resnick LM, Prince MR. Diagnosis of renal artery stenosis: combining gadolinium-enhanced three-dimensional magnetic resonance angiography with functional magnetic resonance pulse sequences. Am J Hypertens 2003;16: 1079–82.
7. Nelemans PJ, Leiner T, de Vet HC, van Engelshoven JM. Peripheral arterial disease: meta-analysis of the diagnostic performance of MR angiography. Radiology 2000;217:105–14.
8. Meaney JF, Prince MR, Nostrant TT, Stanley JC. Gadolinium-enhanced MR angiography of visceral arteries in patients with suspected chronic mesenteric ischemia. J Magn Reson Imaging 1997;7:171–6.
9. Remonda L, Heid O, Schroth G. Carotid artery stenosis, occlusion, and pseudo-occlusion: first-pass, gadolinium-enhanced, three-dimensional MR angiography—preliminary study. Radiology 1998; 209:95–102.
10. Kaewlai R, Abujudeh H. Nephrogenic systemic fibrosis. Am J Roentgenol 2012;199(1):W17–23.
11. Khoo MM, Deeab D, Gedroyc WM, et al. Renal artery stenosis: comparative assessment by unenhanced renal artery MRA versus contrast-enhanced MRA. Eur Radiol 2011;21(7):1470–6.
12. Miyazaki M, Akahane M. Non-contrast enhanced MR angiography: established techniques. J Magn Reson Imaging 2012;35(1): 1–19.
13. Chung JH, Ghoshhajra BB, Rojas CA, et al. CT angiography of the thoracic aorta. Radiol Clin North Am 2010;48(2):249–64.
14. Lee EY, Siegel MJ, Hildebolt CF, et al. MDCT evaluation of thoracic aortic anomalies in pediatric patients and young adults: comparison of axial, multiplanar, and 3D images. Am J Roentgenol 2004;182:777–84.

15. Lake DR, Kavanagh JJ, Ravenel JG, et al. Computed tomography and pulmonary embolus: a review. Semin Ultrasound CT MR 2005;26:270–80.

16. Becattini C, Agnelli G, Vedovati MC, et al. Multidetector computed tomography for acute pulmonary embolism: diagnosis and risk stratification in a single test. Eur Heart J 2011;32(13):1657–63.

17. Meaney JF, Weg JG, Chenevert TL, et al. Diagnosis of pulmonary embolism with magnetic resonance angiography. N Engl J Med 1997;336:1422–7.

18. Stein PD, Chenevert TL, Fowler SE, et al, PIOPED III (Prospective Investigation of Pulmonary Embolism Diagnosis III) Investigators. Gadolinium-enhanced magnetic resonance angiography for pulmonary embolism: a multicenter prospective study (PIOPED III). Ann Intern Med 2010;152(7):434–43.

19. Tolia AJ, Landis R, Lamparello P, et al. Type II endoleaks after endovascular repair of abdominal aortic aneurysms: natural history. Radiology 2005;235:683–6.

20. Hanninen EL, Denecke T, Stelter L, et al. Preoperative evaluation of living kidney donors using multirow detector computed tomography: comparison with digital subtraction angiography and intraoperative findings. Transpl Int 2005;18:1134–41.

21. Martin ML, Tay KH, Flak B, et al. Multidetector CT angiography of the aortoiliac system and lower extremities: a prospective comparison with digital subtraction angiography. Am J Roentgenol 2003;180:1085–91.

22. Ota H, Takase K, Igarashi K, et al. MDCT compared with digital subtraction angiography for assessment of lower extremity arterial occlusive disease: importance of reviewing cross-sectional images. Am J Roentgenol 2004;182:201–9.

23. Meaney JF, Ridgway JP, Chakraverty S, et al. Stepping-table gadolinium-enhanced digital subtraction MR angiography of the aorta and lower extremity arteries: preliminary experience. Radiology 1999;211:59–67.

24. Lin W, An H, Chen Y, et al. Practical consideration for 3T imaging. Magn Reson Imaging Clin N Am 2003;11:615–39.

25. Smilowitz NR, Kirtane AJ, Guiry M, et al. Practices and complications of vascular closure devices and manual compression in patients undergoing elective transfemoral coronary procedures. Am J Cardiol 2012;110(2):177–82.

26. Lupi A, Rognoni A, Secco GG, et al. Different spectrum of vascular complications after angio-seal deployment or manual compression. J Invasive Cardiol 2012;24(3):90–6.

27. Burke MN, Hermiller J, Jaff MR. StarClose vascular closure system (VCS) is safe and effective in patients who ambulate early following successful femoral artery access closure—results from the RISE clinical trial. Catheter Cardiovasc Interv 2012;80(1):45–52.

28. Hallett JW Jr, Wolk SW, Cherry KJ Jr, et al. The femoral neuralgia syndrome after arterial catheter trauma. J Vasc Surg 1990;11:702–6.

CHAPTER 3

AORTIC INTERVENTION

Christopher J. Hammond • Anthony A. Nicholson

INTRODUCTION

Open surgical treatment of aortic pathology is often technically demanding for the surgeon and invasive for the patient, being associated with a significant physiological insult. Surgery for the thoracic aorta requires thoracotomy or median sternotomy, aortic cross-clamping, often single lung ventilation and sometimes cardiopulmonary bypass or circulatory arrest. Surgery for the abdominal aorta requires laparotomy, or extensive retroperitoneal dissection, medial visceral rotation and aortic cross-clamping. The aortic tissue is usually diseased and may be friable (especially in the case of dissection and intramural haematoma (IMH)) or calcified and brittle. In either situation, working with, dissecting and suturing the aorta is challenging.

The cohort of patients requiring aortic intervention is usually that least able to withstand it. In most cases, aortic pathology is associated with generalised cardiovascular disease, including ischaemic heart disease, cerebrovascular, renovascular and peripheral vascular disease as well as other comorbidites such as respiratory impairment. Mortality rates for elective open surgery for thoracic and abdominal aneurysms are in the region of 8 and 5%, respectively,[1,2] and morbidity is significant.

These considerations have driven the development of minimally invasive endovascular therapies for aortic disease. Endovascular repair of the aorta using covered stents (stent-grafts) was first described in 1991[3] and is generally associated with a smaller physiological insult and lower mortality than open surgical repair.[2,4] However, there are a number of unique limitations (particularly relating to anatomy) and complications. Although the current generation of stent-grafts is easier to insert and performs better in the long term than their predecessors,

they are by no means a panacea for all aortic pathology. A multidisciplinary approach to aortic disease is vital and should include cardiothoracic and vascular surgeons, interventional radiologists, vascular anaesthetists and device specialists (e.g. company representatives). This multidisciplinary approach should ensure that the patient receives the most appropriate treatment, be it open surgery, endovascular repair or medical management.

This chapter will discuss the endovascular management of aortic pathology and in particular the indications, anatomical and technical considerations and complications of the technique.

STENT-GRAFTS AND BASIC PRINCIPLES OF STENT-GRAFTING

A stent-graft (Fig. 3-1) is composed of a fabric tube, usually woven polyester or expanded polytetrafluoroethylene (Gore-Tex). Circular or crown-shaped metal struts ('ring stents'), usually made of nitinol or Elgiloy, are attached to the tube by either suturing or gluing. The exact design of the ring stent varies from manufacturer to manufacturer, but in all cases serves to provide support for the fabric and provide firm apposition of the stent-graft to the wall of the aorta. Some devices have uncovered stents at one end to provide additional support and anchorage above or below the covered portion of the device. The stent-graft is held in place by the radial force of the ring stents, which produce friction against the aortic wall and prevent distal device migration. Additionally, some devices have small hooks (usually at the top end of the fabric or on an uncovered stent) which engage with the aortic wall to prevent migration (Fig. 3-1B). Most manufacturers make a range of stent-graft

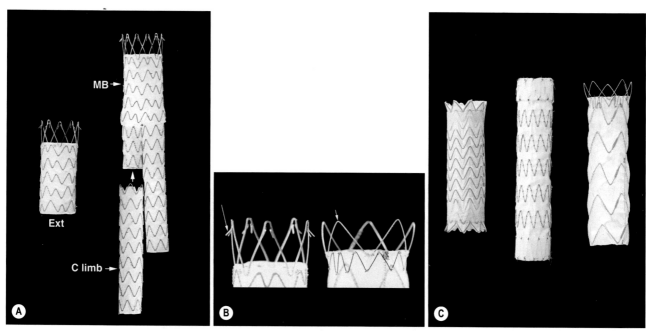

FIGURE 3-1 ■ **Stent-grafts.** (A) Typical bifurcated stent-graft, consisting of a main body (MB) with a short and a long limb, a contralateral limb (C limb), which is docked into the short limb stump (short arrow) during deployment inside the aneurysm sac, and a proximal extension cuff (Ext), which can be deployed within the main body to extend the seal cephalad if necessary. Note the ring stents (zig-zag lines) which are sutured to the fabric and the proximal bare metal (uncovered) stent which acts to increase device fixation. (B) Types of proximal bare stent. The device on the left has a bare metal proximal stent to which small hooks have been soldered (long arrow). The device on the right has a bare metal proximal stent (short arrow) but no hooks. (C) Three thoracic stent-grafts. Gore-TAG (left), Cook TX2 (middle) and Medtronic Talent (right). Note the differences in ring stent design, fabric and presence (or absence) of hooks.

diameters and lengths to allow 'off the shelf' device selection. Complex devices (such as fenestrated or branched devices or devices in sizes outside the normally manufactured ranges) can be ordered but are expensive and there is a lead-time associated with their manufacture. Currently (July 2013), the approximate cost of a typical single thoracic aortic stent-graft (Fig. 3-1C) is £10k. A bifurcated abdominal aortic device costs about £6k and a custom-made device can cost £15k or more.

Good quality high-resolution imaging is required to choose the correct stent-graft for a particular aneurysm. This is usually achieved with thin-section contrast-enhanced arterial phase computed tomography (CT) to include the whole of the diseased section of the aorta and the access vessels (see below) in a volumetric acquisition. Magnetic resonance (MR) angiography is sometimes utilised. Multiplanar reformatting software is essential to allow measurement of true axial diameters and vessel length. Expert systems are available to automate this process, though many clinicians prefer to do it by hand.

To achieve a good 'seal' between the device and the aortic wall, the stent-graft is usually oversized relative to the aorta by 10–20%. The aorta at the point of seal (sometimes called the 'neck') should be relatively disease free and straight-sided. Most stent-grafts require a neck length of 8–15 mm to achieve a seal. Shorter necks (Fig. 3-2A) and diseased necks (e.g. those containing marked atheroma or thrombus, Fig. 3-2B) risk a suboptimal seal and leakage between the device and the aortic wall. A neck which is sharply angulated relative to the more distal

aorta (Fig. 3-2C) risks the stent-graft not deploying truly perpendicular to the aortic wall. This can increase the risk of suboptimal apposition and leak, though modern devices are designed to accept a greater degree of neck angulation than earlier designs, and some devices are specifically marketed for greater neck angulation. This requires specific design features to prevent graft lumen collapse. Finally, markedly barrel or conical shaped necks (Fig. 3-2D) increase the risk of poor seal as the degree of oversize needed to achieve a seal at the narrower portion of the neck may not be sufficient to achieve seal at the wider portion. The considerations outlined above for the 'neck' apply equally to the distal sealing point, often called the 'landing zone'.

Approximately 40% of abdominal aortic aneurysms are unsuitable for conventional (as opposed to fenestrated or branched) endovascular repair because of adverse morphology.[5] A description of the degree to which an operator can compromise on an 'ideal' neck (minimal angulation, straight-sided, long and disease free) is beyond the scope of this chapter though there are many reports of operators deploying devices in 'off-label' morphologies (where the characteristics of the aorta are outwith the published 'indications for use' (IFU) limits of the device) with satisfactory results.[6,7]

Stent-grafts are supplied preloaded on a deployment system. They are usually constrained within a sheath, which, at deployment, is gradually withdrawn, allowing the stent to expand under its own radial force. Many delivery systems have mechanisms to allow partial

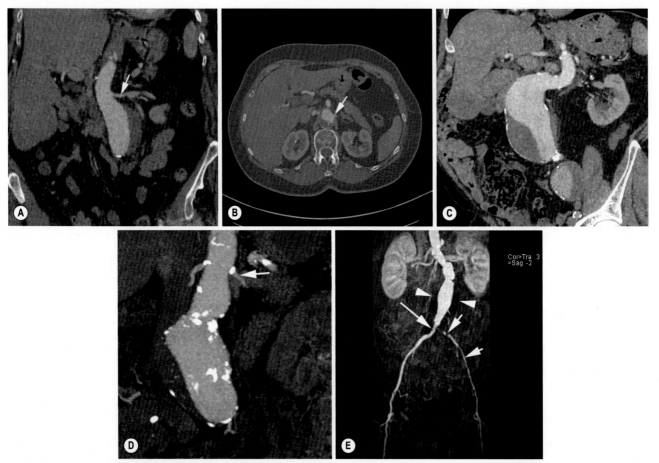

FIGURE 3-2 ▪ **Adverse anatomy for EVAR.** (A) Short neck between the renal artery (short arrow) and the aneurysm. (B) Significant atheroma/thrombus in the aneurysm neck (posteriorly) at the level of the renal artery (short arrow). (C) Markedly angulated neck with 90° bends between the suprarenal aorta and the neck (which runs horizontally in the image) and between the neck and the aneurysm itself. (D) Conical neck below the renal artery (short arrow). (E) Stenosed access vessels precluding passage of a device delivery system. There is a right common iliac artery origin stenosis (long arrow) and multifocal left iliac stenoses (short arrows). The true diameter of the AAA (between the arrowheads) is discernible from the dark bands of thrombus outwith the flowing lumen.

deployment and repositioning before final release. The 'windsock' effect of systolic pressure during the cardiac cycle forcing a partially deployed device distally from its intended deployment position is occasionally problematic, though usually only in the proximal thoracic aorta. Some thoracic delivery systems have mechanisms to constrain the proximal portion of the stent-graft until the remainder of the device is fully deployed to minimise this windsock effect. Where the proximal positioning of a thoracic stent-graft is critical (e.g. in short or angulated necks) overdrive cardiac pacing or pharmacological manipulation to lower blood pressure may be used as the device is deployed.

Once completely released, a device cannot be retrieved or repositioned without open surgery.

Deployment systems vary in diameter between 14 and 25Fr (approximately 4–9 mm). Patients in whom the access vessels (usually the common femoral and iliac arteries) are narrower than the diameter of the delivery system required (Fig. 3-2E) cannot undergo endovascular repair without adjunctive procedures such as previous angioplasty or stenting of the stenosed segment or the placement of a temporary surgical conduit to allow the

device to be inserted from above any stenosis. Heavily calcified or tortuous access vessels may also preclude endovascular repair as they will not straighten sufficiently to allow passage of the delivery system. Attempts to force a large delivery system through suboptimal access can result in access vessel rupture or avulsion with potentially disastrous consequences.

Table 3-1 summarises the absolute and relative contraindications to endovascular repair of aortic pathology with conventional stent-grafts. The characteristics of some currently manufactured stent-grafts are summarised in Table 3-2.

SURVEILLANCE IMAGING AND COMPLICATIONS

Endovascular repair of aortic pathology is associated with a number of novel complications that may occur months or years following the procedure. For this reason, patients undergoing endovascular repair undergo a programme of surveillance imaging over a number of years (and sometimes indefinitely) following the procedure. The exact

TABLE 3-1 Absolute and Relative Contraindications to Endovascular Repair of Aortic Pathology

Contraindication	Comment
Absolute	
Patient preference for open surgical repair	
Limited life expectancy	Where the risks of intervention outweigh the benefits
Poor cardiopulmonary reserve or other comorbid condition	Where the risks of intervention outweigh the benefits
Significant (>50%) or circumferential thrombus at seal zone	
Unstable patients	Where they are deemed unable to withstand the small delay associated with imaging of the pathology
Ascending aortic pathology	Unless there is absolutely no surgical alternative
Relative	
Contrast allergy	Procedures can be performed with carbon dioxide angiography or intravascular ultrasound as imaging guidance
Renal insufficiency	Procedures can be performed with carbon dioxide angiography or intravascular ultrasound as imaging guidance
Suboptimal proximal seal zone ('neck') • Angulation • Length • Shape	Proceed accepting an increased risk of endoleak, or use fenestrated or branched device
Poor access vessels • Stenosis • Tortuosity • Calcification	Can be mitigated with angioplasty or proximal surgical conduit
Children	Where physiological growth may result in loss of seal and device dislocation
Young patients	As long-term durability of endovascular repair has not yet been established
Not Contraindications	
Rupture	
Malignancy	
Mycotic aneurysms	

details of the surveillance vary from institution to institution though most will involve cross-sectional imaging initially (arterial phase CT or MR angiography at 1 or 3 months, or both) and regularly (at least annually) thereafter for a number of years. Plain radiographs of the device are also obtained to assess for ring stent fracture, device dislocation and migration. Ultrasound (US) and contrast-enhanced US may be used to detect sac expansion and endoleak. Some authors have advocated replacing CT with US as early as 1 year post-abdominal EVAR (within certain strict criteria) to minimise radiation, dose of iodinated contrast agent, cost and inconvenience to the patient.[8] Such programmes of less intensive surveillance will evolve as device performance improves with successive stent-graft generations.

The novel complications of endovascular repair are endoleak, device migration and dislocation, kinking and occlusion (Fig. 3-3).

Endoleak

This is defined as continuing flow of blood into the diseased segment of aorta outside the lumen of the stent-graft. There are five types of endoleak described.

Type 1 Endoleak (Fig. 3-3A)

Poor sealing between the device and the aortic wall, at both the proximal and distal seals (the neck and distal 'landing zone'), can result in leakage of blood between the aortic wall and the device and incomplete exclusion of the treated segment of the aorta from the circulation. This is a type 1 endoleak. It is often associated with adverse neck morphology[9,10] and sometimes with device migration over time. Errors in device sizing can also be a cause. Type 1 endoleak is associated with poor long-term outcome, with ongoing sac pressurisation, expansion and rupture.[11] It typically requires treatment. Therapeutic options include insertion of proximal or distal extension cuffs, balloon moulding or restenting of the seal zones, open surgical buttressing, device explantation and repair or attempts at transcatheter embolisation of the endoleak.

Type 2 Endoleak (Figs. 3-3B and C)

Small side branches of the aorta (e.g. the intercostal, lumbar or inferior mesenteric arteries) are not usually occluded during endovascular repair. This allows the possibility of retrograde flow of blood into the diseased segment of aorta via these side branches—a type 2 endoleak. These endoleaks often cease spontaneously. They do not require treatment in the absence of aneurysm sac or false lumen expansion.[11] Such expansion is uncommon, but, if it occurs, it can cause alteration in the morphology of the proximal or distal stent-graft seal zones with eventual loss of seal and type 1 endoleak (which would require treatment). Therefore type 2

TABLE 3-2   **Summary of Characteristics of Some Currently Manufactured Aortic Stent-Grafts**

Name	Endurant AAA	Excluder C3	Anaconda	AorFix	Zenith LP	Zenith Flex	Valiant Thoracic	TAG Conformable	TX2
Manufacturer	Medtronic	Gore	VascuTek Terumo	Lombard Medical	Cook	Cook	Medtronic	Gore	Cook
Date to Market	2012 (2nd gen)	2010	2007	1999	2010	1999	2009	2009	2009
Intended Deployment Site	Abdominal	Abdominal	Abdominal	Abdominal	Abdominal	Abdominal	Thoracic	Thoracic	Thoracic
Fabric	Polyester	ePTFE	Polyester	Polyester	Polyester	Polyester	Polyester	ePTFE	Polyester
Stent Material	Nitinol	Nitinol	Nitinol	Nitinol	Nitinol	Stainless steel	Nitinol	Nitinol	Stainless steel
Bare Stent—Distal	No	No	No	No	No	No	Yes (on some components)	No	Yes (distal components only)
Bare Stent—Proximal	Yes	No	No	No	Yes	Yes	Yes (on some components)	Yes (partially uncovered)	No
Hooks	On proximal bare stent	On proximal ring stent	On proximal ring stent	On proximal ring stent	On proximal bare stent	On proximal bare stent	No	No	On proximal ring stent and distal bare stent
IFU(*)									
Minimum Neck Length (mm)	10	15	15	20	15	15	15	20	20
Maximum Neck Angulation (°)	60	60	Not defined. Used up to 90	90	60	60	Not defined	Not defined	Not defined
Delivery System Diameter (Fr**)	18–20	18–20	20–23	22	16	18–22	22–25	18–24	20–22
Device Size Range (mm)	23–36	23–31	21–34	24–31	22–36	22–36	22–46	21–45	22–42
Comments			'Fish mouth' deployment system with marked repositionability. Magnet system for cannulation of contralateral limb	CE marked for 90° necks	Low profile version of Flex		Tip capture delivery system		Two-piece system (proximal and distal components). Trifold delivery system

*IFU = Indications for use.
**Diameter (mm) = French size /π.

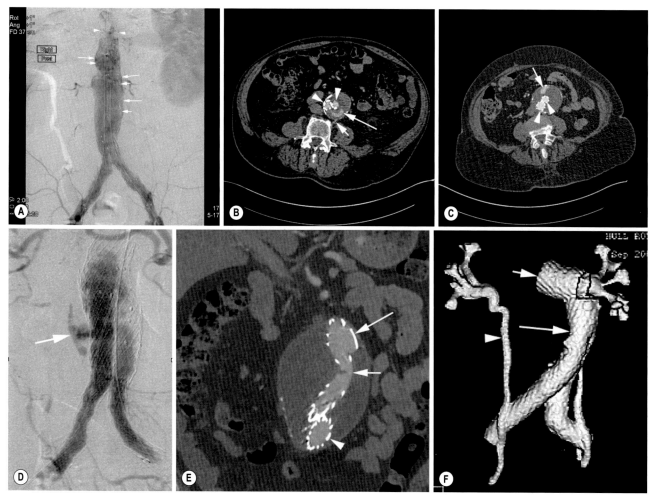

FIGURE 3-3 ■ **Complications of EVAR.** (A) Type 1 endoleak. Pigtail aortogram immediately following stent-graft deployment. The outer margins of the stent-graft are indicated by the lateral edges of the ring stents (short arrows). Contrast can be seen outside the stent-graft in the aneurysm sac and neck (long arrows). The lumbar vessels were filling antegradely, indicating this was not a type 2 leak. The proximal markers on the stent-graft fabric (arrowheads) are evident just below the proximal bare metal stent. (B) Type 2 endoleak from a lumbar vessel. A pool of contrast (long arrow) is evident posteriorly in the aneurysm sac outside the stent-graft limbs (arrowheads). It lies in close association with a prominent lumbar vessel (short arrow). (C) Type 2 endoleak from the inferior mesenteric artery. A pool of contrast (arrow) is evident anteriorly in the aneurysm sac outside the stent-graft limbs (arrowheads). It lies in close association with the inferior mesenteric artery (not shown). (D) Type 3 endoleak. A defect in the graft fabric has resulted in leakage of contrast from the graft lumen into the aneurysm sac (arrow). (E) Limb kinking. A fold of stent-graft fabric (short arrow), causing significant stenosis in one of the limbs of a bifurcated device (reformatted oblique image), is evident. The other limb (arrowhead) and proximal main body (long arrow) are unremarkable as they course through the image plane. (F) Device dislocation. Morphological changes in the aneurysm post EVAR have resulted in marked dislocation of a proximal extension cuff (short arrow) out of the main body (long arrow) of this bifurcated device. The renal collecting systems have been opacified by iodinated contrast media at the time of scan (arrowhead).

endoleaks with ongoing expansion are treated, usually with embolisation. Routine embolisation of prominent side branches before stent-graft deployment is time-consuming and has not been shown to alter rates of subsequent sac expansion.[12] The exceptions to this are the left subclavian artery and the internal iliac artery, both of which are moderately large vessels with prominent collateral circulation and, untreated, are a source of significant type 2 endoleak.

Type 3 Endoleak (Fig. 3-3D)

Graft defects and fabric tears are rare with modern devices but for modular devices (such as bifurcated

abdominal aortic stent-grafts, or long segment thoracic aortic devices) the seal between components can be incomplete or dislocation of one component from another can occur. The associated type 3 endoleak causes repressurisation of the diseased segment of aorta and (for aneurysmal disease) sac expansion and rupture. It requires treatment, usually by balloon moulding any joints, relining defects with a secondary device or operative repair.

Types 4 and 5 Endoleak

Type 4 endoleak refers to transient graft 'porosity'—equivalent to the 'sweating' sometimes seen with knitted open surgical grafts. It is rare with modern stent-graft fabric and does not require treatment. Type 5 endoleak refers to ongoing aneurysm sac expansion in the absence of any other demonstrable endoleak. It may be due to unidentified very low volume or intermittent endoleak, osmotic effects of dissolving atheroma and thrombus or low-grade infection. Treatment, if required (e.g. if the proximal or distal seal is threatened), can be difficult and complex.

Device Migration, Dislocation, Kinking and Occlusion

Each cardiac cycle produces a force estimated to be approximately 10 N (equivalent to 1 kg) tending to push the graft distally in the aorta. This can result in graft migration over time, especially where the proximal seal zone is short or diseased when device apposition to the wall of the aorta is suboptimal. Device migration can result in limb kinking (Fig. 3-3E), which predisposes to occlusion or thrombus formation and distal embolisation. Migration can also result in type 1 or 3 endoleak (if the device migrates out of the neck, or the migration results in a change in device geometry and dislocation of modular components—Fig. 3-3F). Longer-term morphological changes in the treated aortic segment can alter device geometry and cause kinking and dislocation in the absence of migration.

Device kinking and migration are rare with modern devices, occurring in approximately 1 and 2% of patients, respectively.[5] If there is little risk of complication associated with the migration or kinking (e.g. a small amount of migration in a long neck or a minor kink unlikely to cause haemodynamically significant stenosis), no treatment is required. However, if needed, treatment can be complex. Options include extension stent-grafting, device reinforcement with stent-grafts or uncovered stents, surgical buttressing of the neck or device explantation and open repair.

INFRASTRUCTURE AND STAFFING[13]

The management of patients with aortic disease is complex and should not be undertaken without adequate supportive infrastructure, staffing, processes and governance. The decision on how (and whether) to treat relies on detailed anatomical, physiological and clinical information. Electively, patients should undergo a formal assessment of their general cardiovascular fitness (such as a cardiopulmonary exercise test (CPX)) with treatment and optimisation, where possible, of any underlying pathology. Once clinical information and data on aortic morphology and cardiovascular fitness are available, the patient should be discussed at a multidisciplinary team meeting and a plan for treatment constructed. Written information should be provided to the patient about their aortic pathology and the proposed treatment. In an emergency such detailed work-up is clearly impossible, though there is occasionally time to optimise the patient's physiology to an extent.

Endovascular aortic repair should be carried out by experienced staff in a sterile environment of theatre standard with optimal imaging facilities and equipment to convert rapidly to open repair in an emergency. The ideal is an angiography theatre with fixed C-arm image intensification and theatre-grade air change and lighting, anaesthetic and surgical equipment, piped gases and suction and facilities for rapid (level 1) infusion and cell salvage.

Postoperative care in an intensive-care or high-dependency unit should be available if needed with facilities for invasive ventilation and renal support. Vascular surgical, anaesthetic and radiological support should be available on a 24/7 basis. Written protocols for accelerated postoperative recovery, mobilisation and discharge are desirable. Data should be submitted to national or international registries (such as the National Vascular Database (NVD) in the UK).

There is evidence of improved outcomes for open abdominal aortic aneurysm (AAA) repair at centres that undertake a greater volume of work.[14] This is almost certainly as much to do with pre- and post-procedural process as it is to do with individual surgical competence. There is likely to be a similar relationship for endovascular repair of all aortic lesions.[15] Centralisation of services for aortic repair is being undertaken currently in the UK.

THORACIC AORTIC INTERVENTION
Anatomical Considerations

For the purposes of endovascular repair, thoracic aortic pathology is best classified according to its location relative to the left subclavian artery (the Stanford classification, described originally for thoracic aortic dissection— see Fig. 3-4). Pathology affecting the aortic root and ascending aorta (Stanford A disease) is generally unsuitable for endovascular repair due to the frequent

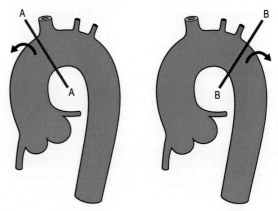

FIGURE 3-4 ■ **Stanford classification of aortic dissection.** Dissection is classified according to the site of the primary entry tear (curved arrows). If the tear lies proximal to the brachiocephalic artery, it is type A. If it lies distal to the left subclavian artery it is type B.

involvement of the aortic valve (which may also need repair) and close association of critical branch vessels (the coronary arteries and great vessels). There are occasional situations where endovascular intervention is preferable, though at present these must be considered experimental.[16]

Disease affecting the aorta distal to the left subclavian artery (Stanford B disease) is amenable to endovascular repair, assuming there is enough disease-free aorta proximally to achieve a seal (usually 15–20 mm). The left subclavian artery can be covered by the device to increase the available useable neck proximal to the diseased aorta without significant morbidity[17] and an even more proximal seal can be achieved with prior carotid–carotid bypass (which allows a seal proximal to the left common carotid origin) or complete arch debranching (with all the great vessels transposed onto the more proximal ascending aorta—Fig. 3-5), which allows coverage around the entire arch, distal to the reimplanted inominate artery. These techniques make distal- and mid-arch disease amenable to endovascular repair, though they increase the invasiveness and complexity of the intervention. Carotid–carotid bypass can be performed via incisions in the neck but complete arch debranching requires median sternotomy (though not cardiopulmonary bypass).

Angulation is a particular problem in the aortic arch and proximal descending thoracic aorta where the arch is not a smooth curve (like a Norman arch) but rather is peaked with an apex (like a Gothic arch; Fig. 3-6). This can lead to type 1 endoleak, particularly around the inner curve of the aorta. If there is a marked 'stand-off' between the device and the inner curve of the aorta the stent-graft can be folded in on itself by the action of blood flowing around the stent-graft rather than through it. Device placement such that the seal zone is (where possible) in a straight segment of aorta a few centimetres either proximal or distal to the point of angulation will avoid issues of poor seal and stand-off, but frequently such placement is impossible and a compromise must be struck between neck length and angulation. Modern devices conform to angled aortic morphology more readily than their predecessors but marked angulation remains a problem which can preclude thoracic aortic endovascular repair.

The blood supply to the spinal cord arises from the anterior spinal artery, a branch of the vertebral artery which usually arises from the first part of the subclavian artery. Additionally there is supply directly from the intercostal arteries as they arise from the descending thoracic aorta and enter the spinal canal as radicular (or medullary) arteries with the dorsal nerve roots. There is frequently a dominant radicular artery—the artery of Adamkiewicz—arising between T8 and L1, usually on the left. Repair of thoracic aortic pathology (whether open or endovascular) carries a risk of coverage (and therefore occlusion) of some or all of this spinal supply with resultant spinal cord ischaemia and diplegia. Open repair offers the possibility of intercostal vessel reimplantation but endovascular repair does not. The overall risk of diplegia with endovascular repair of thoracic aortic aneurysm is in the region of 3%.[18] The risks are higher

if the left subclavian is covered, if longer lengths of the thoracic aorta are covered and if there has been prior abdominal aortic repair.[19] Cerebrospinal fluid drainage preserves spinal cord blood flow during aortic cross-clamping and minimises rebound hyperaemia thereafter in animal models.[20] A prophylactic lumbar cerebrospinal fluid drain is protective during open and endovascular repair of thoracic aortic aneurysm (TAA) where the risks of cord ischaemia are thought to be high.[21,22]

THORACIC AORTIC ANEURYSM

The incidence of TAA is approximately 10 per 100,000 people per year,[23] with the incidence increasing as the population ages. Most (70%) involve the ascending aorta. They present frequently as incidental findings on chest X-rays (CXRs) or other imaging, or may cause hoarseness, stridor, dypnoea, dysphagia or pain due to local mass effects. Rupture presents with chest pain and shock and patients with rupture rarely survive to hospital.

The risk of rupture of a TAA is determined by size, site, rate of growth and association with genetic syndromes such as Marfan's. Untreated, most TAAs will eventually rupture[24] but the annual risk of rupture is difficult to accurately quantify. A retrospective review of outcomes of patients with TAA demonstrated annual rupture risk to be 0.3% for TAAs 4–4.9 cm in diameter, 1.7% for TAAs 5–5.9 cm in diameter and 3.6% for TAAs 6 cm or above. Similar annual risks of dissection in TAAs were noted.[25] These estimates are compound risks for all TAAs (ascending, arch and descending aortic sites). Descending thoracic aortic site was an additional (independent) predictor of rupture and descending thoracic aortic aneurysms were larger at presentation.

Repair should be considered when the risks of rupture exceed the risks of intervention. Guidelines from a joint US task force suggest that endovascular repair be considered when an asymptomatic descending aortic TAA reaches 5.5 cm.[26] A higher threshold (6 cm) is suggested for open repair given its greater risks.[26] There have been no clinical trials to demonstrate that observation only is safe up to a given aortic diameter for TAA (unlike the UK small aneurysm trial[27] for abdominal aortic aneurysm (AAA)—see below).

Rapidly expanding aneurysms or symptomatic aneurysms usually require treatment whatever their size. Pseudoaneuryms, saccular aneurysms and mycotic aneurysms are perceived to be at a greater risk of rupture than fusiform degenerative aneurysms and generally require early intervention.

Outcomes of Endovascular Repair and Comparison with Surgery

The aims of endovascular repair of a TAA are a proximal and distal seal in disease-free segments of the aorta and complete exclusion of the aneurysm sac from the circulation. Frequently the length of the aneurysm may require

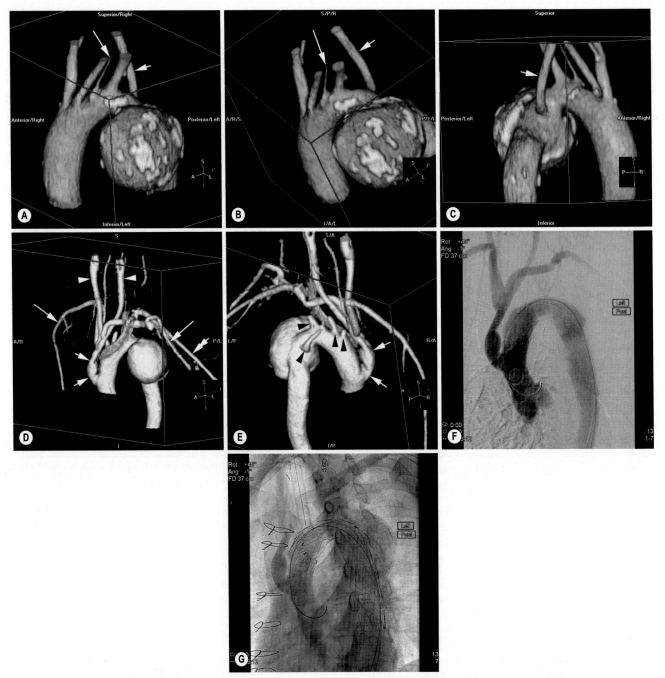

FIGURE 3-5 ■ **Proximal arch aneurysm treated with complete aortic debranching and stent-grafting.** (A–C) Surface-shaded volumetric CT reconstruction of the aortic arch in left anterior oblique (A), left superior anterior oblique (B) and right posterior oblique (C) projections. The great vessels can be seen arising from the superior surface of the arch. Additionally there is an aberrant left vertebral artery arising directly from the arch (long arrow) and an aberrant right subclavian arising from the aneurysmal proximal descending thoracic aorta (short arrow). (D, E) Surface-shaded volumetric MRA reconstruction following arch debranching in left anterior oblique (D) and right superior posterior oblique projections (E). A 'Y' graft (short arrows) has been constructed between the ascending aorta and the distal great vessels (arrowheads: common carotid arteries; long arrows: subclavian arteries). Gadolinium has been injected into the left arm, resulting in dense opacification of the left subclavian vein (double arrowhead). The ligated stumps of the great vessels (black arrowheads) are evident on the posterior view (E). Subtracted (F) and unsubtracted (G) angiographic images following stent-graft placement over the origins of the ligated great vessels, to the origin of the bypass graft.

several devices to be 'telescoped' one into the other to provide coverage. This may require considerable overlap of components to prevent subsequent dislocation and type 3 endoleak.

Registry data indicate that the overall 30-day mortality for endovascular repair of TAA is in the region of 2–5%.[28–30] Complications include stroke (4–7%), spinal cord ischaemia (2–4%), access vessel damage (2–5%), myocardial infarction (2–4%) and respiratory failure (5%). Endoleaks usually occur early and are seen in 10–20%, and device migration occurs in approximately 3%, though the requirement for secondary intervention

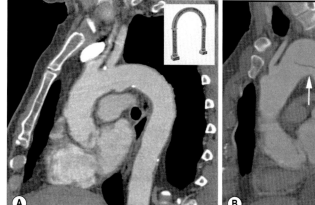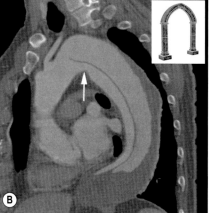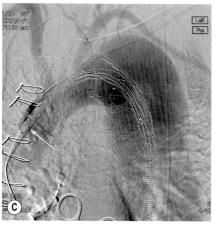

FIGURE 3-6 ■ **Aortic arch configurations for thoracic EVAR.** (A) Norman arch configuration with a shallow ulcer on the inner curve at its apex. Note the smooth curve around the arch without a focal angle (inset: architectural drawing of a Norman arch). (B) Gothic arch configuration with an aortic dissection. Note the angle (arrow) at the apex of the arch (inset: architectural drawing of a Gothic arch). (C) Complication of stent-grafting into a short neck around the apex of a Gothic arch. The device has dislocated out of the short neck at the point of arch angulation, resulting in a significant type 1 endoleak. A new device is being deployed (arrow: delivery system nosecone), extending the stent-graft more proximally in the arch (covering the left subclavian artery) to seal the leak. (Architectural images courtesy of Redwood Stone, West Horrington, Well, UK.)

to treat these problems is low (6–8%).[1] Aneurysm-related mortality by 1 year following endovascular repair of TAA is low (2%). Overall 1-year survival is 80%.[28]

Elective surgical mortality is approximately 10%,[31] dependent on the type of the repair necessary. There are no randomised studies comparing open surgical and endovascular repair of TAAs. Data from non-randomised studies indicate a lower all-cause mortality at 30 days and lower aneurysm-related (but not all-cause) mortality at 12 months for patients treated with endovascular repair.[1] The long-term durability of stent-grafts in the management of thoracic aortic disease is unknown, but 15 years of worldwide experience gives no reason to doubt their structural integrity in the lifespan of the patient. Newer generations of stent-graft might perform better long term than their predecessors, but this is unproven. In the UK, the National Institute for Health and Clinical Excellence (NICE) recommendation is that endovascular repair of TAA is a suitable alternative to surgery in appropriately selected patients.[32]

ACUTE AORTIC SYNDROME

Acute aortic syndrome is a general term used to encompass three aortic lesions with similar presentation: aortic dissection, intramural haematoma (IMH) and penetrating atherosclerotic ulcer (PAU). The exact pathological relationship between these entities is unclear. In aortic dissection, intimal disruption that allows blood to track through a dissection plane in the media can be identified. However, the initiating event for this may be a direct tear in the intima (due to shear stresses on the aortic wall) or intramural haemorrhage (from vasa vasorum) weakening the intima at the site of the tear. Thrombosis of the false lumen of a dissection may give rise to appearances identical to IMH or IMH may be due to microscopic dissection-like intimal tears. Bleeding at the base of a PAU could give rise to IMH or act as a focus for dissection.

Clinical presentation of acute aortic syndromes is usually with abrupt onset of severe chest pain. The classical description is of 'tearing interscapular' pain but pain may be anterior, abdominal or migratory. The symptom complex overlaps with many other potential diagnoses (e.g. myocardial infarction) and diagnosis relies significantly on index of suspicion. A small proportion of patients have a clinically silent dissection. Associated presenting features may be cerebrovascular accident, renal failure and acutely ischaemic bowel or limbs (due to branch vessel occlusion), myocardial infarction and acute aortic regurgitation (due to involvement of the aortic root or coronary ostia), pericardial tamponade, massive haemothorax and profound shock (due to rupture) or progression to aneurysm formation. These complicating features are more common with dissection than with IMH.[33]

Definitive diagnosis is usually made by cross-sectional imaging or transoesophageal ultrasound. A normal CXR does not exclude aortic dissection, IMH or PAU, although it may confirm an alternative diagnosis in patients with low clinical risk.

Of patients presenting with acute aortic syndrome, three-quarters have dissection, with 10–20% having IMH and a small proportion having PAU. Dissection involves the ascending aorta and arch in three-quarters of cases. IMH involves the descending thoracic aorta more frequently and tends to occur in older patients. PAU usually occurs in markedly atheromatous aortic segments, usually the descending thoracic aorta. Whatever the exact pathological relationship between these entities, the principles of management are broadly similar.

THORACIC AORTIC DISSECTION

The incidence of thoracic aortic dissection is about 5–10 per 100,000 people per year and is increasing with an ageing population. Dissection is associated with hypertension (especially if uncontrolled), inherited disorders of elastin such as Marfan's syndrome and certain vasculitides. TAA is a risk factor for dissection and vice versa.

Classification of dissection is important for management. It is classified according to its age (acute: less than 14 days old; subacute: 14 days–2 months; chronic: older than 2 months), the presence of associated complications and location (Stanford A or B).

Untreated, the prognosis of aortic dissection is poor, with an approximately 1% mortality per hour for the first 48 h after presentation. The mortality for type A dissection is worse than that for type B: uncomplicated type B dissection is associated with a 30-day mortality of 10%, though complications occur in 30% and are associated with significantly higher mortality (20% by 48 h, 30% by 30 days).[34]

Management

All patients with aortic dissection should be managed in a high-dependency environment with invasive monitoring. They should have aggressive management of heart rate (HR) and blood pressure to reduce aortic wall stress (HR <60 bpm, sBP <120 mmHg)[35]—though this can sometimes be difficult, requiring a combination of agents. Intravenous β-blockade and nitrates are commonly titrated to an adequate response. Pain control is essential.

As discussed above, disease affecting the ascending aorta is generally unsuitable for endovascular repair and definitive management should be surgical.

For Stanford type B dissections (involving the descending aorta, beyond the left subclavian artery) close clinical observation and serial imaging is mandatory as the requirement for definitive management is determined by the development of complications. A recent randomised trial demonstrated no additional benefit of endovascular repair of uncomplicated Stanford type B dissection over best medical therapy[36] and prophylactic surgical or endovascular repair in the absence of complications is not indicated.

Complicated Type B Dissection

The aim of endovascular management of complicated type B dissection is to treat the complications of the pathology (branch vessel occlusion and end-organ ischaemia) and prevent aneurysm formation and rupture.

Restoration of branch vessel flow is achieved by closure (i.e. coverage with a stent-graft) of the dissection entry tear with the aim of depressurising the false lumen and allowing true lumen re-expansion. Where branch vessels have been occluded dynamically (where the dissection flap has prolapsed across their aortic true lumen ostium—Fig. 3-7A), depressurisation of the false lumen allows the flap to move away from the ostium, with restoration of flow. Where the dissection has extended into a branch vessel (static occlusion—Fig. 3-7B) or where dynamic obstruction is not adequately relieved, additional branch vessel stenting or the deliberate formation of holes in the flap ('fenestration') may be needed.

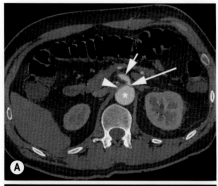

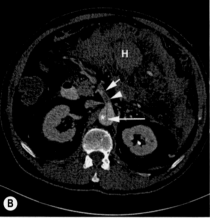

FIGURE 3-7 ■ **Static and dynamic branch vessel occlusion.** (A) Dynamic branch vessel occlusion. The true lumen (arrowhead) is markedly compressed by the false lumen (asterisk). The dissection flap (long arrow) is seen to prolapse across the ostium of the superior mesenteric artery (SMA) (short arrow), compromising its inflow (though the SMA is still filling). The patient had abdominal pain, rising lactate and thickening of small bowel loops (not shown) consistent with small bowel ischaemia. (B) Static vessel occlusion. The dissection flap (long arrow) has extended into the SMA (short arrow) and there has been thrombosis of the false lumen in the SMA (arrowhead). The true lumen (asterisk) is obliterated distally in the SMA by the combination of the dissection and the thrombus. A large intraperitoneal haematoma is evident (H) due to bleeding from infarcted bowel.

Not infrequently there are several tears ('fenestrations') in the dissection flap. Coverage of all these fenestrations necessitates stent-grafting a longer length of aorta with increased risk of diplegia, though (theoretically at least) with a greater chance of false lumen collapse. Whether all fenestrations or just the 'primary' entry tear should be covered is debatable. If the dissection extends below the diaphragm there are often fenestrations at the level of the renal arteries or in the infrarenal aorta. Stent-graft placement from the thorax into the abdominal aorta is clearly impossible, as it would necessitate splanchnic and renal artery coverage. In this situation the proximal entry tear (or tears) in the thoracic aorta only are covered in the hope that this will alter the haemodynamics enough to allow abdominal true lumen re-expansion.

Ideally the false lumen should collapse entirely (and be obliterated) or should at least thrombose (Fig. 3-8). False lumen thrombosis protects against rupture and aneurysm formation and is associated with good

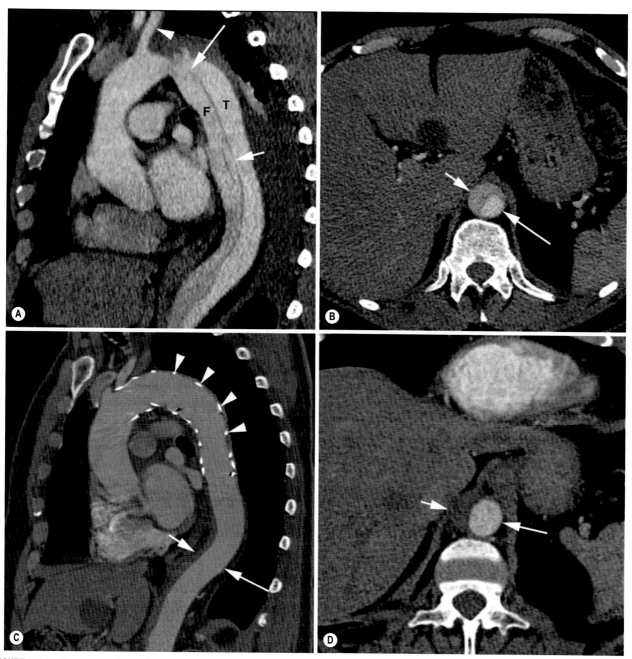

FIGURE 3-8 ■ **Coverage of proximal entry tear of a dissection with false lumen thrombosis and collapse.** (A) Acute type B dissection. The entry tear (long arrow), a more distal fenestration (short arrow) and the dissection flap are clearly visualised. Arrowhead: left common carotid artery; F: false lumen; T: true lumen. (B) Representative aortic cross-section at the level of the diaphragmatic crura. The true lumen (long arrow) and false lumen (short arrow) both opacify with contrast, indicating patency. (C) Following stent-graft (arrowheads) placement in the true lumen, covering (and sealing) the proximal entry tear. The false lumen (short arrow) has thrombosed and partially collapsed. The true lumen (long arrow) remains patent. (D) Representative aortic cross-section (same level as B), demonstrating thrombosis of the false lumen (short arrow) and retained patency of the true lumen (long arrow).

long-term outcome.[37] Ongoing false lumen perfusion after stent-graft coverage of the entry tear (Fig. 3-9) can occur via uncovered fenestrations, retrogradely from the distal end of the dissection or via backbleeding from branch vessels.

Other techniques to eradicate the false lumen include scissoring or 'cheese-wiring' the flap or using large uncovered stents to pin it back in place. Often a combination of techniques is used.

Stent-grafts for treating acute dissection should not be oversized relative to the vessel to be treated (in contrast to sizing for TAA) as the vessel wall is extremely friable. Aggressive oversizing and the use of balloon moulding can result in aortic rupture or proximal or distal extension

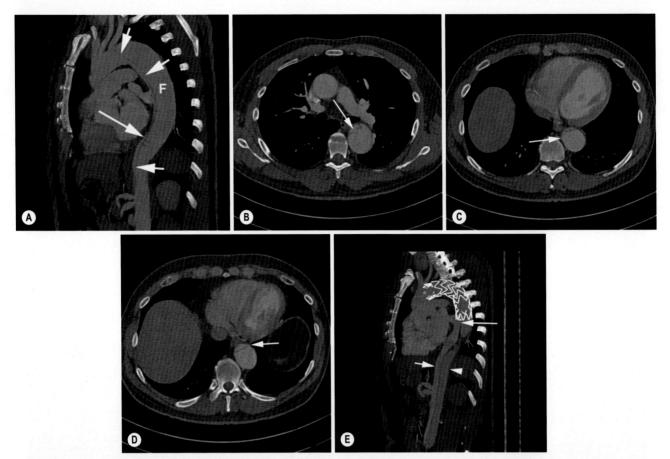

FIGURE 3-9 ■ **Coverage of proximal entry tear of a dissection with failure of false lumen thrombosis and ongoing perfusion.** (A) Acute type B dissection. The true lumen (long arrow) is significantly compromised by the false lumen (F). In addition to the proximal entry tear, several other fenestrations (short arrows) are evident in the dissection flap. (B–D) Representative aortic cross-sections in the mid (B) and distal (C, D) thoracic aorta demonstrating the fenestrations (arrows) in the flap. The true lumen is compromised by the false lumen. (E) Following stent-graft placement in the true lumen covering (and sealing) the proximal entry tear. The false lumen persists due to ongoing perfusion via a large fenestration just distal to the stent-graft (long arrow), and the other smaller fenestrations demonstrated on the pre-EVAR CT (A–D). Short arrow: true lumen; arrowhead: false lumen.

of the dissection, potentially converting a type B dissection into a type A.[38]

Chronic Dissection and Aneurysmal Development

Thoracic aortic dissection may be associated with aneurysmal development of the aorta at presentation, or it may develop over time following acute dissection. Dissection may also occur de novo in a pre-existing TAA. Management (as for TAA) requires exclusion of the aneurysmal segment of aorta from the circulation by obtaining a proximal and distal seal above and below the aneurysmal segment. This is difficult if the aneurysm is extensive (and especially if it extends below the diaphragm). Moreover, with time, the dissection flap becomes stiffer and fibrous, and is more difficult to displace. It may prevent a stent-graft from opening fully. Not infrequently there has been previous placement of stent-grafts in the aorta (e.g. as treatment for the acute phase of the dissection), which can make subsequent device placement challenging as multiple layers of metalwork and device markers can become confusing.

Outcomes of Endovascular Repair and Comparison with Surgery

A recent meta-analysis of 609 patients undergoing endovascular repair of type B aortic dissection indicated rates of 30-day mortality of 5%, in-hospital major complication of 11% and aortic rupture (during mean follow-up of 20 months) of 2%. False lumen thrombosis was seen in 75% of patients.[39] For studies with follow-up to 2 years, the overall survival was 90%. This compares favourably with surgical outcomes (in-hospital mortality: 34%; in-hospital major complication: 40%).[40] NICE recommendations are that endovascular repair of thoracic aortic dissection is a suitable alternative to surgery in appropriately selected patients.[32]

ACUTE INTRAMURAL HAEMATOMA AND PENETRATING ULCER

The management of these lesions is broadly similar to that of acute aortic dissection. Aggressive medical management should be instituted. Type A lesions require surgery. Complicated type B PAU (with or without associated IMH) should be treated similarly to aortic dissection, with the PAU being considered the 'entry tear'. Complicated type B IMH without an identifiable intimal defect represents a therapeutic challenge as there is no 'target' for limited stent-graft coverage even though the IMH itself may be extensive. It may be necessary to cover the entire involved aorta.

TRAUMATIC LESIONS OF THE THORACIC AORTA

Blunt traumatic lesions of the thoracic aorta account for approximately 15% of road traffic accident fatalities in the UK.[41] The most common site of blunt injury is at the aortic isthmus, at the site of the ligamentum arteriosum, probably because of differential torsional and shear forces acting on the relatively mobile arch and the less mobile descending thoracic aorta during sudden deceleration or acceleration. Other mechanisms such as osseous pinch or hydrostatic injury have been proposed.

A range of appearances is seen on imaging for traumatic aortic injury from minor flaps of intima to traumatic dissection, intramural haematoma or abrupt (sometimes circumferential) changes in aortic contour[42] (Fig. 3-10). Mediastinal haematoma may be evident, though it is unlikely to be aortic in origin (arising instead from damaged mediastinal vessels). A full-thickness tear in the aorta, with high-pressure bleeding into the loose connective tissue of the mediastinum, is unlikely to seal spontaneously and will result in exsanguination and death, usually at-scene. It follows therefore that most patients who survive to imaging will have some form of incomplete aortic injury (IAI), with at least one layer of the aortic wall (often the adventitia) intact.

Untreated, the prognosis of patients with IAI is very poor, with an approximately 30% mortality within 6 h and 50% mortality at 24 h.[43] There are invariably significant associated injuries and prognosis reflects the compound effects of diffuse and significant trauma to multiple organs and organ systems, rather than being due to the aortic injury alone.

The observation that early mortality in patients with IAI was high led to a doctrine of early aortic repair as paramount whatever the priorities for management of associated injuries. More recently, extrapolating from medical management of type B aortic dissection, several studies have demonstrated that immediate aggressive blood pressure control (mBP<80 mmHg) markedly reduces the risks of rupture,[44,45] allowing time for treatment of other life-threatening injuries and control of haemorrhage, sepsis, hypothermia and acidosis. Control of blood pressure in this manner may allow definitive aortic repair to be safely delayed by days or weeks.[44,45] Sometimes blood pressure control may be incompatible with requirements for treatment of other injuries (especially the maintenance of cerebral perfusion pressure in head injury), in which case earlier definitive repair is indicated. Senior clinical consultation is essential in these complex cases[46] to ensure sequencing of therapeutic interventions is optimised and timely.

The mortality associated with endovascular repair of IAI is significantly less than that for open surgical repair (7 vs 15%).[47] Rates of significant morbidity are also lower (diplegia: 0 and 6%; stroke 1 and 5%, respectively) with identical rates of technical success.[47] However, the long-term performance of stent-grafts in these (often young) patients is unknown. American College of Cardiology guidelines on management of thoracic aortic disease[26] state that endovascular repair of IAI 'be considered'. There are currently no guidelines in the UK.

Penetrating Injury to the Thoracic Aorta

Full-thickness penetrating injury to the thoracic aorta usually results in death at-scene. IAI is uncommon but if it occurs, it can be managed similarly to blunt injury.

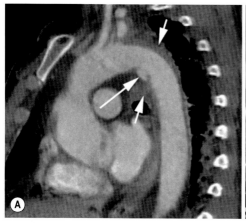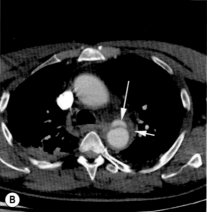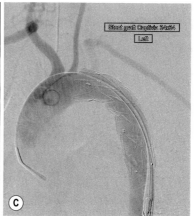

FIGURE 3-10 ■ **Aortic trauma.** (A, B) Typical appearances of blunt traumatic incomplete aortic injury with irregularity of the external aortic contour in the region of the ligamentum arteriosum (long arrow) and periaortic blood (short arrow) from damage to vasa-vasorum and mediastinal vessels. (C) Stent-graft repair with coverage of the site of aortic injury with a short device.

Iatrogenic injury (usually the result of misplaced attempts at central venous cannulation) is survivable if recognised immediately and ideally before the device is removed.

AORTIC COARCTATION

Most cases of aortic coarctation are diagnosed in childhood and early repair is associated with improved outcome and rates of complication.[48] Endovascular treatment of coarctation in childhood is problematic as access vessels are small and stent deployment can interfere with the later growth of the treated aortic segment, leading to recoarctation despite initial technical success. Angioplasty (without stenting) is possible, though it cannot deal with elastic vessel recoil. In general, endovascular management of coarctation is therefore reserved for older children and adults.

Outcomes after endovascular repair for coarctation (Fig. 3-11) are good with technical success rates in excess of 90%.[49] Peri-procedural mortality is low (2–3%) for both endovascular and open-surgical repair.[50,51] Rates of restenosis are approximately 10% following primary surgical repair and 5% following stent placement.[50,51] Redo surgery is complex and in this situation endovascular repair may be preferable.

ABDOMINAL AORTIC ANEURYSM

Abdominal aortic aneurysm (AAA) is a disease of the elderly with a prevalence of 8% in the over 60s. The male : female ratio is 7 : 1. AAA is six times more common than TAA. Most are occult and are only diagnosed incidentally during investigation of other disorders or when they rupture. Occasionally, AAAs present with symptoms other than rupture—usually abdominal or back pain.

The risk of AAA rupture is a function of size: a 5.5-cm AAA has an annual risk of rupture of about 6%, but for an 8-cm AAA the risk it is 25%.[52,53] Symptomatic AAAs are at greater risk of rupture and usually require urgent intervention.

The aetiology of AAA is unclear. There is a strong familial tendency, and most patients are smokers or ex-smokers. Patients often have atherosclerotic disease elsewhere. An inflammatory infiltrate is seen in the walls of large AAAs though whether this arises in response to atheromatous deposits or merely as a response to common risk factors is unknown. In a small proportion of AAAs (5–10%) the inflammatory infiltrate is marked. These patients tend to be younger, and are more often symptomatic, though the risks of rupture for a given size are lower. Unlike 'atherosclerotic' AAA there is often elevation of serum inflammatory markers and a cuff of peri-aortic 'haziness' on CT.

Anatomical Considerations in AAA repair

Most AAA stent-graft systems comprise a main body with a long limb on one side and a short limb (or 'gate') on the other (see Fig. 3-1). Once the main body is deployed,

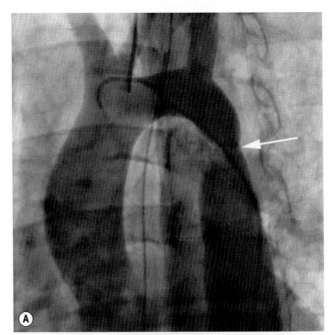

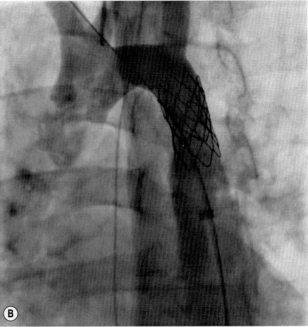

FIGURE 3-11 ■ **Aortic coarctation.** (A) Aortic coarctation (arrow). Note the hypertrophied great vessels (particularly the left subclavian) which supply collateral pathways (e.g. via the internal thoracic artery and intercostals) to beyond the coarctation. (B) Coarctation (same patient as A) treated with a balloon mounted stent.

the short limb is catheterised from the opposite side. A second limb is then inserted over a wire into the short limb of the main body, sealing inside the main body at a flow divider. Innovative single-piece stent-graft designs are available (for example, with limbs that are pulled into place) though these have, as yet, not been widely adopted.

As stated earlier, the anatomy of the proximal 'neck' is critical for the efficacy of any endovascular repair. For AAA the 'neck' refers to the segment of aorta between the lowest renal artery and the aneurysm. Short, angled or thrombus-filled necks increase the risk of endoleak and device failure. Proximal bare stents can be deployed across the renal arteries to achieve a more secure fixation in short necks.

The distal 'landing zone' in AAA repair is usually the common iliac artery. However, where this vessel is also aneurysmal, or is short, extension to the external iliac artery is necessary, usually with previous proximal embolisation of the internal iliac artery (IIA) to prevent a significant type 2 endoleak via back-filling. Embolisation of the IIA on one side is associated with buttock claudication in up to 31% and erectile dysfunction in up to 17%.[54] Risks of buttock claudication are higher if the IIA embolisation is necessary bilaterally. Iliac branched devices which preserve IIA patency are available.

Risks and Timing of Repair

Scheduling intervention to aortic aneurysms is a balance between the risks of intervention (be it open surgery or EVAR) and the risks of rupture. The patient's overall fitness needs to be carefully considered as this affects both the risks of intervention and the likelihood of the patient surviving long enough beyond the intervention to see the benefit of it. The UK Small Aneurysm Study[27] demonstrated that surgical treatment of AAAs smaller than 5.5 cm (on US) was associated with a greater overall mortality than conservative management and this has underpinned the practice of 'watchful waiting' with serial imaging of AAAs smaller than 5.5 cm. Intuitively, any new method of treating AAA with an improved perioperative mortality over that of open surgery (6%)[2,4] would alter the balance of risks between watching and intervening, so that treatment could be offered safely for smaller AAAs. Endovascular repair of AAA is associated with a 30-day mortality approximately one-third that of open repair (2%),[2,4] though whether this means smaller aneurysms should be treated with EVAR remains unproven. A recent randomised trial to test this hypothesis in AAAs 4–5 cm in diameter demonstrated equal mortality for EVAR and surveillance groups though the study was probably underpowered to detect a difference.[55]

Outcomes of Endovascular Repair and Comparison with Surgery

There are two randomised trials that compared EVAR with open surgical repair of AAA: the UK EVAR 1 trial and the Dutch DREAM Trial.[2,4] Both these trials demonstrated a threefold reduction in 30-day mortality with EVAR (2 vs 6% for open repair). At 4 years aneurysm-based mortality was also reduced in patients randomised to EVAR though all-cause mortality (principally due to non-aneurysm-related cardiovascular death) was the same in both EVAR and open repair groups.[5]

Critics of endovascular repair note that there is an increased rate of secondary interventions in the EVAR group (20 vs 6% for open surgery by 4 years, mostly for type 1 or 2 endoleak), that not all patients are anatomically suitable for EVAR, that an economic analysis of the

EVAR 1 trial's data suggests that by 4 years EVAR is more expensive than open repair (£13,257 vs £9946) and that the durability of EVAR in the medium-to-long term is unknown. However, both of the randomised trials of EVAR versus open surgery were carried out relatively early in the development of endovascular aneurysm repair (EVAR 1 recruited from 1999 to 2003). Since they reported, rates of secondary intervention have fallen[56] due to the improved performance of newer generations of devices and a greater awareness of what is and is not suitable anatomy for EVAR. More conformable, fenestrated and scalloped devices increase the applicability of an endovascular approach in challenging anatomy, meaning more patients are treatable with EVAR. Device costs are falling and, as less intensive follow-up protocols are advocated,[8] the cost of follow-up (a significant proportion of the cost of EVAR) is decreasing. Finally, though long-term durability of EVAR remains unproven, the significant cumulative cardiovascular mortality of the cohort of patients with large AAA[57] renders this consideration rather moot.

ENDOVASCULAR REPAIR OF RUPTURED AAA

The mortality of ruptured AAA (rAAA) exceeds 85%. About half of patients with ruptured aneurysms die in the community and of those arriving alive in hospital only a quarter will survive to discharge. These figures have changed little over the past 50 years.[58] The incidence of rAAA is increasing.[59]

Emergency endovascular repair (eEVAR) of rAAA (Fig. 3-12) necessitates taking a haemodynamically compromised patient to CT (to allow device sizing and procedural planning) before the point of definitive care, introducing a small delay with potential adverse effects on mortality. About half of all patients with rAAA have aneurysm morphology suitable for endovascular repair.[60] On the other hand, the theoretical benefit of a minimally invasive repair over open surgery is enhanced in a critically ill patient. The trade-off between these three factors (delay, suitability and invasiveness) is fundamental in determining the possible role of eEVAR in rAAA. In practice, logistical issues (such as availability of skilled staff) will also be critical, especially out-of-hours.

Meta-analyses of pooled data from numerous small studies of eEVAR have demonstrated in-hospital mortality of about 20%.[60,61] Open repair of rAAA is associated with 30-day mortality of about 40%.[58,62] The transfusion requirements, intensive care and hospital stay and cost of eEVAR also appear to be lower.[61,63,64] Some of the improved outcomes seen with eEVAR may be accounted for by publication[61] and selection bias (more stable patients being transferred to CT for EVAR work-up, whilst the less stable ones are taken immediately to open surgery). There is, as yet, no level 1 evidence comparing eEVAR with open repair for rAAA, though a multicentre randomised controlled trial (IMPROVE)[65] is due to report in November 2013 and it would not be surprising if eEVAR became the treatment of choice for rAAA once the results of this trial are known.

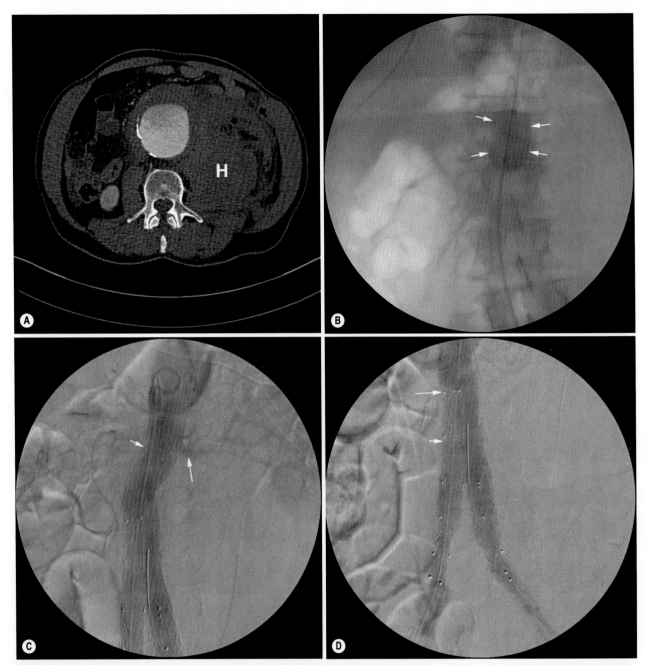

FIGURE 3-12 ■ Emergency EVAR for ruptured AAA. (A) Typical appearances of a ruptured AAA with a sizable left retroperitoneal haematoma (H) and a 7-cm AAA. (B) Suprarenal aortic occlusion balloon (arrows) has been placed (percutaneously) via a common femoral artery approach as a temporising measure to prevent further bleeding while the patient is prepared and the stent-grafts chosen and readied. (C, D) Completion angiograms following emergency stent-graft repair demonstrating complete exclusion of the AAA from the circulation and good flow into the common iliac arteries bilaterally. (C) Long arrow: left renal artery; short arrow: marker on upper edge of stent-graft fabric. (D) Long arrow: upper markers of contralateral limb aligned with flow divider of the main body; short arrow: ring marking lower extent of contralateral limb stump or 'gate'. The patient was discharged 3 days later.

THORACO-ABDOMINAL ANEURYSMS

So far this chapter has dealt specifically with aneurysms arising solely above or below the renal and mesenteric arteries. Thoraco-abdominal aneurysms cross these anatomical arterial boundaries and present very significant challenges for both open and endovascular repair. Thoraco-abdominal aneurysms are classified into four types depending on their anatomical location and extent. They are invariably fatal when they rupture but (as with TAA) there are no studies to guide timing of intervention.

The peri-procedural mortality of open repair is around 19%.[66] This usually involves replacement of the affected portions of the aorta with a synthetic graft, with reimplantation of branch vessels either individually or as

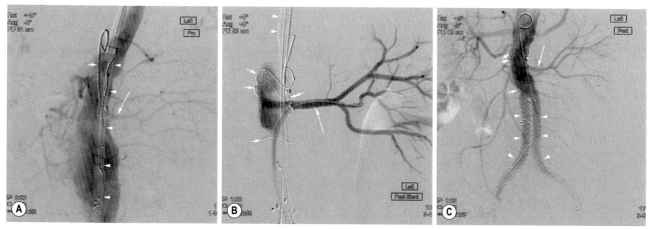

FIGURE 3-13 ■ **Branched stent-graft repair.** AAA with a short conical neck, unsuitable for repair with a conventional device, being repaired with a custom-built branched device (same patient as in Fig. 3-2A). (A) Main body of the device about to be deployed. Long arrow: left renal artery; short arrow: pigtail catheter; arrowheads: delivery system sheath within which the constrained main body is evident. (B) Angiogram following main body and branch vessel stent-graft deployment. The main body (short arrows) has been deployed above the left renal artery. A ring of high-density markers can be seen in the main body wall (double arrowhead) surrounding a custom-made fenestration (hole). A short covered stent (long arrow) has been placed through this into the left renal artery, preserving flow into it. Arrowheads: main body delivery system nose cone. (C) Completion angiogram following branched stent-graft repair. The proximal seal is above the left renal artery but below the right. Flow into the left renal artery is preserved via the fenestration and covered stent (long arrow). There is good flow into the common iliac arteries via iliac extensions (arrowheads). The aneurysm is completely excluded from the circulation. Short arrows: main body.

'islands' of native aorta from which several vessels arise. Cardiopulmonary bypass is sometimes necessary. A 'hybrid' repair involves insertion of a stent-graft to exclude the aneurysm, with the mesenteric and renal arteries then surgically reimplanted onto a conduit from the iliac arteries. The peri-procedural mortality of hybrid repair is in the region of 15–20%.[66]

Endovascular grafts that have a means of preserving flow into the visceral vessels have been developed, principally to allow treatment of complex juxtarenal AAAs. Such devices have fenestrations (holes) or branches to allow aortic side branch perfusion (Fig. 3-13). Series of fenestrated stent-grafts to treat thoraco-abdominal aneurysms have been published with encouraging intermediate-term mortality (about 5%),[66] though these results are predominantly from three institutions (worldwide) with expertise in the technique and may not be generalisable more widely.[67]

AORTIC STENOSES AND OCCLUSIONS

Haemodynamically significant stenoses of the infrarenal aorta are rare. Surgical options include localised aortic endarterectomy or bypass. Endovascular options include 'kissing balloon' angioplasty, 'kissing' aortic to common iliac artery stents or primary aortic stenting (first described in 1985[68]). These procedures are significantly less invasive than open aortic surgery, usually requiring a single night's stay in hospital. In some institutions they are performed as day cases. Primary stenting has 5-year patency rates of 80–100% for aortic stenosis and 60% for stenoses extending into the iliac ateries.[69,70] Complications are uncommon.[69]

SUMMARY AND CONCLUSION

Management of aortic disease is complex, requiring the involvement of vascular radiologists, vascular surgeons and anaesthetists skilled in the management of vascular patients. Stent-grafts offer a minimally invasive option for aortic repair though they are associated with some novel complications and clinical and imaging follow-up is essential. The evidence suggests that, in general, endovascular repair is associated with lower procedural mortality, though at the expense of greater rates of secondary interventions over time, than open surgical repair. There remains a cohort of patients who are unsuitable for endovascular repair, principally because of morphological constraints. Emergency EVAR for aortic trauma and spontaneous rupture is promising, with particularly low mortality relative to open surgery.

As stent-graft technology develops, the results and applicability of endovascular repair of aortic pathology would be expected to improve further. Branched and fenestrated technologies are particularly exciting developments. It is possible that, in the near future, the majority of aortic pathology is treated with an endovascular technique, with open surgery being the exception rather than the rule.

REFERENCES

1. Fairman RM, Criado F, Farber M, et al. Pivotal results of the Medtronic Vascular Talent Thoracic Stent Graft System: the VALOR trial. J Vasc Surg 2008;48:546–54.
2. Greenhalgh RM. Comparison of endovascular aneurysm repair with open repair in patients with abdominal aortic aneurysm (EVAR trial 1), 30-day operative mortality results: randomised controlled trial. Lancet 2004;364:843–8.

3. Parodi JC, Palmaz JC, Barone HD. Transfemoral intraluminal graft implantation for abdominal aortic aneurysms. Ann Vasc Surg 1991;5:491–9.
4. Blankensteijn JD, de Jong SE, Prinssen M, et al. Two-year outcomes after conventional or endovascular repair of abdominal aortic aneurysms. N Engl J Med 2005;352:2398–405.
5. EVAR trial participants. Endovascular aneurysm repair versus open repair in patients with abdominal aortic aneurysm (EVAR trial 1): randomised controlled trial. Lancet 2005;365:2179–86.
6. Torsello G, Troisi N, Donas KP, Austermann M. Evaluation of the Endurant stent graft under instructions for use vs off-label conditions for endovascular aortic aneurysm repair. J Vasc Surg 2011;54:300–6.
7. Cox DE, Jacobs DL, Motaganahalli RL, et al. Outcomes of endovascular AAA repair in patients with hostile neck anatomy using adjunctive balloon-expandable stents. Vasc Endovascular Surg 2006;40:35–40.
8. Chaer RA, Gushchin A, Rhee R, et al. Duplex ultrasound as the sole long-term surveillance method post-endovascular aneurysm repair: a safe alternative for stable aneurysms. J Vasc Surg 2009; 49:845–9; discussion 849–50.
9. Sampaio SM, Panneton JM, Mozes GI, et al. Proximal type I endoleak after endovascular abdominal aortic aneurysm repair: predictive factors. Ann Vasc Surg 2004;18:621–8.
10. Stanley BM, Semmens JB, Mai Q, et al. Evaluation of patient selection guidelines for endoluminal AAA repair with the Zenith stent-graft: the Australasian experience. J Endovasc Ther 2001;8:457–64.
11. van Marrewijk C, Buth J, Harris PL, et al. Significance of endoleaks after endovascular repair of abdominal aortic aneurysm: The EUROSTAR experience. J Vasc Surg 2002;35:461–73.
12. Nevala T, Biancari F, Manninen H, et al. Inferior mesenteric artery embolization before endovascular repair of an abdominal aortic aneurysm: effect on type II endoleak and aneurysm shrinkage. J Vasc Interv Radiol 2010;21:181–5.
13. Vascular Society of Great Britain and Northern Ireland. Framework for improving the results of elective AAA repair. Available at: <http://www.vascularsociety.org.uk/library/quality-improvement.html>. Accessed 29 February 2012.
14. Holt PJ, Poloniecki JD, Loftus IM, et al. Epidemiological study of the relationship between volume and outcome after abdominal aortic aneurysm surgery in the UK from 2000 to 2005. Br J Surg 2007;94:441–8.
15. McPhee J, Eslami MH, Arous EJ, et al. Endovascular treatment of ruptured abdominal aortic aneurysms in the United States (2001–2006): a significant survival benefit over open repair is independently associated with increased institutional volume. J Vasc Surg 2009;49:817–26.
16. Ye C, Chang G, Li S, et al. Endovascular stent-graft treatment for Stanford type A aortic dissection. Eur J Vasc Endovasc Surg 2011;42:787–94.
17. Riesenman PJ, Farber MA, Mendes RR, et al. Coverage of the left subclavian artery during thoracic endovascular aortic repair. J Vasc Surg 2007;45:90–4; discussion 94–5.
18. Bavaria JE, Appoo JJ, Makaroun MS, et al. Endovascular stent grafting versus open surgical repair of descending thoracic aortic aneurysms in low-risk patients: a multicenter comparative trial. J Thorac Cardiovasc Surg 2007;133:369–77.
19. Buth J, Harris PL, Hobo R, et al. Neurologic complications associated with endovascular repair of thoracic aortic pathology: incidence and risk factors. a study from the European Collaborators on Stent/Graft Techniques for Aortic Aneurysm Repair (EUROSTAR) registry. J Vasc Surg 2007;46:1103–10; discussion 1110–11.
20. Bower TC, Murray MJ, Gloviczki P, et al. Effects of thoracic aortic occlusion and cerebrospinal fluid drainage on regional spinal cord blood flow in dogs: correlation with neurologic outcome. J Vasc Surg 1989;9:135–44.
21. Coselli JS, LeMaire SA, Köksoy C, et al. Cerebrospinal fluid drainage reduces paraplegia after thoracoabdominal aortic aneurysm repair: results of a randomized clinical trial. J Vasc Surg 2002; 35:631–9.
22. Hnath JC, Mehta M, Taggert JB, et al. Strategies to improve spinal cord ischemia in endovascular thoracic aortic repair: outcomes of a prospective cerebrospinal fluid drainage protocol. J Vasc Surg 2008;48:836–40.
23. Clouse WD, Hallett JW, Schaff HV, et al. Improved prognosis of thoracic aortic aneurysms: a population-based study. JAMA 1998; 280:1926–9.
24. Pressler V, McNamara JJ. Aneurysm of the thoracic aorta. Review of 260 cases. J Thorac Cardiovasc Surg 1985;89:50–4.
25. Davies RR, Goldstein LJ, Coady MA, et al. Yearly rupture or dissection rates for thoracic aortic aneurysms: simple prediction based on size. Ann Thorac Surg 2002;73:17–27; discussion 27–8.
26. Hiratzka LF, Bakris GL, Beckman JA, et al. ACCF/AHA/AATS/ACR/ASA/SCA/SCAI/SIR/STS/SVM Guidelines for the diagnosis and management of patients with thoracic aortic disease. A Report of the American College of Cardiology Foundation/American Heart Association Task Force on Practice Guidelines, American Association for Thoracic Surgery, American College of Radiology, American Stroke Association, Society of Cardiovascular Anesthesiologists, Society for Cardiovascular Angiography and Interventions, Society of Interventional Radiology, Society of Thoracic Surgeons, and Society for Vascular Medicine. J Am Coll Cardiol 2010;55:e27–129.
27. The UK Small Aneurysm Trial Participants. Mortality results for randomised controlled trial of early elective surgery or ultrasonographic surveillance for small abdominal aortic aneurysms. Lancet 1998;352:1649–55.
28. Leurs LJ, Bell R, Degrieck Y, et al. Endovascular treatment of thoracic aortic diseases: combined experience from the EUROSTAR and United Kingdom Thoracic Endograft registries. J Vasc Surg 2004;40:670–9; discussion 679–80.
29. Makaroun MS, Dillavou ED, Kee ST, et al. Endovascular treatment of thoracic aortic aneurysms: results of the phase II multicenter trial of the GORE TAG thoracic endoprosthesis. J Vasc Surg 2005;41:1–9.
30. Fattori R, Nienaber CA, Rousseau H, et al. Results of endovascular repair of the thoracic aorta with the Talent Thoracic stent graft: the Talent Thoracic Retrospective Registry. J Thorac Cardiovasc Surg 2006;132:332–9.
31. The Society of Cardiothoracic Surgeons of Great Britain and Ireland. Sixth National Adult Cardiac Surgical Database Report 2008. Available at: <http://www.scts.org/_userfiles/resources/Sixth NACSDreport2008withcovers.pdf>. Accessed 1 March 2012.
32. National Institute for Health and Clinical Excellence. Endovascular stent-graft placement in thoracic aortic aneurysms and dissections. Available at: <http://www.nice.org.uk/nicemedia/live/11013/30553/30553.pdf>. Accessed 1 March 2012.
33. von Kodolitsch Y, Csösz SK, Koschyk DH, et al. Intramural hematoma of the aorta: predictors of progression to dissection and rupture. Circulation 2003;107:1158–63.
34. Nienaber CA, Eagle KA. Aortic dissection: new frontiers in diagnosis and management: Part I: from etiology to diagnostic strategies. Circulation 2003;108:628–35.
35. Tsai TT, Nienaber CA, Eagle KA. Acute aortic syndromes. Circulation 2005;112:3802–13.
36. Nienaber CA, Rousseau H, Eggebrecht H, et al. Randomized comparison of strategies for type B aortic dissection: the INvestigation of STEnt Grafts in Aortic Dissection (INSTEAD) trial. Circulation 2009;120:2519–28.
37. Bernard Y, Zimmermann H, Chocron S, et al. False lumen patency as a predictor of late outcome in aortic dissection. Am J Cardiol 2001;87:1378–82.
38. Eggebrecht H, Schmermund A, Herold U, et al. Rapid progression of discrete type A intramural hematoma: prevention of a 'procedure-related' complication by intraoperative transesophageal echocardiography. J Endovasc Ther 2005;12:252–7.
39. Eggebrecht H, Nienaber CA, Neuhäuser M, et al. Endovascular stent-graft placement in aortic dissection: a meta-analysis. Eur Heart J 2006;27:489–98.
40. Fattori R, Tsai TT, Myrmel T, et al. Complicated acute type B dissection: is surgery still the best option?: a report from the International Registry of Acute Aortic Dissection. JACC Cardiovasc Interv 2008;1:395–402.
41. Williams JS, Graff JA, Uku JM, Steinig JP. Aortic injury in vehicular trauma. Ann Thorac Surg 1994;57:726–30.
42. McPherson SJ. Thoracic aortic and great vessel trauma and its management. Semin Intervent Radiol 2007;24:180–96.
43. Parmley LF, Mattingly TW, Manion WC, Jahnke EJ. Nonpenetrating traumatic injury of the aorta. Circulation 1958;17:1086–101.

44. Pate JW, Fabian TC, Walker W. Traumatic rupture of the aortic isthmus: an emergency? World J Surg 1995;19:119–25.
45. Rousseau H, Dambrin C, Marcheix B, et al. Acute traumatic aortic rupture: a comparison of surgical and stent-graft repair. J Thorac Cardiovasc Surg 2005;129:1050–5.
46. NCEPOD trauma report. Trauma: who cares? 2007. Available at: <http://www.ncepod.org.uk/2007t.htm>. Accessed 3 March 2012.
47. Tang GL, Tehrani HY, Usman A, et al. Reduced mortality, paraplegia, and stroke with stent graft repair of blunt aortic transections: a modern meta-analysis. J Vasc Surg 2008;47:671–5.
48. Presbitero P, Demarie D, Villani M, et al. Long term results (15–30 years) of surgical repair of aortic coarctation. Br Heart J 1987; 57:462–7.
49. Shah L, Hijazi Z, Sandhu S, et al. Use of endovascular stents for the treatment of coarctation of the aorta in children and adults: immediate and midterm results. J Invasive Cardiol 2005;17:614–18.
50. Pilla CB, Fontes VF, Pedra CA. Endovascular stenting for aortic coarctation. Expert Rev Cardiovasc Ther 2005;3:879–90.
51. Cohen M, Fuster V, Steele PM, et al. Coarctation of the aorta. Long-term follow-up and prediction of outcome after surgical correction. Circulation 1989;80:840–5.
52. Johansson G, Nydahl S, Olofsson P, Swedenborg J. Survival in patients with abdominal aortic aneurysms. Comparison between operative and nonoperative management. Eur J Vasc Surg 1990; 4:497–502.
53. Katz DJ, Stanley JC, Zelenock GB. Operative mortality rates for intact and ruptured abdominal aortic aneurysms in Michigan: an eleven-year statewide experience. J Vasc Surg 1994;19:804–15; discussion 816–17.
54. Rayt HS, Bown MJ, Lambert KV, et al. Buttock claudication and erectile dysfunction after internal iliac artery embolization in patients prior to endovascular aortic aneurysm repair. Cardiovasc Intervent Radiol 2008;31:728–34.
55. Ouriel K, Clair DG, Kent KC, Zarins CK. Positive Impact of Endovascular Options for treating Aneurysms Early (PIVOTAL) Investigators. Endovascular repair compared with surveillance for patients with small abdominal aortic aneurysms. J Vasc Surg 2010; 51:1081–7.
56. Nordon IM, Karthikesalingam A, Hinchliffe RJ, et al. Secondary interventions following endovascular aneurysm repair (EVAR) and the enduring value of graft surveillance. Eur J Vasc Endovasc Surg 2010;39:547–54.
57. Ohrlander T, Dencker M, Dias NV, et al. Cardiovascular predictors for long-term mortality after EVAR for AAA. Vasc Med 2011; 16:422–7.
58. Bown MJ, Sutton AJ, Bell PR, Sayers RD. A meta-analysis of 50 years of ruptured abdominal aortic aneurysm repair. Br J Surg 2002;89:714–30.
59. Acosta S, Ogren M, Bengtsson H, et al. Increasing incidence of ruptured abdominal aortic aneurysm: a population-based study. J Vasc Surg 2006;44:237–43.
60. Mastracci TM, Garrido-Olivares L, Cinà CS, Clase CM. Endovascular repair of ruptured abdominal aortic aneurysms: a systematic review and meta-analysis. J Vasc Surg 2008;47:214–21.
61. Visser JJ, van Sambeek MR, Hamza TH, et al. Ruptured abdominal aortic aneurysm: endovascular repair versus open surgery-systematic review. Radiology 2007;245:122–9.
62. Aylin P, Bottle A, Majeed A. Use of administrative data or clinical databases as predictors of risk of death in hospital: comparison of models. BMJ 2007;334:1044.
63. Visser JJ, van Sambeek MR, Hunink MG, et al. Acute abdominal aortic aneurysms: cost analysis of endovascular repair and open surgery in hemodynamically stable patients with 1-year follow-up. Radiology 2006;240:681–9.
64. Cochrane Database of Systematic Reviews. Endovascular treatment for ruptured abdominal aortic aneurysm. Available at: <http://dx.doi.org/10.1002/14651858.CD005261.pub2>.
65. Improve trial webpage. Available at: <http://www.improvetrial.org/>. Accessed 9 April 2012.
66. Greenberg RK, Lytle B. Endovascular repair of thoracoabdominal aneurysms. Circulation 2008;117:2288–96.
67. Reilly LM, Chuter TA. Endovascular repair of thoracoabdominal aneurysms: design options, device construct, patient selection and complications. J Cardiovasc Surg 2009;50:447–60.
68. Palmaz JC, Sibbitt RR, Reuter SR, et al. Expandable intraluminal graft: a preliminary study. Work in progress. Radiology 1985; 156:73–7.
69. Tapping CR, Ahmed M, Scott PM, et al. Primary infrarenal aortic stenting with or without iliac stenting for isolated and aortoiliac stenoses: single-centre experience with long-term follow-up. Cardiovasc Intervent Radiol 2013;36:62–8.
70. Schwindt AG, Panuccio G, Donas KP, et al. Endovascular treatment as first line approach for infrarenal aortic occlusive disease. J Vasc Surg 2011;53:1550–6.

CHAPTER 4

PERIPHERAL VASCULAR DISEASE INTERVENTION

Robert A. Morgan • Anna-Maria Belli • Joo-Young Chun

Since the first edition of this textbook, vascular radiology has changed beyond recognition. It was only 30 years ago that the role of radiology in the vascular system was mainly to provide diagnostic images using invasive angiography. Since the development of interventional techniques in the late 1980s, interventional radiologists have assumed a major role not only in the diagnosis of vascular disorders but also in their treatment.

The other main advance in vascular radiology has been the development of non-invasive imaging such as duplex ultrasound, multidetector computed tomographic angiography (MDCTA) and magnetic resonance angiography (MRA). The current range of diagnostic and interventional techniques is too extensive to be described fully in a general textbook of radiology. The aim of this chapter is to provide a brief overview of salient features of diagnostic angiography and to describe the role of the main interventional techniques in the vascular system. A description of non-invasive angiographic imaging is described in Chapter 2 and a discussion of aortic and renal arterial disease is covered in Chapter 3 and Chapter 8.

INTERVENTIONAL RADIOLOGY TECHNIQUES

The following are brief descriptions of the main therapeutic procedures used by vascular interventional radiologists.

Angioplasty

Percutaneous transluminal angioplasty (PTA) refers to treatment of a vascular stenosis or occlusion with a balloon catheter, which is introduced into the blood vessel and advanced to the site of the lesion. The balloon is inflated for a short period of time. After deflating the balloon, a check angiogram is performed to assess the success of the procedure (Fig. 4-1).

Stenting

This refers to the placement of a metallic mesh tube across a vascular stenosis or occlusion. There are two main types of stent: balloon expandable stents are mounted on a balloon catheter and deployed by inflating the balloon; self-expanding stents are compressed on a delivery catheter and released by withdrawing an outer sheath, allowing them to expand by their own radial force (Fig. 4-2).

Stents may be used as the primary method of treatment or may be reserved for use if PTA is unsuccessful, depending on the location and type of lesion.

Embolisation

Embolisation refers to the occlusion of a blood vessel by delivery of embolic material through a catheter. Embolisation has a wide range of applications, including the treatment of haemorrhage, aneurysms, vascular malformations and the treatment and palliation of cancer, particularly primary and secondary hepatic malignancy.

There are a large variety of embolic agents, including metallic springs (coils), particulate matter, gelatin sponge, glue and liquids such as absolute alcohol. The choice depends on the anatomical site, the nature of the lesion and the personal preference of the operator.

Some embolic agents, such as gelatin sponge, are considered temporary, and can be used to control

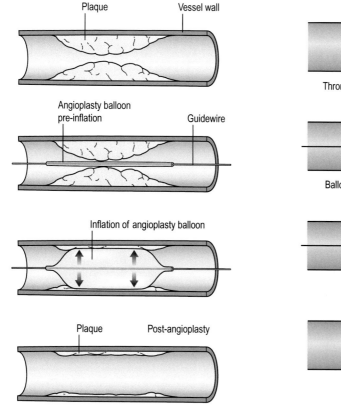

FIGURE 4-1 ■ **Diagram of angioplasty.**

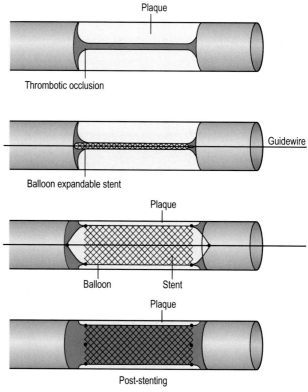

FIGURE 4-2 ■ **Diagram of stenting.**

haemorrhage when recanalisation of the parent vessel may be desirable once the 'acute' lesion has healed, e.g. traumatic injury to the internal iliac artery following pelvic trauma. Permanent particulate emboli are made from various agents, but polyvinyl alcohol (PVA) is the best known example. These agents are not radio-opaque and must be suspended in contrast medium. They cause occlusion by 'silting up' the blood supply. The level of occlusion depends on the size and type of particles chosen. Particulate emboli are used in the treatment of benign and malignant tumours, such as uterine leiomyoma and renal angiomyolipoma (Fig. 4-3). They may be used in combination with chemotherapeutic agents (drug-eluting beads) in hepatic chemoembolisation. Coils are used in situations analogous to tying of a vessel surgically, but knowledge of vascular anatomy is important for avoiding retrograde filling of a lesion from collateral vessels. They are used widely in the embolisation of haemorrhage (Fig. 4-4) and the exclusion of aneurysms and pseudoaneurysms.

Liquid embolic agents include sclerosants such as absolute alcohol, sodium tetradecyl sulphate (STD), glue (e.g. n-butyl-2-cyanoacylate) and newer agents such as Onyx. Sclerosants are useful in venous embolisation, e.g. varicoceles and low-flow vascular malformations. Glue and Onyx are particularly useful in dealing with high-flow arteriovenous malformations and visceral artery aneurysms.

Thrombolysis

This refers to the dissolution of blood clots within an artery or vein by the injection or infusion of a thrombolytic (clot-dissolving) drug directly into the thrombus through a catheter, which has been advanced directly into the thrombus. Although successful thrombolysis may be achieved within a short time, it is not uncommon for the lytic agent to be infused over 24–48 h. Patients undergo periodic check angiography to assess the progress of the treatment. In most cases, successful clearance of the thrombus reveals an underlying causative lesion, which should be treated by angioplasty or stenting during the same procedure. Thrombolysis was a very popular technique for the treatment of acute lower limb ischaemia about 10–15 years ago. It is less often used now but it is still performed in selected cases.

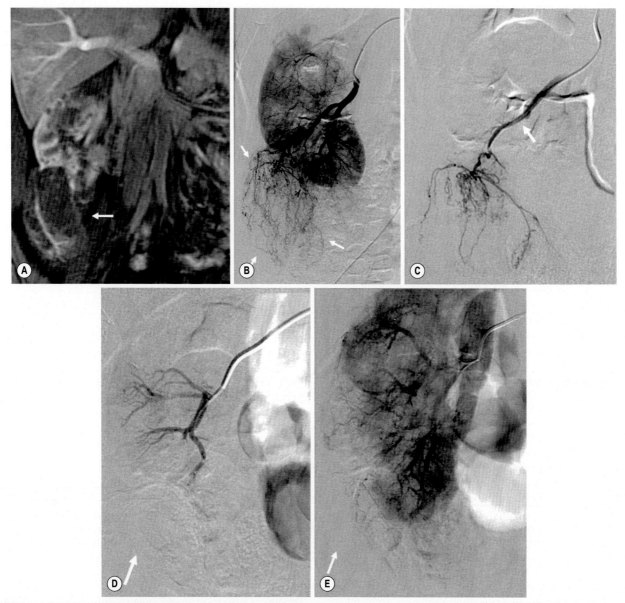

FIGURE 4-3 ■ **Embolisation of angiomyolipoma (AML).** (A) Large AML in the lower pole of right kidney in a patient with tuberous sclerosis (arrow). (B) Right renal angiogram demonstrating tumour vascularity within the AML (arrows). (C) Super-selective catheterisation of an interpolar segmental artery that supplies the AML with a coaxial microcatheter (arrow). (D, E) Angiograms after embolisation with PVA demonstrating devascularisation of the AML (arrows).

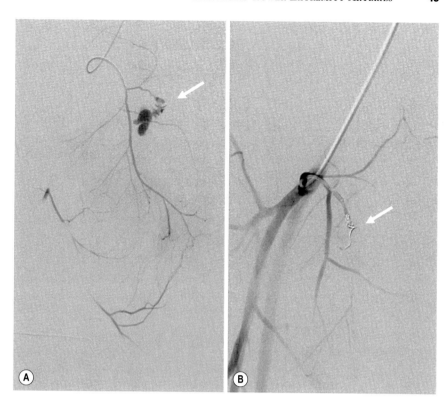

FIGURE 4-4 ■ **Embolisation of bleeding lower limb artery.** (A) Femoral angiogram in a patient who incurred penetrating traumatic arterial injury to the upper thigh. There is active extravasation of contrast medium from a branch of the profunda femoris artery (arrow). (B) The bleeding has ceased after selective embolisation with metal coils (arrow).

ARTERIAL SYSTEM

PELVIC AND LOWER EXTREMITY ARTERIES

Angiographic Anatomy (Fig. 4-5)

At the level of L4, the aorta divides into the common iliac arteries, which pass in front of the iliac veins and give off no major branches. At the level of the mid sacrum, they divide into the external and internal iliac arteries. The internal iliac arteries supply the pelvis and surrounding musculature. They divide into anterior divisions, which supply the viscera, and posterior divisions, which mainly supply the musculature. The external iliac artery has no major branches, although it gives rise to the inferior epigastric artery at the junction with the common femoral artery. At the level of the inguinal ligament, the external iliac artery becomes the common femoral artery—a short vessel that gives rise to the profunda femoris (or deep femoral artery), which supplies the muscles of the thigh; and the superficial femoral artery (SFA), which has no major branches and passes distally. At the level of the adductor canal, the SFA becomes the popliteal artery, which gives rise to the vessels of the calf, which are the anterior and posterior tibial arteries and the peroneal artery. At the level of the ankle, the anterior tibial artery becomes the dorsalis pedis artery and the posterior tibial artery becomes the medial and lateral plantar arteries. The anterior tibial artery is the most lateral calf vessel, whereas the posterior tibial

artery is the most medial. In the forefoot, the plantar arch is formed by the lateral plantar branch of the posterior tibial artery and the dorsalis pedis artery. Anatomical variations of the lower extremity arteries are outside the scope of this chapter.

Arterial Disease Affecting the Lower Extremity

The most common condition affecting the arteries of the lower extremity is tissue ischaemia due to occlusive disease. Occlusive disease may be acute, acute-on-chronic (where acute occlusion occurs in the presence of a previous chronic stenosis or occlusion) or chronic occlusion. Most patients present with symptoms of chronic occlusive disease, usually caused by atherosclerosis. Less common causes include thromboembolism, acute thrombotic occlusion, microembolism, entrapment syndromes, cystic adventitial disease, trauma and vasculitis, including vasospastic disorders and Buerger's disease.

The clinical presentation varies, depending on the type, location and number of the arterial lesions. Patients may be asymptomatic, may suffer from pain on walking (intermittent claudication), pain while at rest, or tissue loss in the form of either ulceration or gangrene. In general, patients with intermittent claudication are not treated with invasive procedures unless their claudication distance is very short or their symptoms substantially limit their lifestyle. Patients with rest pain and tissue loss

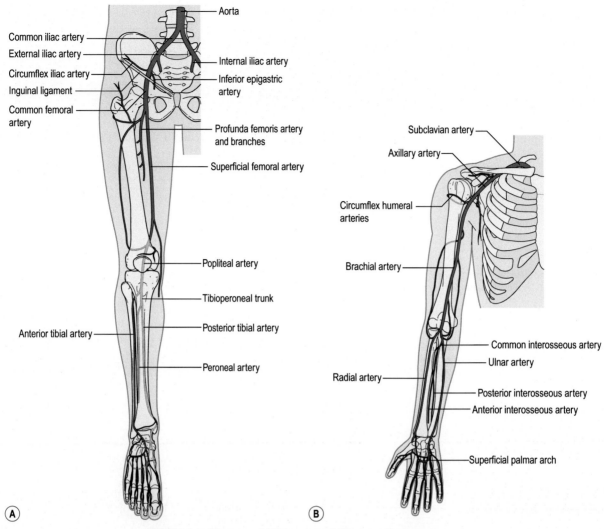

FIGURE 4-5 ■ Diagram of (A) lower and (B) upper limb anatomy.

are at risk of limb loss and must be treated by angioplasty, stenting or surgery.

Angiographic Diagnosis

Most pathological processes affecting the lower extremity arteries cause stenosis, occlusion or dilatation, i.e. aneurysm formation. Atherosclerosis may affect the arteries at any level, from the iliac arteries to the small vessels of the foot. While it is true that a stenosis or occlusion is almost always due to atherosclerosis, it is important to consider other possible causes. The clinical history may often be of help in this respect. For example, a patient who develops acute severe pain in the lower leg with no previous history or symptoms has probably sustained an acute embolus in the femoral or popliteal arteries, rather than a long-standing atherosclerotic occlusion. Patients with diabetes develop arterial occlusive disease, which involves mainly the distal vessels of the calf and feet. Patients with a history of radiotherapy to the pelvis for the treatment of carcinoma of the cervix may develop occlusive lesions of the common and external iliac arteries due to ischaemic vasculitis induced by the radiation.

Treatment of Chronic Limb Ischaemia

Iliac Artery Disease

Stenosis. In the treatment of stenotic lesions, PTA has a technical success rate approximating 100% (Fig. 4-6). Stents are used when PTA is immediately unsuccessful or when lesions recur soon after a previous angioplasty. There is no evidence that primary stenting is better than a policy of angioplasty with selective stenting for PTA failure.[1,2] Five-year patency rates are around 64–75%,[3] which, although lower than those of surgical aortobifemoral bypass, are acceptable considering the minimally invasive nature of this treatment.

Patients with diffusely stenosed iliac arteries respond less well to PTA. These patients are often treated with stents, although there is no definite evidence to support this policy.

Occlusions. Occlusions of the iliac artery are usually amenable to endovascular treatment, with a technical success rate of recanalisation of around 80% (Fig. 4-7). Most operators favour primary stent insertion because angioplasty carries a 7–24% risk of significant distal

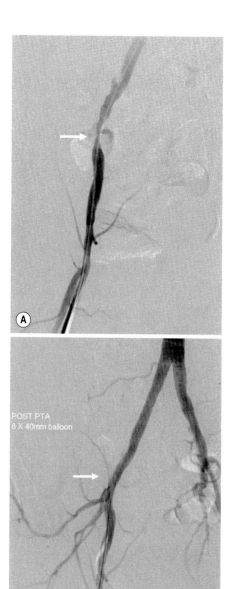

FIGURE 4-6 ▧ **Iliac angioplasty.** (A) Flush angiogram from the distal aorta shows a tight stenosis at the right iliac bifurcation (arrow). (B) Improved lumen following 8-mm balloon angioplasty (arrow).

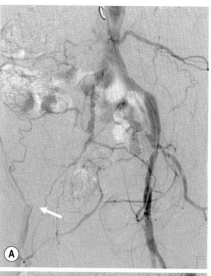

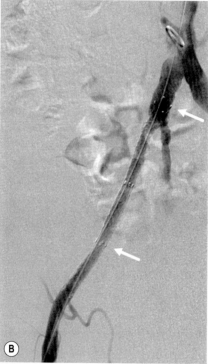

FIGURE 4-7 ▧ **Iliac stenting.** (A) A pelvic angiogram showing occlusion of the external iliac artery with reconstitution distally via collateral vessels (arrow). (B) A guidewire has been passed retrograde through the occlusion from the right and two 8-mm self-expanding stents deployed. This has resulted in successful recanalisation of the occluded segment. The proximal and distal extents of the stents are indicated (arrows).

embolisation.[4] The durability of endovascular treatment of iliac artery occlusion is similar to that for iliac artery stenosis.

Common Femoral Artery and Profunda Femoris

Stenoses of the common femoral artery are amenable to PTA. Access to these lesions is usually gained from the contralateral groin involving catheter and guidewire manipulation across the aortic bifurcation. However, common femoral endarterectomy is a straightforward procedure and may be performed under local anaesthesia. Surgery is considered a better option than PTA at this site when lesions are calcified and eccentric. If the SFA is patent or salvageable by intervention, PTA of a stenosis in the profunda artery is usually not carried out. However, if the SFA is occluded, then any stenosis of the main profunda trunk should be treated by PTA or at the time of endarterectomy. The success and durability rates of PTA are similar to those for the SFA (see below).

Occlusions of the common femoral artery and profunda femoris are generally treated surgically.

Superficial Femoral Artery

Stenosis. Angioplasty is the first-line treatment for stenosis of the superficial femoral artery. Patency is around 55% at 5 years,[3] which is lower than for surgical bypass using vein grafts. However, most patients are treated by PTA because of the lower rate of complications compared with surgery. Angioplasty can be repeated if lesions recur. An additional advantage of angioplasty is that it spares the long saphenous vein, which is commonly used for femoropopliteal bypass, but which is also used for coronary artery bypass. The results of angioplasty are less satisfactory if the vessel is diffusely stenosed or if the number of calf run-off vessels is reduced. The technical success of stenting is higher than for angioplasty, but studies have found no convincing long-term benefit for stents versus PTA. More recently, drug-eluting balloons and stents have been introduced. These devices are coated with immunosuppressive and anti-proliferative drugs (e.g. sirolimus and paclitaxel) that have been shown to limit neointimal hyperplasia, and therefore inhibit vessel restenosis. Early evidence suggests improved patency of femoropopliteal lesions after treatment using either of these devices when compared with standard PTA balloons and bare metal stents.[5-7]

Occlusions. SFA occlusions are usually treated by PTA (Fig. 4-8) followed by selective stent placement in cases where angioplasty is unsuccessful. Many radiologists use a technique called subintimal angioplasty in which a catheter and guidewire are manipulated outside the lumen of the vessel underneath the intima and into the subintimal space. Unless the vessel is heavily calcified, it is usually easy to advance the catheter and guidewire down the occluded vessel via the subintimal space. When the guidewire reaches the level of the patent vessel below the occlusion, it re-enters the lumen. After replacing the catheter with a balloon catheter, the subintimal space is dilated in the usual manner. Overall, the results for endovascular management of SFA occlusions are lower than for stenoses.[3] Although there is no conclusive evidence, primary stenting is often preferred for the treatment of occlusions. Drug-eluting balloons and stents may be used for these lesions if the long-term outcomes of these devices replicate early published data. In general, endovascular treatment is favoured over surgery in view of its lower morbidity and repeatability.

Popliteal Artery

The principles of treatment, results and durability are similar to those in the SFA. In general, the more distal the lesion, the more likely it is to produce symptoms of critical limb ischaemia. If treatment of these lesions fails, the limb may be lost. In general, lesions in the popliteal artery are only treated if the patient has critical limb ischaemia or very short distance claudication.

Calf Vessels

Angioplasty has become the main method of treatment for focal or diffuse lesions (stenosis or occlusions) of the

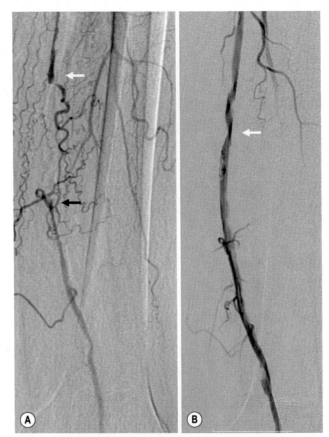

FIGURE 4-8 ■ Subintimal angioplasty. (A) Occlusion of the SFA (white arrow). There is reconstitution of the distal SFA via collaterals (black arrow). (B) The occlusion has been crossed subintimally with a hydrophilic guidewire and a 5-mm PTA performed (white arrow), restoring flow.

tibial and peroneal arteries (Fig. 4-9). In view of the size of these vessels, it is necessary to use small-calibre catheters and guidewires. Interventions in the calf vessels are performed in the setting of critical limb ischaemia, i.e. rest pain or tissue loss. The primary patency and limb salvage rates are 49 and 82% at 3 years, respectively.[8] More recently, bare metal stents, drug-eluting stents and drug-eluting balloons have been introduced to the market for use in the tibial arteries.[9] The data regarding their efficacy remain limited and studies are ongoing. Endovascular intervention in the pedal circulation is now being performed more frequently, with reasonable outcomes, but limited data.

Treatment of Acute Lower Limb Ischaemia

Patients with acute limb ischaemia usually present with severe rest pain. In many cases, the limb is threatened and patients may develop paraesthesia or motor dysfunction. In such circumstances urgent treatment is required to prevent limb loss. In the 1990s, this condition was often treated by intra-arterial thrombolysis. However,

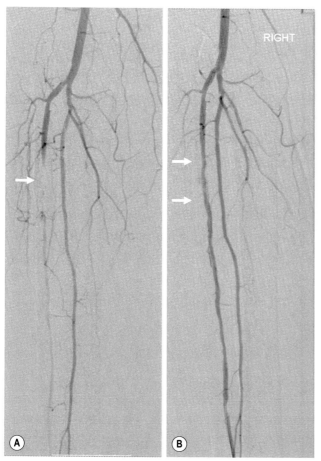

FIGURE 4-9 ■ Tibial artery angioplasty. (A) Angiogram of the tibial vessels in a patient with critical limb ischaemia. There is occlusion of the proximal anterior tibial artery (arrow) with reconstitution via collaterals. The posterior tibial artery is occluded. (B) Appearance after angioplasty with a 2.5-mm balloon with improved distal flow (arrows).

because of the overall lack of data showing a benefit for thrombolysis compared with surgery and a high rate of haemorrhagic complication, the technique is now used less frequently, although it is still employed on a selected patient basis.[10,11]

Some patients presenting with acute limb ischaemia have emboli lodged in the popliteal artery. They can be treated by percutaneous aspiration of the thrombus using wide-bore catheters placed directly into the thrombus via the femoral artery. A variety of mechanical thrombectomy devices for fragmenting thrombus either as an adjunct or instead of thrombolysis in patients with a large thrombus load are also available.

UPPER EXTREMITY ARTERIES

Anatomy

The subclavian artery extends to the lateral border of the first rib and continues as the axillary artery. The axillary artery extends to the lower border of the Teres major muscle, where it becomes the brachial artery. At the elbow, the brachial artery gives rise to the radial artery and ulnar arteries. At the wrist, the radial artery gives rise to the deep carpal arch that anastomoses with branches of the ulnar artery. The ulnar artery gives rise to the superficial carpal arch. The digital arteries originate from both arches.

Pathology

Most lesions involving the arteries of the upper limb are caused by atherosclerosis. However, other processes form a greater proportion of lesions compared with the legs, including Takayasu's arteritis, giant cell arteritis, thoracic outlet syndrome and thromboembolism.

Endovascular Treatment

Stenoses and occlusions of the subclavian artery (Fig. 4-10) usually occur at the origin, and are amenable to angioplasty and/or stent insertion with technical success

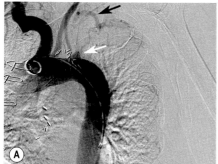 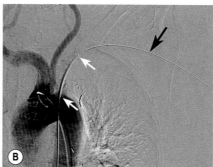 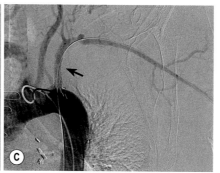

FIGURE 4-10 ■ Subclavian artery occlusion. (A) Left anterior oblique projection flush aortogram performed via a pigtail catheter in the ascending aorta. There is left subclavian artery occlusion in this patient who presented with arm claudication. Note that the left vertebral artery (the third vessel from the right) arises directly from the aortic arch, rather than off the left subclavian. The stump of the left subclavian is marked (white arrow). There is reconstitution of the distal left subclavian artery (black arrow). (B) A guidewire (black arrow) has been placed across the occlusion from the left brachial artery. A balloon expandable stent (white arrows) is seen in position ready for deployment. (C) After deployment of a 7-mm stent (arrow). Continuous flow has been restored.

rates of around 95% (less for occlusions). There are no convincing data on the superiority of stents versus angioplasty (although most interventionalists treat these lesions with stents).

Thromboembolism is a common cause of acute upper extremity ischaemia that is almost always treated surgically. Thrombolysis is rarely performed, because of significant haemorrhagic and embolic stroke complications.

The role of angioplasty or stenting in the treatment of stenotic or occlusive lesions distal to the subclavian arteries is very limited, with very little evidence for it.

GASTROINTESTINAL SYSTEM

The coeliac axis and the superior mesenteric artery (SMA) usually arise at the level of T12 and L1,

respectively. The inferior mesenteric artery (IMA) arises at the level of L3. The coeliac axis and SMA anastomose with each other via the pancreaticoduodenal arcades, while the superior and inferior mesenteric arteries anastomose via the middle colic branch of the SMA and left colic branch of the IMA, just proximal to the splenic flexure.

Angiography (Fig. 4-11)

The main problems affecting the gastrointestinal circulation are haemorrhage, occlusive disease and aneurysms.

Mesenteric Haemorrhage

Upper gastrointestinal (GI) haemorrhage is defined as bleeding proximal to the duodenojejunal flexure. It is

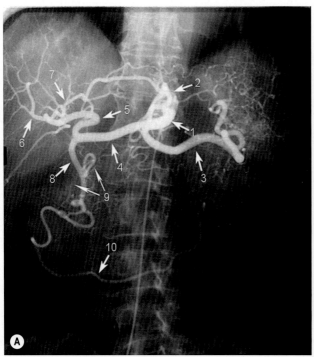

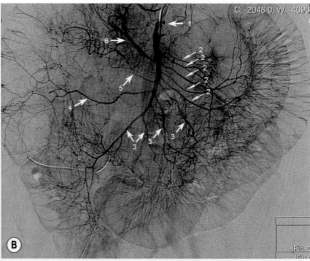

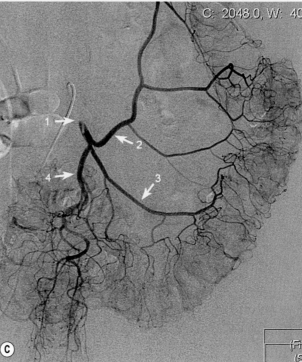

FIGURE 4-11 ■ **Mesenteric anatomy.** (A) Coeliac artery: 1 = coeliac axis, 2 = left gastric artery, 3 = splenic artery, 4 = common hepatic artery, 5 = proper hepatic artery, 6 = right hepatic artery, 7 = left hepatic artery, 8 = gastroduodenal artery, 9 = superior pancreaticoduodenal arteries, 10 = right gastroepiploic arteries. (B) Superior mesenteric artery: 1 = sidewinder catheter in the superior mesenteric artery, 2 = jejunal arteries, 3 = ileal arteries, 4 = ileocolic artery, 5 = right colic artery, 6 = middle colic artery. (C) Inferior mesenteric artery: 1 = catheter in the inferior mesenteric artery, 2 = left colic artery, 3 = sigmoid artery, 4 = superior rectal artery.

commonly caused by peptic ulceration, inflammatory disease such as pancreatitis, or as a complication of endoscopic, surgical or percutaneous biliary procedures. Lower GI haemorrhage is less common and is usually due to angiodysplasia, diverticular disease, neoplasms or haemorrhoids.

MDCTA has transformed the diagnostic algorithm for acute GI hemorrhage as it allows fast, accurate and non-invasive detection and localisation of bleeding. MDCTA may be performed as the first-line investigation or after a negative endoscopy. MDCTA has a high sensitivity for detecting active arterial bleeding, with a threshold bleeding rate of approximately 0.35 mL/min.[12] A triphasic scan protocol that includes unenhanced, arterial and portal-venous phase imaging should be used (Figs. 4-12A, B). Active bleeding is diagnosed when extravasated contrast material is seen within the bowel lumen during the arterial phase, which increases or pools during the portal-venous phase. Unenhanced images ensure that high-attenuation materials such as clips, suture material and faecoliths are not mistaken for acute bleeding. CTA may detect the cause of bleeding even when there is no active haemorrhage at the time of the scan, by identifying underlying pathology such as pseudoaneurysms. The information from the MDCTA allows the interventional radiologist to plan arterial embolisation by identifying the source branch. This enables faster selective catheterisation of the target vessels, reducing radiation exposure and contrast volume during the procedure.

Catheter angiography can detect active bleeding at a rate of 0.5 mL/min. If there is no active haemorrhage but the site of bleeding is known or clinically suspected because of associated pathology or recent intervention, prophylactic embolisation may be successful. This is easier in the upper GI than the lower GI tract, where collateral supply is less good and precise identification of the bleeding site is required to avoid bowel ischaemia or infarction.

The only direct sign of haemorrhage is contrast medium extravasation into the bowel lumen (Figs. 4-12C–E), but this may not be visible if the bleeding is intermittent or if the rate is too low. Indirect signs indicating the source of haemorrhage include the presence of a pseudoaneurysm, vessel truncation, early venous return, vascular lakes or tumour circulation and irregularity of the vessel wall.

Once the source of haemorrhage is identified, embolisation can be therapeutic, or enable stabilisation of the patient's condition before surgery. Consideration of the anatomical site will dictate the type of agent used and the extent of the embolisation required to avoid tissue

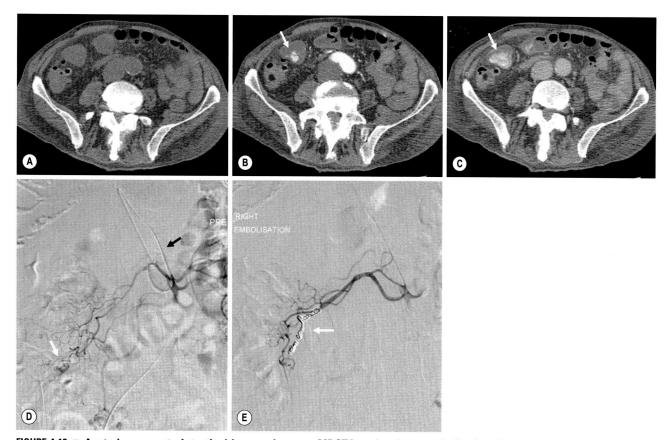

FIGURE 4-12 ■ **Acute lower gastrointestinal haemorrhage on MDCTA and catheter embolisation.** (A) Unenhanced axial CT image shows no evidence of high attenuation in relation to the bowel wall or lumen. (B) Arterial phase shows contrast material extravasation into the lumen of the ascending colon. (C) There is pooling of contrast in the bowel lumen on portal-venous phase. (D) Superselective angiogram performed via a coaxial microcatheter (black arrow). Contrast extravasation is seen from a right colic branch (white arrow). (E) After embolisation with microcoils (white arrow), there is no further bleeding.

ischaemia or infarction. For example, consideration should be given as to whether the vessel is an end artery (when the risk of infarction is greater) or whether there is significant collateral supply. The embolic agent is selected, depending on the anatomy and presence of collateral supply. As a very general rule, particulate emboli are used in the upper GI tract where there is good collateral supply, and coils are placed very distally in the branches of the lower GI tract where the collateral supply is poor.[13,14]

Visceral Artery Aneurysms

These are uncommon. The splenic artery is the vessel most frequently involved, followed by the hepatic artery and SMA. The aneurysms may be found incidentally on imaging, or present due to symptoms or actual rupture. Visceral artery aneurysms (VAA) may be true or pseudoaneurysms and occur as a result of atherosclerosis, arteritis, collagen vascular disorders (true aneurysms), or trauma and infection (pseudoaneurysms) (Fig. 4-13).

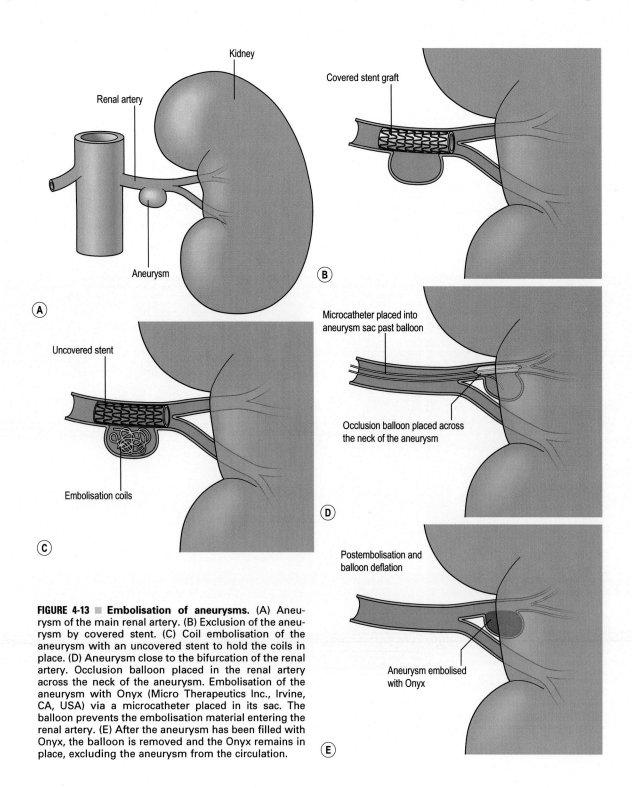

FIGURE 4-13 ■ Embolisation of aneurysms. (A) Aneurysm of the main renal artery. (B) Exclusion of the aneurysm by covered stent. (C) Coil embolisation of the aneurysm with an uncovered stent to hold the coils in place. (D) Aneurysm close to the bifurcation of the renal artery. Occlusion balloon placed in the renal artery across the neck of the aneurysm. Embolisation of the aneurysm with Onyx (Micro Therapeutics Inc., Irvine, CA, USA) via a microcatheter placed in its sac. The balloon prevents the embolisation material entering the renal artery. (E) After the aneurysm has been filled with Onyx, the balloon is removed and the Onyx remains in place, excluding the aneurysm from the circulation.

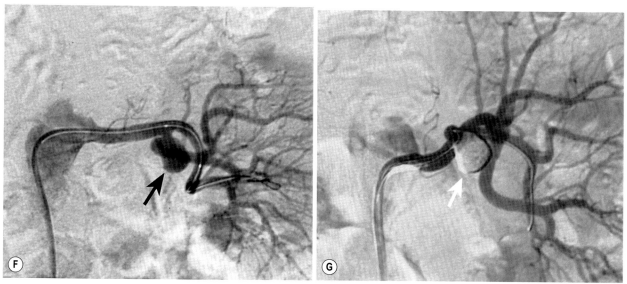

FIGURE 4-13, Continued ▪ (F) Angiogram demonstrating a saccular aneurysm (arrow) of the anterior division of the left renal artery. (G) Appearance after embolisation with Onyx (arrow). Both anterior and posterior divisions remain patent.

Depending on the vascular anatomy, endovascular treatment may involve embolisation (with coils, glue or Onyx), insertion of stent grafts or a combination of these methods.[15] A new type of stent called a flow diverting stent which occludes the neck of the aneurysm whilst maintaining patency of side branches has been developed, but early experience is very limited.

Occlusive Mesenteric Vascular Disease

Nowadays, acute mesenteric ischaemia (AMI) is more frequently diagnosed on CT than at laparotomy. If suspected, and the bowel is deemed viable, targeted thrombolysis is a potential treatment option, although the evidence for this treatment is limited to small case series and reports.

Chronic mesenteric ischaemia (CMI) presents with post-prandial abdominal pain and weight loss. Autopsy series quote mesenteric vessel atherosclerosis in 35–70% of unselected patients.[11] However, clinical symptoms are rare because of the excellent collateral vessels between mesenteric arteries. At least two of the three mesenteric arteries must be significantly stenosed for symptoms to occur.

The main therapeutic options for CMI are surgery and arterial stenting (Fig. 4-14). The diagnosis may be made non-invasively by Doppler ultrasound, CT or MRI. Catheter angiography is reserved for confirmation at the time of intervention. Lateral aortography is the best way to assess the anatomy before intervention. It is important to exclude extrinsic compression of the coeliac axis by the median arcuate ligament of the diaphragm (MALC) as this requires surgery. MALC causes a non-ostial asymmetric narrowing on the superior aspect of the coeliac axis, accentuated on expiratory angiography.

Angioplasty of the mesenteric vessels may be performed using a femoral or brachial approach. Most lesions occur at the vessel origins, and are treated by primary stenting. In general, treatment of one vessel will relieve symptoms, although treating more than one vessel, if technically feasible, might improve long-term outcomes. Technical success is 80–100% in most series.[16]

Bronchial Artery Embolisation

Haemoptysis can be a life-threatening respiratory emergency. Massive haemoptysis is defined as more than 300 mL of blood loss over 24 h and moderate haemoptysis is more than three episodes of 100 mL/day within 1 week. The aetiology is variable and includes tuberculosis, cystic fibrosis, malignancy, bronchiectasis, aspergilloma and lobar pneumonia.

The bronchial arteries are the most common source of bleeding in haemoptysis. They arise anterolaterally from the descending thoracic aorta at the level of the fifth or sixth thoracic vertebrae. Their anatomy is highly variable; the most common configuration is of an intercostobronchial trunk (ICBT) on the right and two bronchial arteries on the left, although other variations are almost as common.

Bronchoscopy can localise the side of haemorrhage when there is bilateral pulmonary disease but care must be taken in interpreting its findings as they may be misleading. MDCTA can identify the source of bleeding and the underlying disease process as well as providing a roadmap of the thoracic vasculature. The images should be carefully reviewed to search for not only abnormal bronchial arteries but also non-bronchial collaterals that can arise from branches of the subclavian artery in upper lobe disease and infradiaphragmatic branches in lower lobe disease.

Bronchial artery embolisation (BAE) is an effective and safe treatment for massive and recurrent haemoptysis. Bronchial arteries are selectively catheterised with

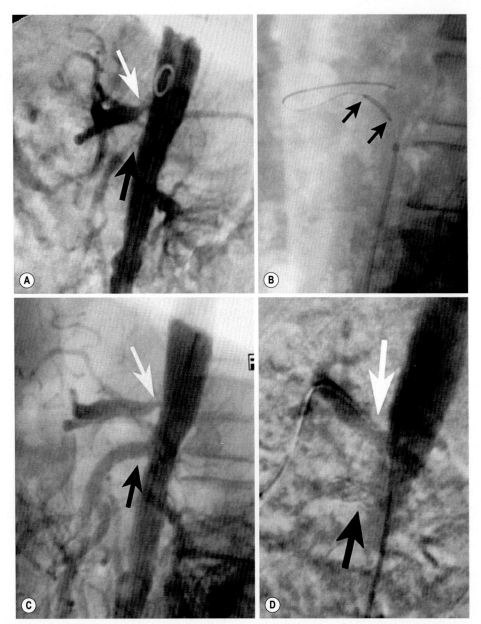

FIGURE 4-14 ■ **Mesenteric revascularisation.** (A) Lateral flush aortogram in a patient who had significant weight loss and post-prandial pain. There are critical stenoses of the coeliac axis (white arrow) and superior mesenteric artery (SMA) (black arrow). The inferior mesenteric artery (IMA) was occluded. (B) Image demonstrating a guidewire in the SMA and a 6-mm balloon expandable stent ready for deployment. The proximal and distal markers of the stent are indicated (arrows). (C) Appearance of the SMA after stent insertion (black arrow). Angioplasty of the coeliac axis had been attempted. The vessel exhibits considerable elastic recoil and continued stenosis at its origin (white arrow). (D) Final angiogram after insertion of stents in the coeliac axis (white arrow) and SMA (black arrow).

pre-shaped catheters, such as cobra and sidewinder. Signs of abnormality include hypertrophy, areas of hyper-vascularity or neovascularity, shunting of blood into the pulmonary artery or vein, aneurysm and contrast extrava-sation (Fig. 4-15). Coaxial microcatheters may be used to obtain a super-selective position to avoid any reflux of embolic material into the aorta or into important side branches, such as the anterior medullary artery that can arise from the right ICBT in 5–10% of cases. Embolisa-tion is usually performed using PVA. It is prudent to check for non-bronchial collaterals which may arise from

the subclavian, axillary and internal mammary arteries in upper lobe disease or from branches of the coeliac axis or inferior phrenic artery in lower lobe disease.

BAE provides immediate relief of symptoms in 73–99% of cases.[17] If bleeding does not stop immediately, repeat angiography and embolisation should be per-formed. The source of haemorrhage lies in the bronchial arteries in 85–90% and in non-bronchial arteries in 10–15% of cases. The pulmonary arteries are rarely the cause of massive haemoptysis. It is important to note that BAE does not address the underlying disease process and

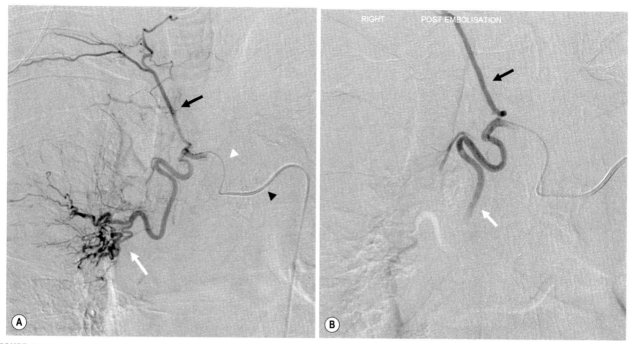

FIGURE 4-15 ■ **Bronchial artery embolisation.** (A) Right bronchial angiogram in a patient with lower lobe bronchiectasis who presented with haemoptysis. The right intercostobronchial trunk has been selectively catheterised with a cobra catheter (black arrow head) and a more stable position achieved with a coaxial microcatheter (white arrow head). An enlarged tortuous right bronchial branch is seen to supply an abnormal hypervascular area of lung corresponding to the bronchiectatic area (white arrow). The intercostal branch is unremarkable (black arrow). (B) Angiogram after superselective embolisation of the right bronchial branch with polyvinyl alcohol particles. The abnormal bronchial branch has been successfully embolised (white arrow) while the intercostal branch remains patent (black arrow).

re-bleeding is likely if the cause of hemoptysis is not treated effectively. Complications of bronchial embolisation include chest pain, dysphagia, broncho-oesophageal fistula, spinal cord ischaemia and stroke.

THE CAROTID ARTERIES

Internal carotid artery stenosis is an important cause of ischaemic stroke and transient ischaemic attack (TIA) (Fig. 4-16). Patients with symptomatic carotid stenosis are at a higher risk of developing further ischaemic cerebral events than patients with asymptomatic stenosis. Standard non-medical treatment is surgical carotid endarterectomy, although carotid stenting is an alternative to surgery.

Two trials (European Carotid Surgery Trial (ECST) and the North American Symptomatic Carotid Endarterectomy Trial (NASCET)) showed benefit in surgically treating patients with 70–99% stenosis. The criteria for treating patients by stenting are the same as for surgery. There remains controversy regarding the management of asymptomatic significant carotid artery disease.

Imaging

The standard imaging methods for delineating the carotid arteries are duplex ultrasound, MDCTA and MRA.

Catheter angiography has little place in the diagnosis of carotid disease except as a problem-solving tool when the non-invasive methods are discordant.

Angiography

Selective carotid angiography is associated with a risk of stroke in 1% of procedures.[18] Selective angiography is performed using one of a variety of pre-shaped catheters, such as the sidewinder, the Berenstein, Headhunter or Mani.

Endovascular Treatment of Carotid Artery Stenosis

The stenting technique differs slightly from procedures at other sites in that cerebral protection devices are usually used to prevent distal emboli, and predilatation is generally performed before stenting.

An overview of the available evidence suggests that stenting is associated with more minor strokes, especially in the elderly, and surgery with more myocardial infarction.[19] The decision to treat symptomatic and asymptomatic carotid stenosis should be made by a multidisciplinary team, which should include an interventional radiologist/neuroradiologist, a vascular surgeon and a physician with a special interest in stroke.

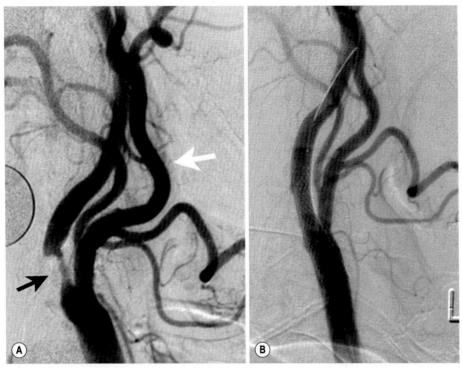

FIGURE 4-16 ■ **Carotid stenting.** (A) Lateral projection angiogram following selective injection into the common carotid artery. There is a tight stenosis at the origin of the internal carotid artery (black arrow). The external carotid artery is marked (white arrow). (B) Angiogram following self-expanding stent deployment.

VENOUS SYSTEM

LOWER EXTREMITY VENOUS SYSTEM

The main pathology affecting the lower extremity venous system is thrombosis. This may be due to factors causing procoagulation such as patient immobility, dehydration and thrombocythaemia; or due to an underlying stenosis/occlusion in the iliac veins. Although some interventionalists advocate catheter-directed thrombolysis as first-line treatment for patients with acute lower limb venous thrombosis, this technique has not yet been widely adopted. Thrombolysis is occasionally performed for patients with limb-threatening ischaemia as a result of acute venous occlusion in the condition of phlegmasia caerulea dolens.

Occasionally, an underlying stenosis or occlusion of the common iliac vein is the underlying cause of thrombosis, which can be treated by stenting. Left lower limb vein thrombosis or oedema due to compression by the right common iliac artery is called May–Thurner syndrome.

UPPER EXTREMITY VENOUS OBSTRUCTION

The main causes of upper limb venous occlusion are thoracic outlet syndrome (Paget–Schroetter syndrome) and occlusive disease related to the presence of dialysis fistulae.

Paget–Schroetter syndrome refers to acute subclavian or axillary vein thrombosis caused by underlying venous obstruction due to muscles or bony structures of the thoracic outlet. Patients presenting with subclavian or axillary vein thrombosis due to thoracic outlet syndrome are usually treated first by thrombolysis. If the thrombus can be cleared by this method, the first rib should be resected to create space for the vein, followed by angioplasty of any residual stenosis.

Patients with high pressure in the upper extremity veins resulting from the presence of dialysis fistulae are prone to develop venous stenoses and occlusions. These can be treated by angioplasty or stenting with high technical success rates. However, recurrence is frequent and long-term durability is very uncommon.

INFERIOR VENA CAVA FILTERS

Inferior vena cava (IVC) filters are placed to prevent fatal pulmonary embolism (PE) in patients with a documented PE, or IVC, iliac or femoropopliteal DVT who cannot be treated with anticoagulants, or in whom anticoagulants have failed to prevent further PE or progression of thrombus.

Other possible indications for IVC filters include protection against PE in pregnant women with proven DVT during Caesarean section or childbirth; in patients

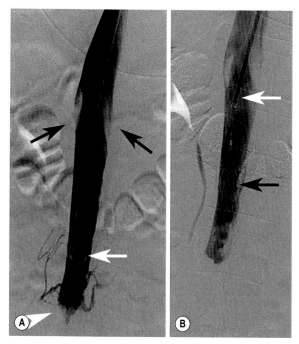

FIGURE 4-17 ■ Inferior vena cava filter. (A) Cavogram performed with a pigtail catheter (white arrow) placed from the right internal jugular vein. Unopacified blood from the renal veins creates a void (black arrows) in the column of contrast medium and thus delineates their position. Thrombus is seen as a filling defect distally (white arrowhead). (B) Post-filter (black arrow) deployment. The delivery catheter is marked (white arrow).

post-severe trauma; and preoperatively in patients with iliofemoral DVT when anticoagulation is contraindicated or pelvic manipulation is expected.

IVC filters may be permanent or optional, meaning they can be retrieved after a period of time, which varies with the individual filter, or left in permanently.

Before placing a filter, the IVC should be assessed by inferior vena cavography, the diameter of the IVC measured to ensure the filter will not migrate and the position of the renal veins documented (Fig. 4-17). The ideal position for the IVC filter is in the infrarenal IVC with the apex of the filter at or just below the level of the renal veins. Filters can be inserted via the femoral or jugular venous route depending on the site and extent of the thrombus. Retrieval is via the jugular route, the right jugular vein being the ideal choice.

Suprarenal positioning of the filter may be necessary when IVC thrombosis extends above the renal veins or there is renal vein thrombosis. Other indications include thrombus above a previously placed filter, pregnant women in whom there will be compression of the infrarenal vena cava, PE following gonadal vein thrombosis and anatomical variants (double IVC).

COMPLICATIONS OF ENDOVASCULAR PROCEDURES

Complications occurring after endovascular procedures are divided into major and minor. Major complications

include death and those complications where intervention is required, while minor complications are usually self-limiting and do not require treatment.

Death occurring after angioplasty or stenting procedures occurs in less than 1% of cases and is usually related to comorbidity rather than to the procedure itself. Other major complications of angioplasty or stenting include vessel rupture, access vessel pseudoaneurysm formation, haemorrhage, distal embolisation and vessel dissection, stent migration and severe reactions to intravascular contrast medium. Major complications occur in around 1% of procedures.[3]

Minor complications of these procedures are self-limiting haematoma, dissection not requiring treatment, minor contrast medium reactions, self-limiting fever and nausea. Thrombolysis is associated with haemorrhage, mainly at the access site, in up to 30% of cases.[20]

REFERENCES

1. Klein WM, van der Graaf Y, Seegers J, et al. Long-term cardiovascular morbidity, mortality, and reintervention after endovascular treatment in patients with iliac artery disease: The Dutch Iliac Stent Trial Study. Radiology 2004;232:491–8.
2. Klein WM, van der Graaf Y, Seegers J, et al. Dutch iliac stent trial: long-term results in patients randomized for primary or selective stent placement. Radiology 2006;238:734–44.
3. Norgren L, Hiatt WR, Dormandy JA, et al. Inter-society consensus for the management of peripheral arterial disease (TASC II). Eur J Vasc Endovasc Surg 2007;33:S1–S75.
4. Belli AM. To stent or not to stent in the iliac artery? Acta Chir Belg 2000;100:251–4.
5. Tepe G, Zeller T, Albrecht T, et al. Local delivery of paclitaxel to inhibit restenosis during angioplasty of the leg. N Engl J Med 2008;358:689–99.
6. Duda SH, Bosiers M, Lammer J, et al. Drug-eluting and bare nitinol stents for the treatment of atherosclerotic lesions in the superficial femoral artery: long-term results from the SIROCCO trial. J Endovasc Ther 2006;13:701–10.
7. Dake MD, Ansel GM, Jaff MR, et al. Paclitaxel-eluting stents show superiority to balloon angioplasty and bare metal stents in femoropopliteal disease: twelve-month Zilver PTX randomized study results. Circ Cardiovasc Interv 2011;4:495–504.
8. Romiti M, Albers M, Brochado-Neto FC, et al. Meta-analysis of infrapopliteal angioplasty for chronic critical limb ischemia. J Vasc Surg 2008;47:975–81.
9. Siablis D, Karnabatidis D, Katsanos K, et al. Infrapopliteal application of sirolimus-eluting versus bare metal stents for critical limb ischemia: analysis of long-term angiographic and clinical outcome. J Vasc Interv Radiol 2009;20:1141–50.
10. Ouriel K, Veith FJ, Sasahara AA. A comparison of recombinant urokinase with vascular surgery as initial treatment for acute arterial occlusion of the legs. Thrombolysis or Peripheral Arterial Surgery (TOPAS) Investigators. N Engl J Med 1998;338:1105–11.
11. Weaver FA, Comerota AJ, Youngblood M, et al. Surgical revascularization versus thrombolysis for nonembolic lower extremity native artery occlusions: Results of a prospective randomized trial. The STILE Investigators. Surgery versus thrombolysis for ischemia of the lower extremity. J Vasc Surg 1996;24:513–21.
12. Roy-Choudhury SH, Karandikar S. Multidetector CT of acute gastrointestinal bleeding. Radiology 2008;246:336.
13. Weldon DT, Burke SJ, Sun S, et al. Interventional management of lower gastrointestinal bleeding. Eur Radiol 2008;18:857–67.
14. Schenker MP, Duszak R Jr, Soulen MC, et al. Upper gastrointestinal hemorrhage and transcatheter embolotherapy: clinical and technical factors impacting success and survival. J Vasc Interv Radiol 2001;12:1263–71.
15. Belli AM, Markose G, Morgan RA. The role of interventional radiology in the management of abdominal visceral artery aneurysms. Cardiovasc Intervent Radiol 2012;35:234–43.

16. Cognet F, Ben Salem D, Dranssart M, et al. Chronic mesenteric ischaemia: imaging and percutaneous treatment. Radiographics 2002;22:863–79.

17. Chun J-Y, Morgan R, Belli A-M. Radiological management of hemoptysis: a comprehensive review of diagnostic imaging and bronchial artery embolization. Cardiovasc Intervent Radiol 2010; 33:240–50.

18. Hankey GJ, Warlow CP, Sellar RJ. Cerebral angiographic risk in mild cerebrovacular disease. Stroke 1990;21:209–22.

19. Macdonald S. Carotid artery stenting trials: conduct, results, critique, and current recommendations. Cardiovasc Intervent Radiol 2012;35:15–29.

20. Ouriel K, Shortell CK, De Weese JA, et al. A comparison of thrombolytic therapy with operative revasculatization in the initial treatment of acute peripheral arterial ischemia. J Vasc Surg 1994;19: 1021–30.

CHAPTER 5

IMAGE-GUIDED BIOPSY AND ABLATION TECHNIQUES

David J. Breen • Elizabeth E. Rutherford • Beth Shepherd

IMAGE-GUIDED BIOPSY

INTRODUCTION

There is an increasing role for imaging in the planning and performing of biopsy procedures. It is becoming unacceptable in modern practice to perform 'blind' liver or renal biopsies when imaging can provide real-time monitoring of needle position and hence reduce complication rates.[1,2] Ongoing technological advances are providing us with new and improved imaging modalities to aid biopsy and there are a number of modality fusion techniques which promise to further improve lesion targeting in the future.

PRINCIPLES OF IMAGE-GUIDED BIOPSY

Percutaneous image-guided needle biopsy is now a standard technique for the diagnosis of most tumours throughout the body and also has a role in the diagnosis of certain infective and inflammatory conditions. It is particularly helpful in the staging of cancer, most notably when the definitive treatment may not involve surgical intervention. Advances in imaging techniques have led to greater precision in the targeting of lesions. Advantages of percutaneous biopsy over surgical excision biopsy include time and cost savings and reduced morbidity. The complication rates associated with percutaneous biopsy vary according to the organ studied, but are generally lower than 0.1%.[3]

CASE SELECTION

Most image-guided biopsies can be performed using local anaesthesia and sedation. General anaesthesia may be preferable in some patients, including children. Pertinent patient history includes bleeding diatheses and anticoagulant usage. Contraindications to biopsy include an uncorrected coagulopathy and lack of a safe needle approach route. The benefits of confirming a suspected diagnosis need to be evaluated against the inherent procedural morbidity.

PRE-PROCEDURAL ASSESSMENT

Pre-procedural assessment aims to reduce complication rates by optimising the patient's physiology and identifying contraindications in a timely fashion. It is also useful in alleviating patient anxiety and discussing post-procedural care to enable the patient to plan time off work, etc. The pre-procedural assessment is also a good time to obtain patients' written consent.

Careful questioning can determine whether a day case procedure is appropriate, taking into account the patient's clinical status and home circumstances. Any language, cultural or religious barriers can also be identified. Regularly updated and referenced departmental patient information leaflets should be available for all common procedures and include links to web-based information and relevant telephone numbers for further advice. These help inform the consent process and provide post-procedural advice as it is well documented that patients retain little of any verbal information they are given.[4]

Another role of pre-procedural assessment is to highlight potential problems related to patient co-morbidity or the nature of the biopsy target. If the patient is on anticoagulants or has a coagulopathy, the timing of the biopsy procedure should be carefully planned around the cessation of anticoagulant medication or admission for correction of coagulation disorders. These patients have an increased risk of post-procedural haemorrhage and may require an extended period of observation. The nature of the target lesion also needs consideration as vascular lesions are at increased risk of bleeding; it may be necessary to establish peripheral venous access and ensure the availability of cross-matched blood. Wherever possible, an obstructed organ should be decompressed prior to biopsy using techniques such as biliary drainage or percutaneous nephrostomy.

Patients should be told how and when they will receive biopsy results and a follow-up outpatient clinic appointment booked prior to discharge.

CORE BIOPSY VS FINE NEEDLE ASPIRATION

Fine needle aspiration (FNA) utilises a small calibre needle (20 to 25G) to obtain a sample of cells from a target organ/lesion for cytological analysis. Core biopsy involves larger calibre needles (14 to 19G) and reveals more structural information, which is often necessary for histological diagnosis (Table 5-1).[5,6] Each method has its own advantages and disadvantages and the decision as to which one to use depends on many factors:

FNA with a small calibre needle may be employed in situations where a structure (e.g. bowel loop) needs to be transgressed as it is interposed between the target lesion and skin. Similarly, where a deep lesion lies in close proximity to critical vascular structures (e.g. a central liver lesion abutting the vena cava), core biopsy may be deemed too hazardous.

Aside from the reduced risk of iatrogenic injury, FNA can be useful in frail or unwell patients who cannot tolerate a prolonged procedure. A further advantage is that cytological slides can be examined immediately to check for adequacy and formal pathology reports can be issued rapidly if required.

The degree of confidence in cytological diagnosis will vary according to the indication; the diagnosis of recurrent malignancy can be more easily made on a cytological sample if previous tumour tissue is available for comparison. For a new diagnosis of malignancy, however, a larger sample of tissue is usually required and hence core biopsy is generally preferred over cytology. This is particularly important where different subtypes of malignancy exist (e.g. lymphoma), and accurate histological typing is necessary to plan treatment.[7-9] Other pathologies requiring histological confirmation include diffuse disease such as cirrhosis and renal parenchymal disease (e.g. glomerulonephritis).

BIOPSY NEEDLES

Needles vary in calibre, tip design, length and mechanism of action and there are a wide range of different products on the market. Needle choice depends on a number of factors including the lesion to be targeted, the number of cores required, the modality chosen for image guidance, personal preference, cost and local availability. They can be broadly classified as follows.

Fine Needle Aspiration Cytology Needles

Cytological samples are usually taken with small calibre needles (20–25G). Different lengths of small calibre needle are available and the needle should be carefully selected according to the depth and size of lesion to be sampled. For abdominal FNA, the target will often be deep and a spinal or other stylet needle is often used. The presence of a needle stylet helps to avoid luminal contamination with tissue before it reaches its target. When using very fine needles, a stylet also aids insertion by stiffening the needle to prevent it deviating from its course.

Core Biopsy Needles

For core biopsy, larger calibre cutting needles are employed (usually 16–18G for abdominal biopsies). The size of biopsy needle chosen depends on the organ being targeted and may also vary according to the number of samples being obtained. For a routine 'background' liver biopsy, a single pass is usually sufficient and so a larger (e.g. 16G) biopsy needle may be chosen. If the operator anticipates that several cores will need to be obtained, e.g. in the case of multiple lesions, then an 18G needle may be more appropriate to reduce the risk of bleeding following multiple liver capsule punctures.

The shape of the tissue core obtained varies according to the design of the chamber within the biopsy needle; various manufacturers have designed biopsy instruments

TABLE 5-1 Needle Gauge and Calibre	
Needle Gauge	**Diameter (mm)**
22	0.72
21	0.82
19	1.10
18	1.26
16	1.67
14	2.13

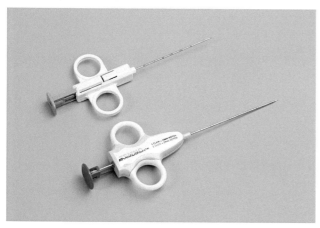

FIGURE 5-1 ■ **Examples of semi-automatic core biopsy instruments.** These allow placement of the central notch at the exact position required with the cutting sheath subsequently fired over the stylet. There is therefore no additional forward excursion of the needle upon firing, so minimising the risk of damage to adjacent structures.

which optimise the volume of tissue obtained for a given needle gauge[10] as there is evidence that increasing needle calibre is related to increased risk of haemorrhage.[11]

Menghini Technique Biopsy Needles, e.g. Surecut

These operate using a suction mechanism but are no longer in common use. They are based on the Menghini principle in which the needle, stylet and syringe form a single unit.

Sheathed Biopsy Needles

Manual, e.g. Tru-Cut

These needles consist of a biopsy chamber that can be opened and closed. After insertion to the correct depth, the needle is opened by manually advancing the inner portion so that the surrounding tissue falls into the biopsy notch. As the outer part of the needle is then advanced, the tissue in the chamber is cut by its leading edge. This requires two hands to operate and so is impractical for ultrasound-guided procedures.

Semi-Sutomatic, e.g. Temno, SuperCore (Fig. 5-1)

Some biopsy instruments allow placement of the central notch at the exact position required and then fire the cutting sheath over the stylet (Fig. 5-2). There is therefore no additional forward excursion of the needle upon firing the cutting part of the needle, so minimising the risk of damage to adjacent structures. This is useful in the case of small lesions or those adjacent to critical structures such as large veins. When the target tissue is fibrous or very firm in texture it can, however, be difficult to manually advance the cutting needle through the lesion without displacing it. This is often overcome by the use

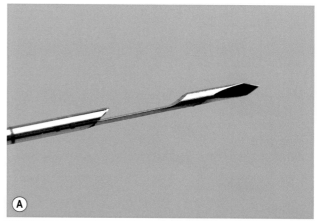

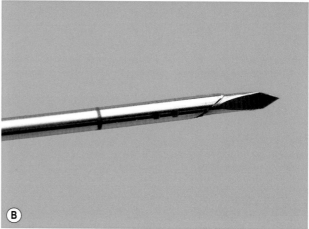

FIGURE 5-2 ■ **The mechanism of a semi-automatic biopsy instrument.** (A) The central notched stylet is advanced to the point required. (B) The cutting sheath is then fired over the stylet with the cored sample of tissue residing in the notch of the stylet.

of spring-loaded fully automated devices that exert more forward force to advance the needle into the target.

Fully Automatic, e.g. Biopty gun, Achieve, Biopince, Bard Max-Core (Fig. 5-3)

These can take the form of metal biopsy guns, which are designed for use with disposable biopsy needles of different gauges, or fully disposable integrated plastic biopsy devices, which have a similar mechanism of action. Whilst the disposable devices are more expensive, they avoid the difficulties associated with sterilisation of the metal biopsy guns and have generally been adopted as the biopsy instrument of choice in many radiology departments. Fully automatic biopsy instruments fire both a central stylet and cutting sheath in a rapid forward motion such that the tissue core is obtained at a preset distance or 'throw' (e.g. 2 cm) ahead of the visualised needle tip. Many of the instruments offer a choice of throw (usually 1 or 2 cm) depending on the size of target lesion or organ. This mechanism of action means that the operator needs to be aware of the size of the lesion to be sampled relative to the throw of the biopsy needle. Often the

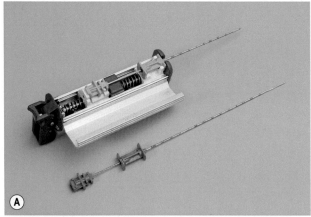

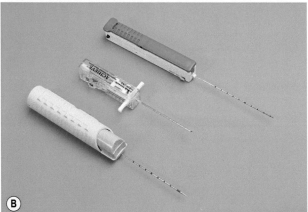

FIGURE 5-3 ■ **Examples of fully automatic core biopsy instruments.** Fully automatic biopsy instruments fire both a central stylet and cutting sheath in a rapid forward motion such that the tissue core is obtained at a preset distance or 'throw' (e.g. 2 cm) ahead of the visualised needle tip. (A) Non-disposable metal biopsy guns, which are designed for use with disposable biopsy needles of different gauges. (B) Fully disposable integrated plastic biopsy devices, which have a similar mechanism of action.

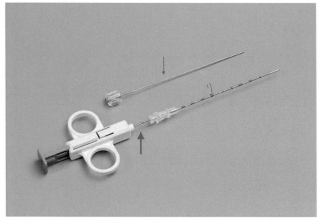

FIGURE 5-4 ■ **Example of a coaxial biopsy system.** The coaxial needle is radiologically guided into the lesion then the central stylet (thin arrow) is removed; a smaller calibre biopsy needle (thick arrow) can then be inserted through the coaxial system to obtain multiple cores.

needle tip can be positioned at the superficial margin of the target lesion to avoid injury to adjacent structures.

COAXIAL TECHNIQUE

Most biopsies are performed by making one or more passes into an organ or mass with a single biopsy needle. Occasionally it may be helpful to employ a system whereby a coaxial needle is radiologically guided into the lesion/mass, the central stylet is removed and then a smaller calibre biopsy needle can be inserted through the coaxial system to obtain multiple cores (Fig. 5-4). This has the advantage of allowing several samples to be taken without re-puncturing the superficial soft tissues or organ capsule, which theoretically reduces the risk of haemorrhage and time taken to target the lesion,[12] although studies have not demonstrated any significant difference in complication rates between coaxial and non-coaxial techniques.[13] The coaxial needle can be angled between samples to increase the volume of tissue sampled. This

technique is commonly employed during CT-guided biopsy, particularly for lung lesions where minimising the number of passes through the pleura, reduces the risk of pneumothorax (Fig. 5-5). It is also used for biopsy of deep abdominal/pelvic masses, as it reduces the radiation dose and trauma involved in re-positioning biopsy needles for each core. There is also a theoretical advantage that coaxial systems reduce the risk of track seeding. A disadvantage is that the calibre of the coaxial needle must be larger than that of the biopsy needle, increasing the overall size of the needle track, with a possible increased risk of damage to adjacent tissues.

IMAGING MODALITIES FOR BIOPSY

Choice of modality for biopsy varies according to the size, location and visibility of the lesion. Most intra-abdominal lesions can be approached using either ultrasound or CT imaging. Modern technology is increasingly allowing a combination of modalities to be used during biopsy procedures (fusion imaging) to aid targeting of lesions. Previously, this required time-consuming manual registration of imaging but newer automated registration/fusion software is considerably reducing the time taken for co-registration of different modalities and it is likely that this technique will become commonplace in the future.

Ultrasound

Ultrasound-guided biopsy is considered an accurate, safe, widely accessible and relatively cheap technique. It has the advantage of real-time visualisation of the needle (particularly important for biopsy of organs such as the liver where the time the biopsy needle remains within liver parenchyma should be limited to minimise haemorrhagic complications). In addition, it allows a multiplanar angled approach that may be more challenging at CT or MR imaging. Ultrasound-guided biopsy procedures have

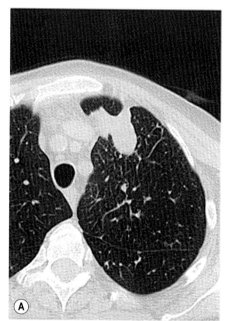

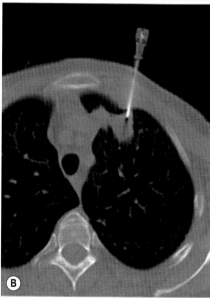

FIGURE 5-5 ■ **A coaxial system has been utilised so there is only one pass through the pleura during lung biopsy.** (A) CT images of the lesion prior to biopsy. (B) A coaxial needle has been placed under CT guidance (seen here on bone windows) through which a biopsy needle can be passed to obtain multiple biopsies.

the advantages of portability and lack of ionising radiation. However, ultrasound-guided biopsies are more operator-dependent than procedures guided by other imaging modalities. Ultrasound platforms and software are becoming increasingly advanced, enabling the operator to benefit from additional information to aid lesion targeting. Intravenous ultrasound contrast agents and elastography data are being used with increasing frequency.

Technology which enables co-registration of real-time ultrasound imaging with CT/MRI studies is becoming more accessible.[14] One example of this is using MRI data to aid ultrasound-guided prostate biopsy. It can be difficult to identify focal prostatic lesions at ultrasound and cancers may be missed despite methods which allow a large number of cores to be acquired. Fusing pre-procedural MRI data with real-time transrectal ultrasound (TRUS) imaging combines the advantages of each modality by allowing the biopsy needle to be introduced into suspicious lesions previously identified with MRI but under real-time TRUS guidance.[15]

CT

CT is generally preferred for biopsies of the lung, bone and spine. CT is also particularly useful for biopsies of deep abdominal lesions where ultrasound visualisation is poor, for example retroperitoneal nodal masses. CT-guided techniques can be extremely accurate with appropriate lesion selection and an experienced user. However, access to scanning time and radiation dose are limiting factors. Additionally non-fluoroscopic CT techniques are not 'real time', as needle position is checked after each adjustment. This theoretically carries a greater risk of damaging local structures compared to true real-time techniques. CT fluoroscopy technology enables biopsies to be performed under real-time CT imaging. This is useful for more challenging procedures (e.g. small target lesions) and may be performed with relatively small radiation doses.[16] CT fusion techniques, for instance with ultrasound, are increasingly used as discussed elsewhere.

MRI

Recent advances in MRI have made it increasingly useful, particularly where an oblique approach is required, e.g. for subdiaphragmatic liver and adrenal masses.[17,18] MRI also provides improved soft tissue detail when imaging certain organs and structures compared with CT or ultrasound and hence can be invaluable in targeting lesions in areas such as the prostate which are difficult to visualise with ultrasound or certain liver lesions which cannot be appreciated on unenhanced CT imaging.[19,20]

MRI-guided breast biopsies are also performed, particularly for lesions that are difficult to localise with mammography or ultrasound. Within the field of musculoskeletal imaging, MRI-guided biopsy is useful for lesions in the bone marrow that cannot be identified with CT. The use of MRI guidance is likely to increase as the technology improves.

The main disadvantage of MRI-guided biopsies is the magnetic environment, which limits equipment usage, making some procedures more complex. This in turn can lead to increased procedural times which may be an issue where MRI capacity is limited. There are also increased costs to consider, and patients may find MRI-guided procedures more uncomfortable due to positioning constraints. Open magnets allow direct access to the patient during the entire procedure, enabling real-time monitoring of needle insertion. A further problem with MRI-guided biopsy is the need for motion correction during the biopsy procedure. In addition, patients may not be able to tolerate MRI due to claustrophobia or have other contraindications such as pacemakers. MRI-safe biopsy equipment is now mass-produced but is expensive and the range is limited.

PET CT

The mechanism by which PET images are obtained is an intrinsic barrier to their use in biopsy, in that images are obtained over a period of time and proximity to the patient during acquisition results in radiation safety issues. However, novel fusion techniques that combine real-time CT with pre-procedural PET/CT to identify lesions that are not easily visualised on conventional CT and are only identified due to their differential FDG uptake have been described.[21]

Fluoroscopy

Plain fluoroscopic biopsy techniques are most frequently used for musculoskeletal lesions, as bony landmarks are easily identified. Fusion techniques are being increasingly developed, for example the use of pre-procedural MRI and CT overlaid on real-time fluoroscopic images; this is useful for sampling multiple targets, including head and neck lesions.[22]

Fluoroscopy is also utilised in transvascular biopsy techniques, where intravascular contrast is used to guide access, e.g. transvenous liver biopsy via the jugular or femoral vein,[23] which is usually performed when liver biopsy is essential but contraindicated percutaneously.

Stereotactic

This technique is mainly limited to the biopsy of breast lesions that are seen on mammography but cannot be visualised with ultrasound. They are performed most commonly for microcalcification and architectural distortion. This technique relies on computer software to interpret angled mammography views to give a three-dimensional location of the lesion.

Endoscopy/Endoscopic Ultrasound (EUS) and Bronchoscopy/Bronchoscopic Ultrasound

More often performed by appropriately trained clinicians than radiologists, direct visualisation biopsies and endoscopic/bronchoscopic ultrasound-guided aspiration or biopsy procedures have an important role in obtaining tissue from areas which are difficult to access percutaneously. EUS can also be combined with elastography to aid lesion identification and biopsy.[24]

TIPS AND TRICKS

'Look Before you Leap'—Procedural Set Up

As with any procedure, time spent reviewing pre-procedural imaging and planning biopsy approach and modality is very well spent. Particularly when performing ultrasound-guided procedures, the operator should try and ensure that the patient's bed is at an appropriate height. Small changes to patient position and room setup can increase or decrease significantly the difficulty of performing the biopsy.

Avoiding Inadequate Samples

In centrally necrotic tumours, it is important to plan a needle trajectory through the periphery of the lesion to obtain useful tissue for histological analysis. Obtaining fibrous or gelatinous material can often result in failure to secure a histological diagnosis. Therefore it is advantageous to identify and subsequently avoid these areas. Often it is possible to assess the likelihood of a diagnosis being reached by visually assessing the sample (e.g. white tissue which sinks in formalin) but if there is doubt, urgent cytological/histological assessment can help to decide whether the biopsy should be repeated.

Improving Needle Tip Visualisation in Ultrasound-Guided Biopsy

This can be technically difficult, particularly when sampling anatomically deep structures or tissues which are particularly echogenic. Accurate needle/transducer alignment is also crucial to good visualisation. The conspicuity of the needle is increased by turning the bevel upwards. 'Jiggling' the needle gently, injecting a tiny volume of air or local anaesthetic, optimising ultrasound platform settings (focal zone, depth, etc.) and use of needle guides can also help to increase needle conspicuity. Many biopsy needles are manufactured with a roughened tip or polymer coating to aid ultrasound scatter/beam reflection.

POST-PROCEDURAL CARE

Good post-procedural care reduces the morbidity associated with percutaneous biopsy by prompt recognition of complications and subsequent instigation of appropriate management. Immediate post-procedural imaging to identify problems can be helpful (e.g. in looking for pneumothorax following lung biopsy) but overall it has a low sensitivity and specificity for identifying complications, the majority of which become evident during the early post-procedural period. Patients should therefore be closely observed to a standard protocol in a dedicated unit with appropriately trained staff. Within the radiology departmental setting, in the initial post-procedural period, patients are best observed in a radiology day case unit. Post-procedural pain is common and usually responds to simple non-steroidal analgesia and reassurance. If opiate analgesia is required, the patient should be clinically assessed for early evidence of complications such as haemorrhage. Standard procedure-specific post-biopsy observation sheets which highlight the management of suspected complications should be used. These are particularly beneficial when patients return to their wards where staff may not have any specialist knowledge of the procedure and its associated risks.

SPECIMEN HANDLING

All core biopsy samples obtained should be very carefully handled to avoid tissue disruption or 'lost samples'. The operator should ensure that clear clinical information is provided on the request form. Specimen handling is aided by the presence of an assistant. Following core biopsy, the needle gate should be opened carefully to reveal the specimen which can be then placed in formalin. The cores obtained should be inspected to make an initial assessment of adequacy: soft tissue generally sinks in the formalin while fat floats to the surface.

COMPLICATIONS AND SAFETY ISSUES

Day case biopsy procedures should be scheduled on morning lists in order to enable an appropriate period of post-biopsy observation. This allows complications to be identified and managed during normal working hours. Higher risk biopsy procedures should be performed in a unit where any associated complications can be managed definitively, in order to avoid the need for emergency patient transfer. For the purposes of clinical governance, those performing biopsy or drainage procedures should audit their complication rates against published standards and monitor their success rate in terms of the percentage of adequate samples for histological evaluation obtained.

Complications are specific to the organ/lesion undergoing biopsy but are more likely to occur in patients who have co-morbidity or abnormal coagulation.

Haemorrhage is the most common major complication after biopsy procedures. If there is clinical suspicion regarding haemorrhage, ultrasound examination can be used to look for free fluid but false negative scans are not unusual and CT imaging is often necessary. The other major general complication of image-guided biopsy is infection (wound infection, deeper abscess formation, septicaemia or peritonitis). Minor complications include post-procedural pain and vasovagal reactions. Procedure-specific complications include haematuria after prostate biopsy and pneumothorax following lung biopsy.

Track Seeding

Seeding the needle track with malignant tumour cells when performing percutaneous needle biopsy is rare and must be differentiated from local tumour recurrence. It has been reported from a number of different tumour sites but certain tumours, such as hepatocellular carcinoma, soft tissue sarcomas, colorectal liver metastases and primary pleural malignancy, have been associated with a higher risk of track seeding.[25] Multidisciplinary team discussion is often appropriate in these cases. Careful consideration should be given to the proposed course of the needle to limit the tissues traversed. Knowledge of proposed surgical/radiotherapy treatment is helpful, particularly in the case of sarcoma biopsy where the needle track should be limited to the same compartment as the target lesion.

CONCLUSION

Image-guided biopsies are increasingly performed as an alternative to open biopsy or resection. Radiologists have a vital role in providing a safe and reliable biopsy service that enables clinicians to make an accurate diagnosis. Although ultrasound and CT are the commonest modalities utilised, the principles of safe biopsy technique can be applied across the modalities. As with all procedures, patient selection and preparation are key considerations and a firm understanding of the benefits and associated risks is essential in the selection and counseling of patients.

Technological advances include the use of MRI and multi-modality fusion imaging. These emerging techniques are enabling biopsies to be undertaken in more challenging patient groups, facilitating the biopsy of lesions that are difficult to identify with conventional imaging and providing more accurate guidance in the biopsy of smaller target lesions.

IMAGE-GUIDED TUMOUR ABLATION

THE CASE FOR TUMOUR ABLATION

Advances in diagnostic imaging have led to ever more frequent identification of small malignant tumours in different organs. It is becoming increasingly difficult to justify traditional, major surgical resection for such small volume disease. An additional consideration is that these tumours are often found in elderly patients who are less likely to tolerate the morbidity of traditional surgical techniques.

Although modern combination chemotherapy is yielding increasingly better results and has improved survival in a number of common cancers, it does not eradicate the disease in the 'surgical' sense. This consideration has stimulated the development of minimally invasive techniques for the treatment of small volume disease. In some cases this is a replacement for surgical resection, as in image-guided ablation of renal tumours, which is increasingly yielding outcomes equivalent to those of partial nephrectomy. In other situations, such as metastatic colorectal disease in the liver, ablation is more likely to be seen as a minimally invasive adjunct to systemic chemotherapy.

This section will set out to discuss the principles of effective tumour ablation and the ablative energies involved. Sound oncological outcomes also require a clear understanding of image guidance as it influences procedural planning and execution, intraprocedural monitoring and perhaps most importantly radiological follow-up of this inherently 'in situ' surgical technique.

THE PRINCIPLES OF TUMOUR ABLATION

Tumour ablation is used mainly in the treatment of small tumours. Image-guided ablation (IGA) sets out to reduce the morbidity of invasive surgery and spare background functioning parenchyma. It has inherent physical limitations but treatment efficacy can be improved by the use of adjunctive techniques such as hydrodissection, (chemo)embolisation and modulation by systemic chemotherapy.

ABLATIVE ENERGIES

The operator must have a firm understanding of the ablative energies currently used and their relative limitations and merits in different environments. Most ablative technologies employ thermal energy to achieve coagulative tissue necrosis through both the target tumour and a surrounding margin of organ parenchyma, in order to reduce the risk of local recurrence. This process of localised thermal destruction is modified in vivo by local tissue interactions, which affect how well the thermal energy is propagated through adjacent tissue. The degree to which the tumour is heated can be modified by heat loss as a result of perfusion-mediated tissue cooling and 'heat-sumping' arising from the cooling effect of blood flow in adjacent vessels of > 3 mm in diameter.[26,27]

The operator must address the shape of the target tumour and aim to incorporate it within a contiguous ablation zone along with an adequate 'resection' margin in the surgical sense. The energy applied must be sufficient not only to denature tumour but also to achieve effective ablation of adjacent normal tissue. An adequate margin is necessary because adjacent parenchyma may harbor microsatellites of disease or small foci of microvascular invasive disease. The aim should be to obtain tissue lethal temperatures in a consistent margin around the tumour without causing thermal injury to adjacent structures.

Radiofrequency Ablation

Radiofrequency ablation (RFA) has evolved rapidly since its first application to tumour ablation in the early 1990s into the most commonly utilised ablative device to date.[26] Monopolar radiofrequency ablation involves the application of high-frequency (460–500 kHz) alternating current to the target tissue using a needle-like applicator. Water molecules, which are inherently polarised, are agitated within the alternating electric field. Large, dispersive grounding pads are attached to the patient's trunk or thighs but the resultant current flux density around the uninsulated probe tip causes 'radiofrequency' agitation of

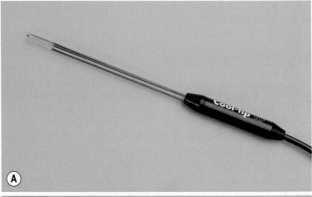

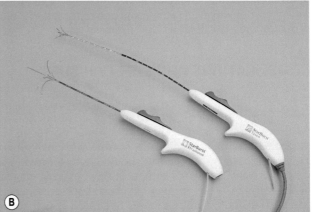

FIGURE 5-6 ■ Radiofrequency ablation (RFA) devices. The manufacturers have developed clustered (A) or expandable probe arrays (B) to overcome the limitations of single-probe RFA.

water molecules and local frictional heating within a few millimetres of the tip of the electrode.

Coagulative necrosis results if the target tissue can be maintained at temperatures above 45°C. RFA can induce temperatures of 100–110°C within a few millimetres of the probe but beyond this zone it relies on conductive heating to raise the temperature of the target tumour. The temperature of the tissue near the edge of the tumour may not be high enough for effective ablation leading to marginal recurrences.

Modern needle applicators can achieve reproducible 3–5 cm spheres of contiguous tissue destruction within 15–20 minutes. Larger ablation volumes can be achieved by 'clustering' needles on a single-hand piece, using expandable multi-tined devices or through multipolar arrays (Fig. 5-6).

Microwave Ablation

Microwave ablation (MWA) employs needle-like probes harbouring a microwave broadcast antenna within the 'feedpoint' towards the tip of the device (Fig. 5-7). These are tuned to interact with soft tissue in the range of 900–2400 MHz. Water molecules oscillate when subjected to microwave (electromagnetic) radiation. There is an inherent physical inefficiency to this process—'lossy dielectrics'—which results in localised tissue heating, often to very high temperatures. This results in effective

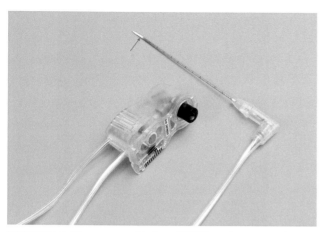

FIGURE 5-7 ■ **Microwave ablation (MWA) probe, 2.45 GHz MW probe with inline pump units.** The probe feedpoint is some 16 mm back from the tip (arrow).

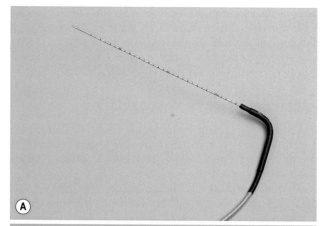

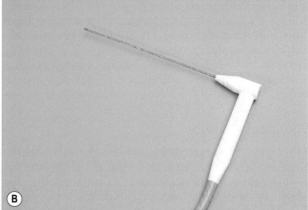

FIGURE 5-8 ■ **Cryoablation (CRA) probes.** Two examples of standard organ cryoprobes.

heating of local tissues, less compromised by tissue limitations and convective tissue cooling than is the case with RFA.[28]

Multiprobe, interactive arrays are available. Alternatively single probes, which operate at 100–180 W, can be repositioned after only 3–5 min to good effect, leading to large volumes of tissue ablation.

Cryoablation

This form of thermal energy has been in variable use for some decades but only in the past few years has there been renewed interest due to the introduction of narrow guage (17G) argon cryoprobes, which have made percutaneous cryoablation (CRA) a practical proposition (Fig. 5-8).[29] In practice several parallel probes (usually 3–4) are placed under image guidance into the tumour, approximately 10 mm from the edge and 15–20 mm apart. The phase change of liquid to gaseous argon can induce temperatures as low as –150 to –170°C in the immediate vicinity of the probes. The cell lethal isotherm lies at –20 to –30°C and is ensured in practice by a double freeze–thaw cycle.[30]

The mechanism of cell injury is multifactorial but intracellular ice formation disrupts cellular organelles whilst extracellular ice formation and osmotic dehydration also aids in achieving cellular disruption. These mechanisms are compounded by microvascular endothelial injury.[29]

The outstanding feature of cryoablation is the physical iceball created through the tissues during the treatment cycle. The evolution of the iceball is more predictable and the phase change to ice is clearly visualised by current ultrasound, CT and MR imaging modalities. This provides a readily visualised 'therapeutic' ovoid iceball.

Focused Ultrasound

Focused ultrasound does not require placement of an invasive probe. Small focal areas of tissue destruction are achieved by focusing sound energy in the 1-MHz range, using an extracorporeal acoustic lens. This has the clear

advantage of avoiding breach of the body wall but the sound energy can be severely attenuated by intervening structures such as bone or gas. The focused energy results in small ovoids of tissue destruction usually of about rice grain size, i.e. 12×3 mm.[31] These areas are stacked together contiguously to create larger ablation zones. This process requires complex motion correction and respiratory gating in organs such as the liver and kidney, and this explains why to date applications have centred on stationary organs such as the prostate or the uterus.

Irreversible Electroporation

Irreversible electroporation (IRE) is a non-thermal ablative technique that acts by the application of millisecond pulses of direct current between monopolar probes or using a single bipolar probe. These bursts of current can temporarily disrupt the electrical potential of the cell membrane and thereby perforate—or 'porate'—the cell membrane. A reversible form of electroporation has been used for some in the laboratory to permit genetic transfection of cells through temporary cell wall permeability. By applying the direct current for slightly longer the cells can be permanently porated—irreversible electroporation—resulting in controlled cell death.[32]

The major disadvantage associated with IRE is the severe muscle contractions induced by the application of direct current pulses. This necessitates the use of a general anaesthetic and muscle relaxants. On occasion cardiac dysrhythmias have been induced by the direct current pulses and as a result the technology is now ECG-synchronised in order to avoid these.[33] Clinical experience with IRE remains in its infancy.

Interstitial Laser Photocoagulation

Interstitial laser photocoagulation (ILP) is known by a number of synonyms including laser interstitial thermotherapy and laser thermal ablation. Laser fibres are coupled to an energy source, commonly neodymium:yttrium aluminium garnet (Nd-YAG), and the fibres emit low energy laser light which interact with chromophobes in the tissue, producing heat. This slow heating can induce useful small zones of tissue destruction over a range of about 10 mm. In practice multiple fibres must be placed using a beam splitter to yield clinically useful volumes of tissue destruction. The unwieldy nature of this device has limited its utilisation in clinical practice although a few centres have produced promising results.[34]

Chemical Ablation

This form of tumour ablation involves the instillation of chemical agents that denature tissue; the main ones are absolute alcohol and acetic acid. Ethanol ablation has been used widely to treat small nodular hepatomas.[35] Excellent results have been achieved in small homogeneous hepatomas. However, in the treatment of larger tumours multiple sessions of ethanol instillation are required because of inhomogeneous distribution of alcohol through the lesion. In recent years multi-tined alcohol infusion needles have been developed and have been advocated by some groups in the treatment of smaller hepatomas, especially in countries with very limited health care budgets.[36]

IMAGE GUIDANCE

This is of defining importance in terms of safety and the achievement of good clinical outcomes. The ablation device must be placed accurately to achieve the desired effect and avoid injury to adjacent structures. In many cases, repositioning of the device is necessary in order to achieve the desired effect. The aim is to destroy the tumour whilst avoiding injury to transgressed or threatened intervening organs.

Pre-Procedural Planning

Ablative techniques are largely aimed at smaller tumours (generally ≤ 5 cm) with the best results obtained in most organ systems for tumours smaller than 3 cm. The aim is to treat the tumour in its entirety without injury to adjacent structures. Injury to structures such as the bowel can be avoided by physical displacement through the use of injected 5% dextrose (Fig. 5-9). The addition of 2% iodinated contrast medium to this fluid can enhance its visualisation. Carbon-dioxide gas insufflation within the

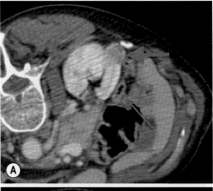
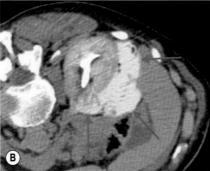

FIGURE 5-9 ■ **Sequence demonstrating the need for hydrodissection during cryoablation of a renal tumour (thick arrow).** (A) Portal venous phase CT; directly adjacent loops of small bowel (thin arrow) that would be at risk if incorporated in the ablation zone. (B) A hydrodissection needle is placed to the interposed retroperitoneum and contrast-tinted saline injected (arrowed), displacing adjacent at risk structures.

retroperitoneum can also be used to displace adjacent bowel for the purpose of renal tumour ablation.[37]

Good positioning of the patient can increase the likelihood of a successful ablation. For example, placing a patient with an adrenal tumour in a lateral decubitus position with the target adrenal lowermost can often help to displace the intervening lung in the deep costodiaphragmatic recess and any adjacent bowel away from the treatment volume.

Procedural Targetting

With current ablative technologies most appropriate tumour targets are in the range of 10–40 mm in diameter. Smaller tumours can be difficult to visualise; for example, small hepatomas clearly visible in the late arterial phase CT within a cirrhotic liver can be very difficult to target using ultrasound guidance. Sound outcomes from IGA require a clear visualisation of the tumour and adjacent structures, ideally in real time. Ultrasound provides real-time imaging but may not be able to demonstrate clearly adjacent threatened bowel. Many operators use a combination of ultrasound and CT. It is possible to combine volumetric CT and ultrasound data on a single display platform, allowing display of real-time ultrasound image and 'cold' CT data in any plane. MR guidance can provide image guidance in multiplanar formats with excellent soft-tissue contrast and is under evaluation with regard to resolution and image feedback speed.[38]

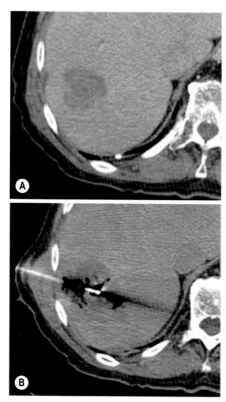

FIGURE 5-10 ■ **Example demonstrating the problem of outgassing following RFA or MWA.** (A) Colorectal metastases in segment 7 for microwave ablation. (B) At initial probe placement and treatment there is considerable 'outgassing' obscuring the target tumour and rendering probe repositioning and treatment dosimetry difficult.

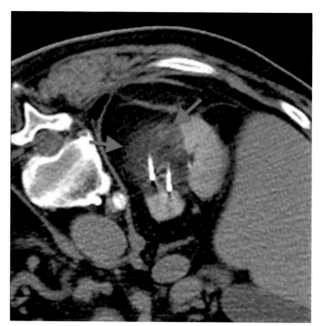

FIGURE 5-11 ■ **Two cryoprobes in a renal tumour demonstrating the formation of the clearly defined low attenuation iceball during the freeze cycle of CRA.**

Peri-Procedural Monitoring

Intraprocedural confirmation of treatment adequacy remains an issue for almost all of the ablation modalities. Visualisation of RFA and MWA procedures is severely compromised by 'outgassing' of the treated lesion (Fig. 5-10), which obscures the target tumour and can impede accurate re-positioning of the probe. Several studies have suggested that contrast-enhanced ultrasound[39] and MR thermometry[38] can guide tumour treatment but each have their limitations in terms of robustness and accuracy.

Cryoablation has the considerable merit of inducing a well-defined and perceivable iceball which can be readily visualised by a number of imaging modalities during the treatment procedure (Fig. 5-11). This feature permits assessment of the effect of treatment with the lethal isotherm of −30°C deemed to reside 5 mm deep to the advancing margin of the iceball.

Post-Procedural Imaging

IGA must assess a 360° global resection margin to confirm treatment adequacy. There is broad acceptance that non-enhancement on CT or MRI during injection of intravenous contrast medium is a surrogate marker of tumour ablation.[40] In some organs such as the kidney and lung other surrogates of complete tumour ablation have been utilised, such as the 'post-treatment' halo artefact seen in the perirenal fat around completely ablated renal tumours[41] and the contiguous ground-glass opacification seen around completely denatured lung tumours.[42]

Follow-up imaging can be delayed for 1–2 weeks after the primary treatment as the ablation zone matures and becomes better defined with immediate post-treatment phenomena such as irregular penumbral arterialisation steadily resolving (though often this can take up to 3 months) and thereby facilitating post-procedural assessment. Degraded blood products within the treatment zone should not be mistaken for residual, viable enhancing tissue. In this respect, subtraction imaging, particularly subtraction T1 volumetric imaging at MR, can help to confirm tumour ablation.

Over time the ablation zone should slowly involute become darker on CT with an increasingly well-defined and sharp margin (Fig. 5-12). In the case of renal tumours and hepatocellular carcinoma, late arterial phase imaging helps to illustrate residual or recurrent disease, which tends to adopt a marginal nodular or crescenteric pattern. Recurrent colorectal metastatic disease can declare itself as an expanding ablation zone with softening of the margins—coined a 'halo' recurrence (Fig. 5-13).

The post-treatment follow-up protocol will clearly be determined by the natural history of the treated tumour. Ablated renal tumours can be indolent and, rarely, recurrent disease can declare itself 2–4 years after the initial treatment. Most local recurrences of colorectal metastases and hepatocellular tumours will be apparent at follow-up within 10 months. As a result most authors advocate follow-up at 3-monthly intervals within the first year, 6-monthly to 2 years and annually out to 5 years.

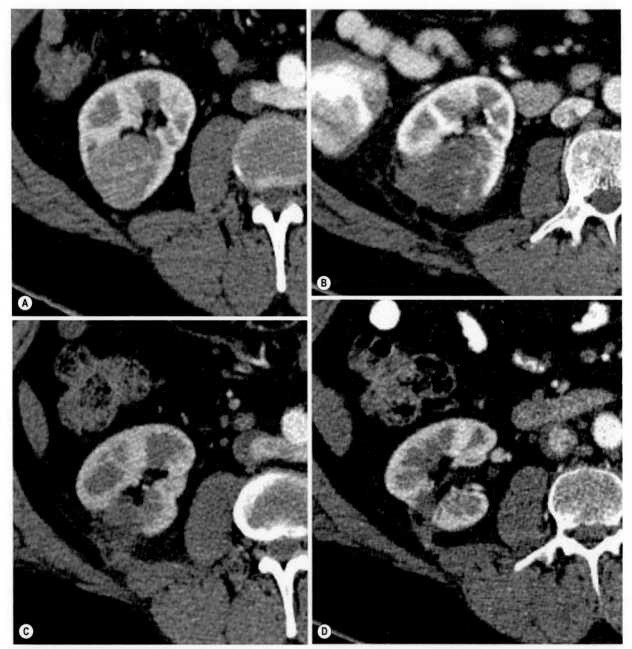

FIGURE 5-12 ■ **Sequential images showing involution of a successfully cryoablated 44-mm renal cell carcinoma on late arterial phase CT.** (A) Pre-treatment. (B) One month post-treatment. (C) Six months post-treatment. (D) Sixteen months post-treatment.

As we become better able to predict treatment success it may be possible to reduce the intensity of follow-up protocols.

Lung tumours are uniquely problematic in that straightforward imaging markers of treatment success are not readily to hand. A circumferential ground-glass opacification after treatment has been advocated as a marker of completion[42] but it is a very indirect surrogate in that it only represents adjacent airspace injury or haemorrhage. Functional imaging such as FDG PET/CT seems set to play a significant role in confirming the absence of tumour metabolism.[43]

UNDERSTANDING AND MODIFYING TUMOUR PATHOPHYSIOLOGY

During RFA, perfusion-mediated tissue cooling, particularly in the adjacent normal parenchyma, can compromise the zone of thermal injury. Similarly 'heat-sumping', in relation to adjacent blood vessels of ≥ 3 mm, can limit the achievement of tissue-lethal temperatures and result in perivascular tumour sparing.

These problems may be overcome through various techniques such as hypotensive anaesthesia, adjacent temporary vessel occlusion and pre-embolisation. Some

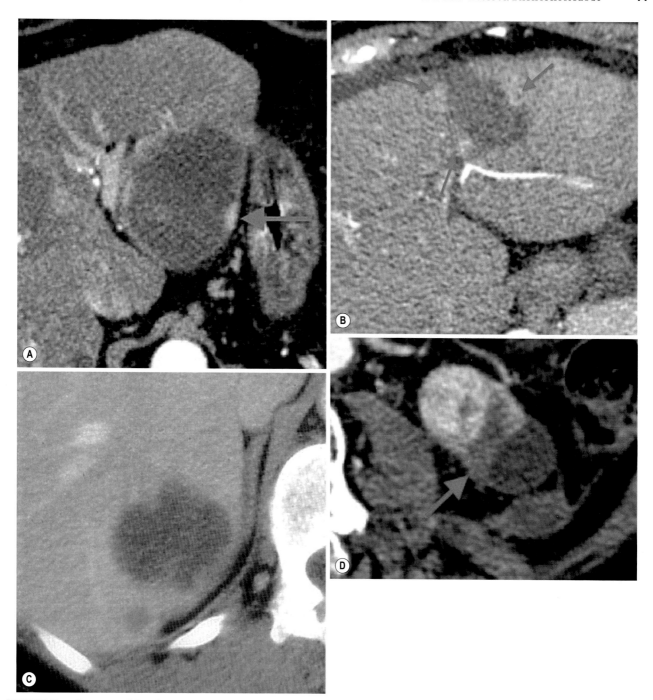

FIGURE 5-13 ■ Patterns of local recurrence can vary according mainly to tumour type. Examples of local recurrence in hepatic tumours but the patterns can apply to all tumour locations. (A) Peripheral nodular recurrence on late arterial phase CT, seen in the subtotal treatment of hepatocellular carcinoma. (B) A patchy peripheral recurrence on late arterial phase CT, sometimes referred to as a 'halo' recurrence. (C) An enlarging (with reference to the ablation zone) low density lesion with increasing ill-defined treatment margin. This form of 'expanding' recurrence is seen with inadequate treatment of a colorectal metastasis. (D) Crescenteric peripheral enhancement on late arterial phase CT indicative of a subtotal treatment.

of these complex treatment modifications have diminished in practice partly through improved case selection for IGA but also through a better understanding of how the tumour pathophysiology can be modified by prior adjuvant chemotherapy bringing tumours within the scope of ablation or the use of anti-angiogenic drugs which appear to modify tumour perfusion and enhance

the therapeutic effect of thermal ablation.[44] A number of studies are currently looking at the modification of tumours by agents such as adjuvant sorafenib.

In the setting of hepatocellular carcinoma thermal ablation has been combined with drug-eluting chemoembolisation with a view to enhancing the efficacy of both techniques.[45] This practice is predicated on the fact that thermal ablation most frequently fails at the margins of the tumour, yet the penumbral zone of partial thermal injury can be utilised to preferentially direct chemoembolic agents to this zone for maximum oncological benefit. The effectiveness and optimal timing of these combined approaches remains to be determined.

SPECIFICS AND CURRENT OUTCOMES

The field of interventional oncology is constantly evolving. A full discussion of the merits and limitations of these factors under each cancer type is beyond the scope of this chapter. This section focuses on some developments.

Renal Cancer

This tumour group in particular represents perhaps one of the most effective applications for IGA. Its use has been prompted by the increasing numbers of small renal tumours detected incidentally. The malignant potential of some of these smaller renal tumours remains the subject of debate with some advocating active surveillance. Yet the treatment paradigm is changed if a simple, minimally invasive and nephron-sparing intervention can be brought to bear where no simple marker of the relative potential behaviour of these tumours currently exists.

The efficacy of RFA for the treatment of sub-35-mm renal tumours has been confirmed with intermediate follow-up at 2–3 years.[46,47] Meta-analysis has suggested that cryoablation may be more effective than RFA with lower rates of local recurrence and subtotal treatment.[48] Experience to date suggests that percutaneous renal cryoablation may achieve results similar to that of surgical resection with lower morbidity.[49]

Hepatocellular Carcinoma

Hepatocellular carcinoma (HCC) is frequently a combination of two disease processes in Western society where HCC almost always arises in the setting of liver cirrhosis. There are multiple treatment options which reflect the stage of hepatocellular carcinoma at presentation but also the functional liver reserve in the setting of cirrhosis. In an attempt to clarify this decision-making process the Barcelona Clinic Liver Cancer Group published a treatment decision algorithm.[50] Chemoembolisation and systemic therapies are reserved for intermediate stage, multifocal disease. The options for more limited disease include ablation, transplantation and resection. Resection of cirrhotic livers carries significantly higher operative complications and is usually reserved for those without frank portal hypertension.

Ablation—mostly using radiofrequency or microwaves—has an increasing role in the management of paucilesional sub-5-cm hepatomas as it carries significantly lower morbidity than resection and has been shown to achieve 61% 5-year overall survival in selected Childs A patients.[51] There is increasing evidence that image-guided ablation is the treatment method of choice for nodular disease of < 2–3 cm in diameter,[52] where the patient is not amenable to transplantation or whilst on the transplant waiting list. For larger disease of 4–6 cm in diameter ablation is being combined with pre- or post-ablation chemoembolisation to good oncological effect.[45]

Colorectal Liver Metastases

Colorectal metastatic disease (MCRC) in the liver is a common problem and whilst current systemic chemotherapy is able to achieve a median survival of 14–26 months,[53] surgical resection in selected patients can achieve 50% 5-year survival.[54] There is increasing interest into whether ablation can replace surgery for isolated small volume metastases, extend the scope of surgery when combined with resection or act as an interventional oncological adjunct to systemic chemotherapy. Outcome data suggest that colorectal metastases are more difficult to ablate than HCC of similar size, with higher local recurrence rates. Most experienced practitioners confine ablation to disease of <25–30 mm in diameter. Data suggests that IGA can achieve median survival of 30–32 months in selected patients.[55,56]

Lung Tumour Ablation

Surgical resection is the preferred treatment for patient with early non-small cell lung carcinomas but is often precluded due to the poor lung function or medical co-morbidities. Conventional external beam radiotherapy is usually offered where feasible but more recently there has been increasing interest in focal stereotactic radiation therapy, percutaneous ablation and combinations of the two procedures. A recent study analysed 64 patients who underwent RFA, CRA or sublobar resection.[57] The 3-year disease-specific survival and disease-free survivals were 87.5 and 50% for RFA, 90.2 and 45.6% for CRA and 90.6 and 60.8% for sublobar resection. A number of studies are increasingly testifying to equable 3-year cancer-specific survivals and there is increasingly studies on how ablation and focal radiotherapy might be best combined.

Small volume lung metastases often occur in older patients who have already undergone previous surgery and may suffer from other medical co-morbidities. Metastases suitable for ablation are usually < 3 per hemithorax, < 35 mm in diameter and located in well-aerated lung, usually at least 2–3 cm remote form the hilar structures. Studies to date have shown radiological confirmation of complete ablation in approximately 80% of colorectal metastases.[58]

Bone Tumour Ablation

Techniques such as RFA and CRA have been increasingly used for the curative treatment of small osteoid osteomas, osteoblastomas and chondroblastomas and in the palliative pain management of larger malignant tumours such as metastases from renal carcinoma. Cryoablation, in particular, is increasingly utilised in this application where visualisation of the therapeutic iceball clearly aids treatment dosimetry. Accruing evidence suggests that cryoablation may have an increasing role in the palliative management of painful metastases.[59]

SUMMARY

Radiological imaging is demonstrating and characterising malignant disease at an ever smaller size. The detection of small volume disease in an often elderly population where organ preservation becomes increasingly more important has stimulated interest in and development of image-guided in situ tumour ablation. Many ablative technologies including RFA, MWA, CRA, IRE and stereotactic radiotherapy are continuously evolving. These minimally invasive technologies and in situ treatments will require precise radiological guidance and diligent imaging follow-up if they are to adopt a central role in the management of small volume cancers.

REFERENCES

1. Al Knawy B, Shiffman M. Percutaneous liver biopsy in clinical practice. Liver Int 2007;27(9):1166–73.
2. Maya ID, Maddela P, Barker J, Allon M. Percutaneous renal biopsy: comparison of blind and real-time ultrasound-guided technique. Semin Dial 2007;20(4):355–8.
3. Livraghi T, Damascelli B, Lombardi C, et al. Risk in fine-needle abdominal biopsy. J Clin Ultrasound 1983;11:77–81.
4. Turner P, Williams C. Informed consent: patients listen and read, but what information do they retain? N Z Med J 2002;115(1164):U218.
5. Haaga JR, LiPuma JP, Bryan PJ, et al. Clinical comparison of small and large calibre cutting needles for biopsy. Radiology 1983;146:665–7.
6. Pagani JJ. Biopsy of focal hepatic lesions. Comparison of 18 and 22 gauge needles. Radiology 1983;147:673–5.
7. Demharter J, Muller P, Wagner T, et al. Percutaneous core-needle biopsy of enlarged lymph nodes in the diagnosis and subclassification of malignant lymphomas. Eur Radiol 2001;11:276–83.
8. Varadarajulu S, Fraig M, Schmulewitz N, et al. Comparison of EUS-guided 19-gauge Trucut needle biopsy with EUS-guided fine-needle aspiration. Endoscopy 2004;36:397–401.
9. Li L, Wu Q-L, Liu L-Z, et al. Value of CT-guided core-needle biopsy in diagnosis and classification of malignant lymphomas using automated biopsy gun. World J Gastroenterol 2005;11(31):4843–7.
10. Diederich S, Padge B, Vossas U, et al. Application of a single needle type for all image-guided biopsies: results of 100 consecutive core biopsies in various organs using a novel tri-axial, end-cut needle. Cancer Imaging 2006;6:43–50.
11. Plecha DM, Goodwin DW, Rowland DY, et al. Liver biopsy: effects of biopsy needle caliber on bleeding and tissue recovery. Radiology 1997;204(1):101–4.
12. Moulton JS, Moore PT. Coaxial percutaneous biopsy technique with automated biopsy devices: value in improving accuracy and negative predictive value. Radiology 1993;186:515–22.
13. Hatfield MK, Beres RA, Sane SS, Zaleski GX. Percutaneous imaging-guided solid organ core needle biopsy: coaxial versus non-coaxial method. Am J Roentgenol 2008;190(2):413–17.
14. Lange T, Papenberg N, Heldmann S, et al. 3D ultrasound-CT registration of the liver using combined landmark-intensity information. Int J Comput Assist Radiol Surg 2009;4(1):79–88.
15. Singh AK, Kruecker J, Xu S, et al. Initial clinical experience with real-time transrectal ultrasonography–magnetic resonance imaging fusion-guided prostate biopsy. BJU Int 2008;101:841–5.
16. Schaefer PJ, Schaefer FK, Heller M, Jahnke T. CT fluoroscopy guided biopsy of small pulmonary and upper abdominal lesions: efficacy with a modified breathing technique. J Vasc Interv Radiol 2007;18(10):1241–8.
17. Schmidt A, Kee S, Sze D, et al. Diagnostic yield of MR-guided liver biopsies compared with CT and US-guided liver biopsies. J Vasc Interv Radiol 1999;10:1323–9.
18. König CW, Pereira PL, Trübenbach J, et al. MR imaging–guided adrenal biopsy using an open low-field-strength scanner and MR fluoroscopy. Am J Roentgenol 2003;180:1567–70.
19. D'Amico AV, Tempany CM, Cormack R, et al. Transperineal magnetic resonance image guided prostate biopsy. J Urol 2000;164:385–7.
20. Stattaus J, Maderwald S, Baba HA, et al. MR-guided liver biopsy with a short, wide-bore 1.5 Tesla MR system. Eur Radiol 2008;18(12):2865–73.
21. Bitencourt AG, Tyng CJ, Pinto PN, et al. Percutaneous biopsy based on PET/CT findings in cancer patients: technique, indications, and results. Clin Nucl Med 2012;37(5):e95–7.
22. Levitt MR, Vaidya SS, Su DK, et al. The 'triple-overlay' technique for percutaneous diagnosis and treatment of lesions of the head and neck: Combined 3D guidance with MRI, cone-beam CT, and fluoroscopy. World Neurosurg 2012;79(3–4):509–14.
23. Khosa F, McNulty JG, Hickey N, et al. Transvenous liver biopsy via the femoral vein. Clin Radiol 2003;58(6):487–91.
24. Giovannini M, Hookey LC, Bories E, et al. Endoscopic ultrasound elastography: the first step towards virtual biopsy? Preliminary results in 49 patients. Endoscopy 2006;38(4):344–8.
25. Robertson EG, Baxter G. Tumour seeding following percutaneous needle biopsy: The real story! Clin Rad 2011;66:1007–14.
26. McGahan JP, Brock JM, Tesluk H, et al. Hepatic ablation with use of radio-frequency electrocautery in the animal model. J Vasc Interv Radiol 1992;3(2):291–7.
27. Goldberg SN, Gazelle GS, Mueller PR. Thermal ablation therapy for focal malignancy: a unified approach to underlying principles, techniques, and diagnostic imaging guidance. Am J Roentgenol 2000;174(2):323–31.
28. Simon CJ, Dupuy DE, Mayo-Smith WW. Microwave ablation: principles and applications. Radiographics 2005;25(Suppl. 1):S69–83.
29. Hoffmann NE, Bischof JC. The cryobiology of cryosurgical injury. Urology 2002;60(2 Suppl. 1):40–9.
30. Baust JG, Gage AA, Robilottto AT, Baust JM. The pathophysiology of thermoablation: optimizing cryoablation. Curr Opin Urol 2009;19(2):127–32.
31. Dubinsky TJ, Cuevas C, Dighe MK, et al. High-intensity focused ultrasound: current potential and oncologic applications. Am J Roentgenol 2008;190(1):191–9.
32. Rubinsky B, Onik G, Mikus P. Irreversible electroporation: a new ablation modality—clinical implications. Technol Cancer Res Treat 2007;6(1):37–48.
33. Deodhar A, Dickfeld T, Single GW, et al. Irreversible electroporation near the heart: ventricular arrhythmias can be prevented with ECG synchronization. Am J Roentgenol 2011;196(3):W330–335.
34. Mack MG, Straub R, Eichler K, et al. Percutaneous MR imaging-guided laser-induced thermotherapy of hepatic metastases. Abdom Imaging 2001;26(4):369–74.
35. Livraghi T, Giorgio A, Marin G, et al. Hepatocellular carcinoma and cirrhosis in 746 patients: long-term results of percutaneous ethanol injection. Radiology 1995;197(1):101–8.
36. Giorgio A, Di Sarno A, De Stefano G, et al. Percutaneous radiofrequency ablation of hepatocellular carcinoma compared to percutaneous ethanol injection in treatment of cirrhotic patients: an Italian randomized controlled trial. Anticancer Res 2011;31(6):2291–5.
37. Tsoumakidou G, Buy X, Garnon J, et al. Percutaneous thermal ablation: how to protect the surrounding organs. Tech Vasc Interv Radiol 2011;14(3):170–6.
38. Clasen S, Pereira PL. Magnetic resonance guidance for radiofrequency ablation of liver tumors. J Magn Reson Imaging 2008;27(2):421–33.
39. Johnson DB, Duchene DA, Taylor GD, et al. Contrast-enhanced ultrasound evaluation of radiofrequency ablation of the kidney: reliable imaging of the thermolesion. J Endourol 2005;19(2):248–52.
40. Goldberg SN, Grassi CJ, Cardella JF, et al. Image-guided tumor ablation: standardization of terminology and reporting criteria. J Vasc Interv Radiol 2009;20(Suppl. 7):S377–90.
41. Schirmang TC, Mayo-Smith WW, Dupuy DE, et al. Kidney neoplasms: renal halo sign after percutaneous radiofrequency ablation–incidence and clinical importance in 101 consecutive patients. Radiology 2009;253(1):263–9.
42. Anderson EM, Lees WR, Gillams AR. Early indicators of treatment success after percutaneous radiofrequency of pulmonary tumors. Cardiovasc Intervent Radiol 2009;32(3):478–83.

43. Purandare NC, Rangarajan V, Shah SA, et al. Therapeutic response to radiofrequency ablation of neoplastic lesions: FDG PET/CT findings. Radiographics 2011;31(1):201–13.

44. Goldberg SN. Science to practice: Which approaches to combination interventional oncologic therapy hold the greatest promise of obtaining maximal clinical benefit? Radiology 2011;261(3):667–9.

45. Lencioni R, Crocetti L, Petruzzi P, et al. Doxorubicin-eluting bead-enhanced radiofrequency ablation of hepatocellular carcinoma: a pilot clinical study. J Hepatol 2008;49(2):217–22.

46. Breen DJ, Rutherford EE, Stedman B, et al. Management of renal tumors by image-guided radiofrequency ablation: experience in 105 tumors. Cardiovasc Intervent Radiol 2007;30(5):936–42.

47. Zagoria RJ, Traver MA, Werle DM, et al. Oncologic efficacy of CT-guided percutaneous radiofrequency ablation of renal cell carcinomas. Am J Roentgenol 2007;189(2):429–36.

48. Kunkle DA, Uzzo RG. Cryoablation or radiofrequency ablation of the small renal mass : a meta-analysis. Cancer 2008;113(10):2671–80.

49. Atwell TD, Callstrom MR, Farrell MA, et al. Percutaneous renal cryoablation: local control at mean 26 months of followup. J Urol 2010;184(4):1291–5.

50. Bruix J, Sherman M; American Association for the Study of Liver Diseases. Management of hepatocellular carcinoma: an update. Hepatology 2011;53(3):1020–2.

51. Lencioni R, Cioni D, Crocetti L, et al. Early-stage hepatocellular carcinoma in patients with cirrhosis: long-term results of percuta-neous image-guided radiofrequency ablation. Radiology 2005;234(3):961–7.

52. Lau WY, Lai EC. The current role of radiofrequency ablation in the management of hepatocellular carcinoma: a systematic review. Ann Surg 2009;249(1):20–5.

53. Garcea G, Ong SL, Maddern GJ. Inoperable colorectal liver metastases: a declining entity? Eur J Cancer 2008;44(17):2555–72.

54. Choti MA, Sitzmann JV, Tiburi MF, et al. Trends in long-term survival following liver resection for hepatic colorectal metastases. Ann Surg 2002;235(6):759–66.

55. Solbiati L, Ierace T, Tonolini M, et al. Radiofrequency thermal ablation of hepatic metastases. Eur J Ultrasound 2001;13(2):149–58.

56. Sørensen SM, Mortensen FV, Nielsen DT. Radiofrequency ablation of colorectal liver metastases: long-term survival. Acta Radiol 2007;48(3):253–8.

57. Zemlyak A, Moore WH, Bilfinger TV. Comparison of survival after sublobar resections and ablative therapies for stage I non-small cell lung cancer. J Am Coll Surg 2010;211(1):68–72.

58. Lencioni R, Crocetti L, Cioni R, et al. Response to radiofrequency ablation of pulmonary tumours: a prospective, intention-to-treat, multicentre clinical trial (the RAPTURE study). Lancet Oncol 2008;9(7):621–8.

59. Callstrom MR, Atwell TD, Charboneau JW, et al. Painful metastases involving bone: percutaneous image-guided cryoablation—prospective trial interim analysis. Radiology 2006;241(2):572–80.

CHAPTER 6

Image-Guided Drainage Techniques

Michael M. Maher • Owen J. O'Connor

CHAPTER OUTLINE

Image-guided drainage is an established technique with a multitude of applications. The indications, techniques and management of image-guided catheter drainage, however, continue to evolve. This chapter provides an overview of the principles of image-guided drainage. We also discuss important technical aspects of specific drainage procedures, how to care for a drainage catheter and potential complications that can arise.

INDICATIONS AND CONTRAINDICATIONS

As a general rule, image-guided drainage is indicated for treatment of an accessible collection in a suitable patient that does not require immediate surgical intervention, to obtain a fluid sample for diagnostic purposes, to relieve symptoms or to inject a sclerosant.[1] Image-guided drainage alone is sometimes sufficient for treatment of a collection, but it can also act as an adjunct or temporising measure before definitive surgical treatment.[2] Drainage of a symptomatic collection such as an abscess is performed in order to drain pus from the cavity, working in conjunction with antibiotics. Infected collections accumulate antibiotics to a limited extent, which generally precludes effective treatment with antibiotics alone unless the collection is very small (1–3 cm).[3] Antibiotic coverage is necessary for many drainage procedures, even if the collection is not infected, to reduce the chance of secondarily infecting the collection. Examples of non-infected symptomatic collections that often require drainage include hydronephrosis caused by ureteric obstruction, bowel obstruction or postoperative seroma, urinoma and haematoma. Diagnostic fluid samples help determine whether a collection is infected and may also help identify the source of a collection. Fluid should be analysed by Gram stain; culture and sensitivity analysis should also be performed. Analysis of the cell count is also useful for quantifying the number of white cells in a sample. Amylase, bilirubin, lymphocytes and creatinine content

can be used to identify collections of pancreatic, biliary, lymphatic and urinary origins, respectively.[4]

There are few absolute contraindications to image-guided drainage. Profound uncorrected coagulopathy, clinical instability and lack of safe access to a collection are among the most common contraindications to image-guided drainage. In practice, many coagulopathies can be corrected to allow drainage. The authors stratify procedure-related bleeding risk into three categories: low, medium and high. Paracentesis, catheter exchange and aspiration are considered low risk. Abdominal and chest procedures are considered medium risk, whereas primary biliary or renal drainages are stratified as high risk. The authors consider correction of abnormal indices for a low-risk procedure if the platelet count is less than 30,000/μL and the international normalised ratio (INR) exceeds 2.5, or for a medium-risk procedure if the platelet count is less than 30,000/μL and the INR exceeds 1.7 or the partial thromboplastin time is 1.5 times normal. Correction is performed prior to a high-risk procedure if the platelet count is less than 50,000/μL and the INR exceeds 1.7 or the partial thromboplastin time is 1.5 times normal. These guidelines need to be tailored to the collection and the patient, taking into account the fact that an untreated abscess has a very high mortality rate, and successful drainage reduces morbidity.[5,6] Encasement by bowel loops and large blood vessels preclude drainage catheter placement. A 19–22G needle can be used to traverse the small bowel for diagnostic sampling but risks infecting a fluid collection with enteric organisms. General anaesthetic or monitored anaesthesiology care is necessary for clinically unstable patients requiring image-guided drainage catheter placement. Lack of maturation of an abscess is a potential reason for close-interval observation before drainage. Peritonitis and a large volume of intraperitoneal air in the setting of a collection are indications for surgical rather than image-guided drainage. Air localised and contained within the vicinity of a collection, generally, does not preclude image-guided drainage, and is usually caused by local gastrointestinal perforation such as from appendicitis or diverticulitis. In cases where there is uncertainty, good communication between the interventional radiologist, referring physician and patient or family is indicated in order to reach consensus.

IMAGING GUIDANCE

Ultrasound and CT are primarily used for image-guided drainage. Modern ultrasound provides excellent real-time visualisation of superficial structures, and good visualisation of viscera or collections. This facilitates careful monitoring of a catheter or needle as it is guided into a collection, irrespective of the plane of angulation. This is preferred in paediatric patients for whom radiation exposure should be minimised and can also be performed at the bedside in an intensive care unit (Fig. 6-1). It is important to maintain the needle or catheter in the plane of imaging when using ultrasound. If possible, a needle-probe angle of 55°–60° should be maintained to optimise reflection of the ultrasound beam and needle or catheter visualisation.[7] The optimal grey-scale image map for ultrasound-guided procedures is different to that of diagnostic ultrasound, and should be sought. Additionally, frequency compound imaging is an ultrasonic imaging technology which can help with needle visualisation during drainage. Compound imaging emits ultrasound at multiple incident beam angles, which increases needle conspicuity because of increased artefact. Compound imaging reduces the pulse repetition frequency, however, which can cause image discontinuity. Ultrasound is often suboptimal for catheter guidance if a collection contains air or if there are bowel loops adjacent to a collection which prevent adequate imaging and increase the risk of bowel injury. Ultrasound guidance can be used in a hybrid manner for drainage purposes (Fig. 6-2). Combined with fluoroscopy, ultrasound can guide access and catheter placement into a large or partially visualised collection before optimal catheter manipulation and positioning by fluoroscopic guidance. Fluoroscopic guidance is also beneficial for guidance of catheters placed using the Seldinger technique and reduces the risk of losing access and kinking the guidewire (Fig. 6-2).

CT-guided fluoroscopy has many proponents since it offers potential real-time guidance and excellent spatial

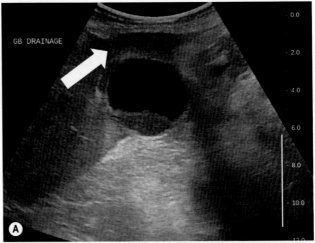

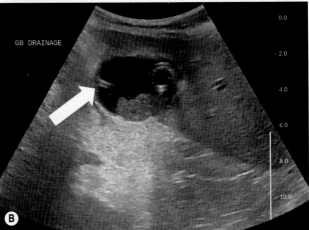

FIGURE 6-1 ■ **Ultrasound-guided drainage of gallbladder for acute cholecystitis in an 85-year-old female in the intensive care unit.** (A) Direct visualisation of catheter placement (arrow) through the liver into the gallbladder was provided with portable ultrasound. (B) The catheter (arrow) was released from the metal stiffener and the position confirmed before aspirating the contents of the gallbladder.

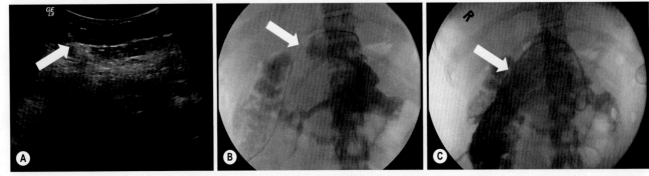

FIGURE 6-2 ■ **Abdominal wall collection drainage following abdominoplasty in a 23-year-old female using ultrasound and fluoroscopy.** (A) There was a large abdominal wall collection on CT. The collection was accessed through the midline with an 18G needle under ultrasound guidance (arrow). (B) A guidewire was directed into the collection using a Kumpe catheter (arrow) after contrast injection under fluoroscopic guidance confirmed position. (C) A multi-sidehole drainage catheter (arrow) was placed into the collection. The collection was successfully treated and no surgery was required.

resolution, which can reduce procedural time. One study has shown a 37% reduction in needle placement time but no significant reduction in room time using CT fluoroscopy for interventional radiology procedures.[8] CT fluoroscopy can be performed *real time* or by using a *quick-check* method. Real-time guidance involves holding the needle or catheter with a clamp and imaging as it is advanced. Quick-check CT guidance is used to image the needle tip after manipulation. Quick-check guidance considerably reduces fluoroscopic time and radiation dose compared with real-time guidance. Conventional CT guidance is favoured over ultrasound for drainage of deep collections with a difficult percutaneous access window.[9] Superior spatial resolution of CT over ultrasound often allows better localisation of the margins of a collection, the thickness of the wall, the adjacent organs and the access route. Tilting the angle of the CT gantry in a cranial or caudal direction is a useful adjunct, which can help image a safe direct route of access into a collection that is not available in the axial plane. This can create an additional level of difficulty for the interventional radiologist; the gantry laser guide is very useful for catheter direction in this circumstance. Room time, available resources, user preference and experience have a determining impact on the choice of image guidance.

PATIENT PREPARATION AND CARE

The authors recommend broad-spectrum antibiotics at least 1 h prior to abscess drainage. This does not preclude culture of material from an abscess since the rind of tissue that surrounds an abscess excludes most abscesses from the normal circulation.

Written informed consent is an important aspect of image-guided drainage. Optimal informed consent entails description of the indications for image-guided drainage, the alternatives, the procedure itself, potential complications and also the expected treatment plan after drainage. Since drainage catheters often remain in place for weeks, it is important that the patient be made aware of this so as to avoid unrealistic expectations. Effective teamwork and open communication between all those involved in the patient's care helps to reduce the risk of error and improves patient safety.[10,11] Normally, nursing sedation and continuous monitoring of vital signs is required for image-guided drainage. Patients should fast for 8 h prior to conscious sedation. The authors normally use fentanyl citrate (Elkins-Sinn, Cherry Hill, NJ, USA) and midazolam (Versed; Hoffmann-La Roche, Nutley, NJ), supplemented by antiemetics where appropriate. General anaesthesia is required for paediatric patients and severely ill or uncooperative patients. The authors advocate 4 h close observation after drainage to assess for complications.

CATHETER INSERTION

The following paragraphs provide an overview of techniques used for generic image-guided drainage. Drainage procedures which require special techniques or

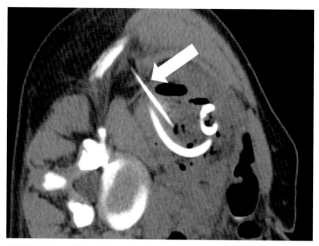

FIGURE 6-3 ■ CT-guided drainage of periappendiceal abscess using tandem-trochar technique in a 54-year-old female. A catheter was placed parallel to the guide needle (arrow) into the right lower quadrant collection with the patient in the left lateral decubitus position.

consideration will be discussed later in the chapter. Percutaneous aspiration is less likely to treat an abscess adequately compared with drain insertion. A collection which communicates with the bowel, biliary or urinary tracts should not be treated by aspiration. Occasionally, a small collection inaccessible to drain insertion, such as an interloop abscess in an immunosuppressed patient with Crohn's disease, may be treated by aspiration; otherwise, drain insertion is favoured.

CT-guided catheter placement is generally performed by one of two methods: tandem-trochar or Seldinger. Tandem-trochar technique relies on the placement of a catheter containing a hollow stiffener and a diamond-pointed stylet, parallel to a guide needle into a collection (Fig. 6-3). Trochar catheters are available from 8 to 16Fr in size. The authors normally use a hydrophilic-coated Ultrathane catheter with a locking loop (Cook, Bloomington, IN, USA) for image-guided drainage. A CT examination, with a radio-opaque grid on the patient's skin enables a safe route for needle and catheter placement to be chosen. The distance from the skin surface to the abscess is measured and a 20G guide needle of appropriate length chosen. The portion of the needle outside the skin needs to be long enough to guide the trajectory of the catheter. Following cleansing and local anaesthetic administration, the needle is placed through the skin into the collection and a sample obtained for culture. This sample also allows assessment of the viscosity of the collection but the collection should not be aspirated further until the catheter is placed. A 10–12Fr catheter is usually necessary if the contents are frank pus; an 8–10Fr catheter may be adequate for less viscous fluid. The distance from the skin to the contents of the collection should be marked on the catheter. Following a skin incision and tissue separation adjacent to the guide needle, the catheter is introduced parallel to the guide needle, to the level of the mark on the catheter. The catheter may then be advanced over the stiffener or the stiffener withdrawn and the retention pigtail formed.

Once adequate catheter position is confirmed, the contents of the collection are evacuated, the catheter is secured to the skin with an adhesive device and a drainage bag is attached. Catheter irrigation at the time of abscess drainage using normal saline can increase drainage yield, disrupt adhesions and improve healing time. However, the volume of normal saline injected must not exceed that of the fluid drained from the collection to prevent cavity distension and reduce the risk of bacteraemia. The tandem-trochar technique is fast and does not require serial dilatation, the metal stiffener affords good catheter directionality. It should be noted that some collections have tough fibrous walls which can deflect the catheter and a malpositioned catheter will generally need to be withdrawn and replaced.

The Seldinger technique allows more controlled catheter placement, especially if there is high risk of catheter transgression of the posterior wall of a collection (Fig. 6-4) and can facilitate better drainage of large multiloculated collections by placement of a multi-sidehole catheter. A 19G ultrathin needle containing a stylet or a sheathed needle is initially placed into the collection. An 0.035-inch guidewire is advanced through the needle or sheath and, once adequate positioning is confirmed, the tract is serially dilated. The Seldinger technique is time consuming and tract dilatation can be painful, especially when traversing muscles. Dilatation also carries increased risk of content spillage during dilator exchange and before catheter placement. Manipulation of a dilator over the wire in a confined space also carries a risk of buckling the guidewire, which can hinder catheter placement.

Ultrasound-guided catheter insertion is performed under direct guidance following skin preparation (Fig. 6-1). A guide needle is not necessary unless one wishes to sample contents of the collection to assess consistency before choosing the catheter size.

CATHETER MANAGEMENT

Drainage catheters should be flushed with normal saline every 8–12 h to maintain catheter patency and optimise drainage. A flush volume of 5 cc towards the patient and 5 cc towards the drainage bag via a three-way stopcock is normally sufficient unless a collection is very small or very large. Daily catheter outputs should be monitored and the contents of the drainage bag noted. This may alert one to evolving issues such as fistulisation or bleeding. In addition, difficulty flushing the catheter, pain on flushing and catheter withdrawal can signal blockage or displacement. Contrast injection into the catheter under fluoroscopic guidance is generally indicated in these circumstances. Catheter removal is considered in a well patient when daily outputs are low, normally on the order of 10 cc or less per day. Before catheter removal it is normally necessary to confirm complete drainage of the collection by CT or ultrasound imaging and confirm that the cavity has collapsed around the catheter and that there is no fistula present by fluoroscopic-guided injection. Catheter removal at this stage should be followed by complete collapse of the cavity. Optimal drainage and complication avoidance are best achieved by active participation of the interventional radiologist in patient rounds.[12]

SPECIFIC DRAINAGE TECHNIQUES

Many image-guided drainages require technical modifications and special consideration. In this section we will discuss pertinent aspects of image-guided drainage procedures of the chest, liver, biliary system, pancreas, gallbladder, urinary tract, gastrointestinal tract, spleen, subphrenic region, peritoneum and deep pelvic territory, and organ traversal for drainage.

Chest

There are many indications for image-guided drainage in the chest, including pleural disease, lung parenchymal, pericardial and mediastinal collections. Pleural collections represent a common clinical problem for which image-guided drainage is recommended to reduce complications encountered as a result of blind drainage.[13]

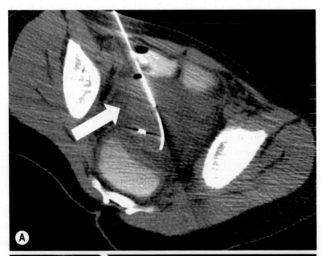

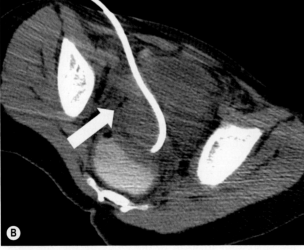

FIGURE 6-4 ■ **CT-guided drainage of periappendiceal abscess using Seldinger technique in a 9-year-old girl.** (A) An 18G needle was used to access the collection (arrow) and a guidewire placed. (B) A 12Fr drainage catheter (arrow) was placed over the guidewire.

Many types of pleural collections exist, and although diagnostic imaging is helpful, aspiration and drainage are often required for treatment and diagnosis. Pleural collections include effusions, haemothorax, empyema and pneumothorax. The success of image-guided drainage depends to a large extent on the contents of a pleural collection. It is, therefore, important for treatment decisions, to characterise the collection at the time of drainage, using biochemical, cytological and microbiological means. Effusions may be transudative or exudative. Light's criteria are 98% sensitive and 80% specific for an exudative effusion if the ratio of pleural fluid protein to serum protein is greater than 0.5, if the ratio of pleural fluid lactate dehydrogenase (LDH) to serum LDH is greater than 0.6 or if the pleural fluid LDH is greater than $\frac{2}{3}$ that of the normal upper limit for serum LDH.[14]

The natural history of an exudative pleural effusion is to evolve from free-flowing fluid to fibrinopurulent material, and later develop an organised fibrous pleural peel. Drainage of an exudative pleural collection should be performed early to prevent progression. Similarly, an infected pleural fluid collection should be drained as early as feasible in order to remove infection, sterilise the cavity, obliterate the pleural space and promote lung re-expansion, which improves drainage of secretions and return of pleural elasticity. Approximately 20% of patients with pneumonia develop an effusion. Since Light's criteria are only reasonably specific for an exudative effusion, confirmation that the effusion is not a transudate is required in cases where there is discrepancy between the clinical and biochemical data. Fluid pH can be useful in these circumstances. The pH of an effusion is a strong predictor of the need for chest tube placement. Based on data from a meta-analysis, a pH less than 7.2 is an indication for chest tube placement.[15]

Image-guided pleural drainage catheters are smaller than surgical drains, measuring up to 16Fr in size, which means they are often better tolerated by patients. A smaller catheter is acceptable for treatment of free-flowing fluid but a large catheter is necessary for a complicated collection. Haemothorax caused by trauma is better treated using surgical drains (36–38Fr), although drainage of small blood-containing postoperative pleural collections may be attempted under imaging guidance. Ultrasound guidance is adequate for uncomplicated collections, but CT is usually needed for drainage of multiloculated pleural collections (Fig. 6-5). It is recommended that, where possible, the dependent portion of the collection be accessed, just above the adjacent rib, away from the paraspinal region where the neurovascular bundle lies lower in the intercostal space, and care should be taken to avoid insertion close to the scapula.[16] The authors favour suturing chest tubes to the skin in order to avoid displacement. Coughing is common as the lung re-expands. For transudative effusions thoracentesis is often preferred over chest tube placement. Aspiration is stopped and the catheter withdrawn when 1.5 L of fluid is aspirated or the patient cannot tolerate further drainage. Imaging is always performed after pleural drainage to assess response and to check for pulmonary oedema and presence of pneumothorax. Daily chest radiographs

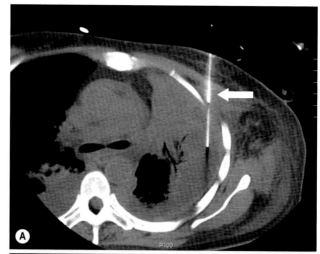

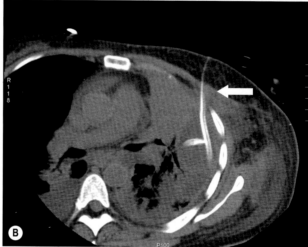

FIGURE 6-5 ■ **CT-guided chest drain insertion for empyema in a 49-year-old male using tandem-trochar technique.** (A) Guide needle (arrow) was placed through an anterior approach into a left chest collection. (B) Chest tube (arrow) placed parallel to guide needle.

are required and interval CT is indicated for assessment of pleural collections treated with a chest tube. It is also important to be aware of a *vacuthorax* phenomenon after pleural drainage so as to avoid unnecessary patient anxiety and harm.[17] This manifests as a pneumothorax with or without fluid on imaging following pleural drainage. Patient's generally have no symptoms from the pneumothorax and usually have an underlying diagnosis of chest malignancy. It is thought that inadequate surfactant causes non-compliance of the lung or the presence of restrictive pleural disease precipitates an asymptomatic hydropneumothorax in this setting, for which chest tube insertion is seldom required. Chest tubes inserted for parapneumonic and complicated effusions often do not drain large quantities of fluid immediately: 20 cm H_2O suction is normally sufficient and a closed underwater seal system is required.

Chest tube removal is considered when there is clinical improvement, improved imaging appearances and absence of bubbling in the one-way valve system (suggests bronchopleural fistula), and outputs have dropped below 1–1.5 cc/kg body weight per day. A chest tube placed for pneumothorax can be removed 24 h after the pneumothorax has resolved. Modified drain management is often necessary as part of pleural collection treatment. For example, air leakage from a drain should prompt search for faulty connections or exposed catheter side-holes; otherwise, a bronchopleural fistula should be suspected. The degree of suction may be carefully reduced to deter further leakage.

A partially treated pleural collection can be further treated by several means. Catheter repositioning and/or exchange for a larger catheter under fluoroscopic guidance may be helpful if the catheter is suboptimally positioned or if an appropriately positioned catheter is not functioning. A partially drained pleural effusion treated with a patent chest tube, placed by image guidance, or an inadequately draining abdominal collection, may benefit by instillation of a fibrinolytic agent, such as tissue plasminogen activator (tPA). The need for this additional measure can often be anticipated on pre-procedure imaging, by the absence of free layering or conformation, loculations, or constrictions, within a fluid collection. Four to six milligrams of tPA mixed in 25–50 cc of normal saline is a suggested dose. After tPA instillation, the patient rotates into prone, supine, right and left lateral positions, each for 15 min at a time, for 1 h, after which time the catheter is unclamped. This process is repeated twice per day for 3 days in order to complete a treatment cycle. A complete treatment cycle can adequately treat a complicated collection in 86% of cases and a repeat cycle for residual fluid is effective in 87% of patients, usually obviating the need for surgery.[18] Therapeutic anticoagulation is a relative contraindication to tPA administration. Haemorrhage has been observed in 33% (4 of 12) of patients treated with tPA receiving therapeutic anticoagulation. Prophylactic anticoagulation is not a contraindication to tPA.

Once adequate treatment of a pleural collection has been achieved, it is sometimes necessary to intervene to obliterate the pleural space, particularly in patients with recurrent pleural effusions. Pleurodesis is utilised to prevent recurrence of effusion or pneumothorax by generating pleural inflammation and fibrosis through instillation of a chemical agent which causes the pleural space to be obliterated. Bleomycin is generally suitable for this purpose. The patient rotates as above for 1 h after instillation and then 20 cm H_2O suction is applied. Mediastinal collections most often occur in the postoperative setting after lung, oesophageal, cardiac and upper abdominal surgery, or after trauma such as severe emesis. Treatment of these collections has traditionally been performed surgically. Recent data indicate that image-guided drainage is feasible and effective. One series reports 100% technical success and 96% clinical success, with avoidance of surgery.[19] Adequate patient positioning and optimum catheter trajectory are key to avoiding complications in this setting. Persistent or worsening lung abscess is another indication for image-guided drainage. Lung abscesses most often occur in the setting of aspiration or immunocompromise, and most respond to antibiotics alone.[20] Occasionally, pericardial effusions require image-guided drainage. Drainage of a pericardial effusion in the absence of tamponade is a topic of debate.

Although technically feasible on almost all occasions, the incidence of cardiac arrhythmias is 26% following drainage, and so catheters should be removed as soon as possible.[21]

Hepatic Parenchyma

Hepatic abscesses generally occur when the liver is unable to sufficiently clear organisms filtered from the portal vein or the biliary tract. It is has been observed that isolated hepatic abscesses are more often of cryptogenic origin due to *Klebsiella pneumoniae*, but that multiple infected collections are usually caused by *Escherichia coli* originating from the biliary tract.[22] More than one hepatic abscess is present in approximately 46–71% of cases.[4] Potential sources of hepatic abscess include trauma, surgery, cancer, bacteraemia and super infection of a pre-existing collection such as a cyst, tumour or haematoma. Catheter-directed drainage is favoured for pyogenic collections, but for an amoebic collection only if it has failed medical management, it is greater than 6–8 cm in diameter or rupture is anticipated. Catheter drainage of an infected tumour should only be performed following careful discussion with the referring physician, surgeon and patient. A catheter placed into an infected tumour in a non-surgical candidate will likely remain permanently. CT or ultrasound guidance is generally adequate for hepatic abscess drainage. Ideally, some normal hepatic parenchyma should be traversed prior to entering the collection (Fig. 6-6). Interval CT to assess response, and interval contrast injection to assess for biliary communication, are normally recommended prior to attempting catheter removal. If possible, pleural transgression should be avoided, but, if traversed, careful observation for the accumulation of pleural fluid is necessary.

Biliary System

Image-guided biliary drainage is technically challenging. As endoscopic techniques have considerably reduced the requirement for percutaneous transhepatic cholangiography and drainage, most such procedures are complicated and are performed for patients who have failed endoscopic treatment or have altered anatomy, often due to surgery. The current indications for biliary drainage include obstructive jaundice, cholangitis, evaluation and treatment of a biliary-enteric anastomosis, access for treatment of stone disease and evaluation of suspected bile duct injury. Any available imaging must be reviewed before the procedure. It is preferable to place the patient supine on the procedure table with the right arm resting above the head and the skin over the right and left lobes of liver should be prepared in a sterile manner. If the patient is haemodynamically stable and does not require general anaesthesia, conscious sedation should be given time to work before traversing the skin, and subsequently titrated to the patient's level of discomfort. Antibiotic prophylaxis should be used, as patients with biliary obstruction are at risk of septicaemia.

Although many technical variations exist, the one- and two-stick techniques are most commonly favoured for biliary drainage. The one-stick system employs a small needle (e.g. 22G Chiba needle), microwire and dilator system to gain access to the biliary tree. Care is required to avoid kinking 0.0018-inch microwires, especially when placing the dilator; this should be directly observed using fluoroscopy. The two-stick system begins with biliary

access and opacification using a small needle, followed by separate biliary access with a larger needle and conventional wire (Fig. 6-7). The lower edge of the right lobe of liver is normally accessed in the mid-axillary line and the needle directed towards the opposite shoulder under fluoroscopic guidance, in order to avoid crossing the pleura. The stylet is removed and contrast material gently injected as the needle is incrementally withdrawn. Bile duct access is indicated by observation of the so-called *dripping wax* appearance, due to contrast dissipating into bile ducts.[23] Once bile duct opacification is achieved, the location of the initial access should be studied. A second puncture, with a sheathed needle, should be made if the initial needle placement is not optimal. Biliary access on the right is preferentially through an inferior duct with a straight course to the hepatic hilum, which may better facilitate future catheter, stent or balloon placement. A fluoroscopic C arm is invaluable for the assessment of the ductal anatomy for these purposes. The proximity of the left lobe bile ducts to the anterior abdominal wall is conducive to ultrasound-guided needle placement and subsequent injection under fluoroscopic guidance. Once access has been gained, obstructions, if present, must be crossed and a catheter advanced to the duodenum. This is best achieved with a combination of an angled catheter and conventional or hydrophilic guidewires. After small bowel access is obtained, an internal–external 8 Fr biliary drain is placed across the obstruction over an Amplatz guidewire. When the patient's condition has improved, biliary stent placement may be considered for treatment of a malignant stricture or serial dilatation followed by trial of catheter clamping and subsequent removal may be considered for benign disease.

Pancreas and Peripancreatic Region

Management of collections in the region of the pancreas can be challenging. Even the terminology used to describe pathology is this region is a topic which receives much attention. The authors recommend using the revised Atlanta criteria in order to optimise communication with referring physicians and possibly better standardise treatment.[24] Access to the region of the head of pancreas is often obtained using an anterior approach

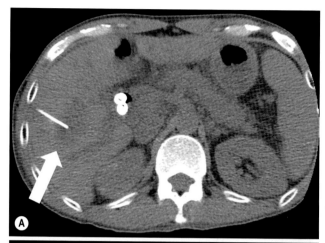
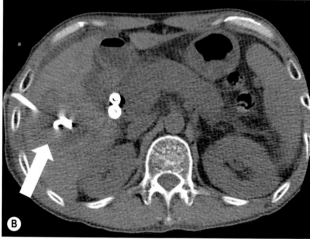

FIGURE 6-6 ■ **Drainage of liver abscess in a 48-year-old male with pancreatic cancer and biliary stents.** (A) A 20G needle has been placed in the collection (arrow). (B) A drainage catheter has been placed in the collection using the tandem-trochar technique (arrow).

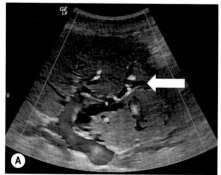
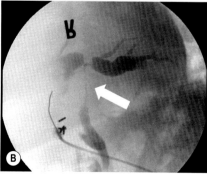
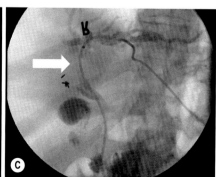

FIGURE 6-7 ■ **Biliary drainage in a 63-year-old male with cholangiocarcinoma using two-stick technique.** (A) Ultrasound used to confirm biliary dilatation (arrow) and guide bile duct access with a 22G Chiba needle. (B) Contrast medium was injected under fluoroscopic guidance to confirm access and demonstrate stenosis of the common hepatic duct, right and left main hepatic ducts (arrow). (C) Left-sided biliary access was obtained, the stenosis was traversed and an internal–external biliary drain was placed (arrow).

through the gastrocolic ligament. Access to the region of the tail of the pancreas is generally through the anterior pararenal space. The liver and stomach are sometimes transgressed in order to access the pancreas but the small and large bowel should not be crossed. Collections secondary to acute pancreatitis may or may not be liquefied. Differentiation can be difficult and may require CT and/or MRI imaging, as well as image-guided sampling. Interstitial oedematous pancreatitis is initially associated with acute pancreatic fluid collections and later with pseudocyst formation. Drainage of a pseudocyst may be indicated in the presence of infection, intractable symptoms such as pain, or obstruction of the gastrointestinal tract or biliary system. Acute pancreatic necrosis can be associated with a sterile acute necrotic collection in or around the pancreas, which can later become infected. Abscess formation is suggested by the presence of gas in a collection or the presence of a thick enhancing wall. Image-guided drainage of an infected acute necrotic collection is often a bridge to surgery, which is best performed after the acute phase of pancreatitis because of the high morbidity of surgery during the first 4 weeks after the onset of pancreatitis (Fig. 6-8). The merits of image-guided drainage for non-infected acute necrotic collections are debatable. The contents of acute necrotic collections are viscous. This necessitates use of large (22–24Fr) or multiple catheters, combined with irrigation, which in effect constitutes percutaneous necrosectomy. Catheter removal may take months because of disconnection of the pancreatic duct in the setting of necrosis.[25] Catheter injection under fluoroscopic guidance is important for the assessment of communication with the pancreatic duct. If ductal communication is noted, endoscopic pancreatic duct stent placement should be attempted, and if leakage persists, transcatheter embolisation may be considered.[26]

Gallbladder

Percutaneous cholecystostomy is used for patients with acute cholecystitis who are poor surgical candidates. It may also be employed to access the biliary tree for decompression or biliary intervention (Fig. 6-1).[27] Percutaneous cholecystostomy has a 2% mortality rate, which is much lower than the mortality of surgical cholecystectomy in very ill patients.[28] Patient selection greatly affects the results. Intensive care unit patients that require cholecystostomy catheters frequently fall into two categories: those that respond to cholecystostomy catheter and those that succumb to their underlying disease. Patients who present to the emergency department with acute cholecystitis may be very ill, but have a better likelihood of treatment response.[29] The authors favour traversing hepatic parenchyma prior to entering the gallbladder where possible to help ensure secure catheter placement and reduce the risk of peritoneal contamination. Catheters placed for calculous cholecystitis generally remain in place until surgery. Catheters placed for acalculous cholecystitis are removed after 6 weeks provided the patent is well, there are no gallstones, the cystic duct is patent and there is an established tract from the gallbladder to the skin. Recurrence rates following

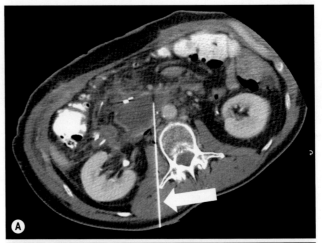
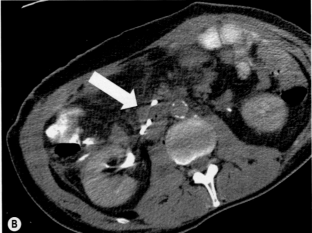

FIGURE 6-8 ■ **Drainage of infected collection in a 41-year-old male with acute pancreatic necrosis.** (A) Needle aspiration (arrow) through a posterior approach with the patient positioned prone confirmed the presence of pus. (B) Catheter was placed using tandem-trochar and the collection decompressed (arrow).

catheter removal are 35 and 7% for acute calculous and acalculous cholecystitis, respectively.[30,31]

Urinary Tract

Percutaneous nephrostomy is performed for urinary tract diversion, access for stone treatment or stent placement (Fig. 6-9). There are several procedure-specific points to be considered.[32] Pre-procedure antibiotics are indicated when there is infection, stones or urinary diversion, in order to help minimise procedure-related sepsis. Brodel's bloodless line of incision is a suitable posterolateral plane through which to access the collecting system. The renal parenchyma in this territory is relatively avascular since it lies at a watershed region at the junction of the anterior two-thirds and posterior third of the kidney. The central component of a lower pole posterior calyx viewed in-plane is a suitable target since this posterolateral oblique approach is orientated along the avascular plane at 20°–30° to the vertical. The procedure is usually guided using fluoroscopy or ultrasound. Direct puncture of the

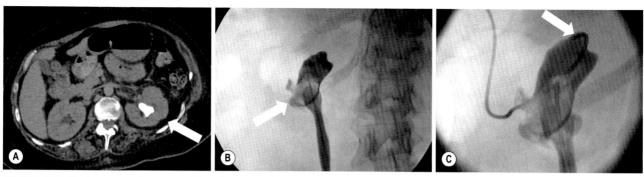

FIGURE 6-9 ■ **Nephrostomy for nephrolithotripsy in a 49-year-old male.** (A) CT demonstrates large left renal stone (arrow). (B) Left renal collecting system opacified using a retrograde ureteric catheter and stone is seen (arrow). (C) A lower pole calyx is traversed to access the renal collecting system and a Kumpe catheter (arrow) used to subsequently direct a guidewire into the ureter for purchase before catheter placement.

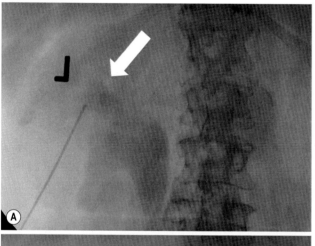

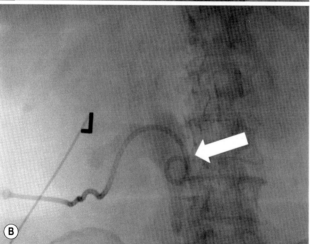

FIGURE 6-10 ■ **Percutaneous nephrostomy using two-stick technique in a 77-year-old female with left renal obstruction due to ureteric stone.** (A) An upper pole calyx (arrow) was accessed with a 22G Chiba needle, a small amount of urine withdrawn and a small volume of contrast injected to opacify the collecting system. (B) A lower pole calyx was traversed to place a percutaneous nephrostomy catheter (arrow).

collecting system under fluoroscopic guidance can be performed at the level of L1/L2, lateral to the transverse process after review of pre-procedure imaging for the location of the kidneys, colon and pleura by noting the position of the twelfth rib (Fig. 6-10). Aspiration is

performed as a 22G needle is withdrawn. Once urine is aspirated, contrast material is injected to opacify the system. The first sample of urine aspirated should be sent for microbiological analysis. It is important to avoid over-distension of the collecting system, in order to reduce the risk of bacteraemia. Carbon dioxide can be used to demonstrate the posterior collecting system calyces in a prone patient. An appropriate posterior calyx may then be accessed using a thin-walled 19G needle or a sheathed 18G needle that will accept an 0.035-inch guidewire. If a ureteric stent is to be inserted, a middle or upper pole calyx should be considered, or a calyx that facilitates future intervention for stone disease if this is the indication for access. Secure wire placement in the collecting system or ureter is important prior to tract dilatation. An 8Fr catheter is normally sufficient and flushing with 10 cc normal saline every 8 h during the early post-procedure period is recommended. Colon transgression should be treated by upper and lower diversion of urine, appropriate antibiotics, withdrawal of the catheter from the kidney into the colon and subsequent removal once a colonocutaneous tract has formed. Normally, blood products clear from urine within 48 h of nephrostomy. Delayed or intermittent haemorrhage, especially after catheter manipulation or exchange can indicate pseudoaneurysm formation. This is sometimes only seen at angiography with the nephrostomy removed. It is best for this to be performed over a guidewire, which is left in place in order to allow catheter replacement for temporary tamponade before definitive treatment. The authors recommend routine nephrostomy exchange approximately every 3 months in patients who require long-term drainage.

Spleen

The American College of Radiology criteria suggest that drainage of an accessible splenic abscess with a rim of surrounding normal tissue is usually feasible.[20] Splenic collections generally occur due to haematogenous spread of infection secondary to endocarditis, sickle cell disease, immunodeficiency or trauma. Safety is a major concern in relation to splenic interventions. Good randomised data are lacking, but anecdotal experience suggests that splenic intervention is generally safe. A recent meta-analysis of splenic biopsy demonstrated sensitivity and specificity of 87 and 96%, respectively.[33] The major complication rate from core needle biopsy with an 18G needle or smaller was 2.2%, which is comparable with liver and renal biopsy. Surgical treatment of an uncharacterised lesion generally entails splenectomy with consequent risk of sepsis from encapsulated organisms and accelerated atherosclerosis.[34] Splenic aspiration or drainage can preserve the spleen and has a high success rate.[35] Peripheral, upper and mid-pole lesions are more easily treated than lower-pole lesions and ideally some normal splenic tissue should be traversed before entering a collection. One of seven patients treated with splenic catheter drainage by Lucey et al. required splenectomy as a result of post-procedural haemorrhage.[35] The remaining six patients, however, were spared splenectomy. Because of the risk of haemorrhage, patients should be admitted overnight following catheter placement. The authors favour the trochar technique, as this avoids dilatation of the tract (which is necessary with the Seldinger technique) and potential peritoneal or pleural contamination (Fig. 6-11). This is particularly important when treating hydatid

disease, as contamination increases the risk of seeding. The absence of leakage can be confirmed by contrast injection and ablation of the inner lining of the cyst can be performed by instillation of alcohol. Fifty per cent of the aspirated fluid volume is replaced with 95% ethyl alcohol, the catheter is clamped for 20 min, and then the alcohol is aspirated.[36] This procedure may be repeated if necessary.

Subphrenic Collections

A subphrenic collection should be approached from a low anterior route where possible to avoid transgressing the pleura, which reduces the risk of pleural infection. The authors favour the Seldinger technique when draining subphrenic collections. Ultrasound guidance allows access into the collection and guidewire manipulation is performed under CT or fluoroscopic guidance. Sometimes the pleura must be crossed to drain a collection (Fig. 6-12). In this circumstance, follow-up chest radiographs and early chest tube insertion for new or enlarging

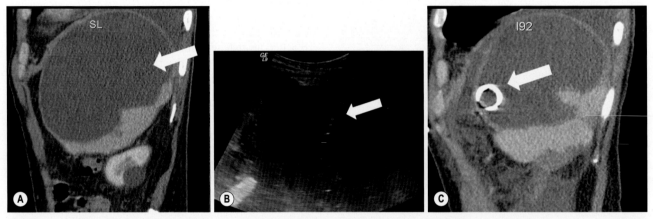

FIGURE 6-11 ■ Ultrasound-guided drainage of symptomatic splenic cyst in a 46-year-old male. (A) Large splenic cystic lesion on CT (arrow). (B) An 8Fr drain inserted (arrow) under ultrasound guidance. (C) Confirmation of drain positioning and degree of decompression after drain insertion (arrow).

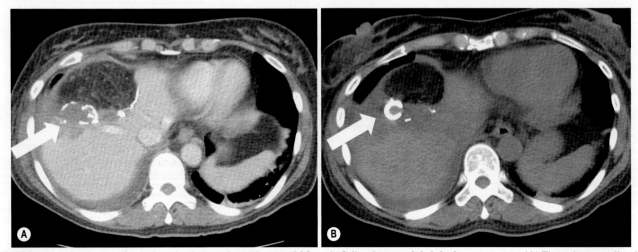

FIGURE 6-12 ■ Drainage of subphrenic abscess in a 62-year-old female following partial right hepatectomy. (A) There is a small collection in the region of the surgical material (arrow). (B) A catheter was placed by tandem-trochar technique into the collection through an anterior approach.

pleural effusions are recommended in order to avoid empyema. Right- and left-sided subphrenic collections should be sampled for bilirubin and amylase, respectively, in order to plan for further management such as biliary or pancreatic drainage.

Gastrointestinal Drainage

Gastrostomy/gastrojejunostomy (G/GJ) catheters are most commonly used to administer enteral feeding to patients with chronic malnutrition or an inability to eat or swallow, usually secondary to neurological impairment or head and neck pathology.[37] G/GJ catheters are also inserted for gastric decompression and palliation in terminal patients, allowing nasogastric tube removal.[38] Radiologic or endoscopic gastrostomy placement is favoured over surgery as these techniques are associated with higher success rates, reduced sedation requirements, fewer complications and less cost.[39] Percutaneous G/GJ requires development of a well-formed tissue tract to avoid leaks after insertion. This is usually accomplished by gastropexy, forming an adhesion of the anterior gastric wall to the anterior abdominal wall. The authors place G/GJ catheters with the patient supine using fluoroscopic or computed tomography (CT) guidance (Fig. 6-13). The stomach is inflated with air using an existing nasogastric tube or by placing a 5Fr Kumpe catheter (Cook, Bloomingdale, IN, USA) under fluoroscopic guidance through the nose into the stomach. The location of the lower left lobe liver edge is identified with ultrasound and marked on the patient's skin and the colon is identified by fluoroscopy using an on-table air or Gastrografin enema. If there is a safe fluoroscopic window to the stomach, the anterior gastric wall is fixed to the anterior abdominal wall using up to four gastropexy sutures. G/GJ catheters are placed in the stomach between the gastropexy sutures over a wire placed through an 18G hollow needle. The use of gastropexy sutures has expanded the range of patients in whom G/GJ can be attempted and, as a result, patients that would have previously been considered unsuitable, such as those with voluminous ascites, may be treated.[40]

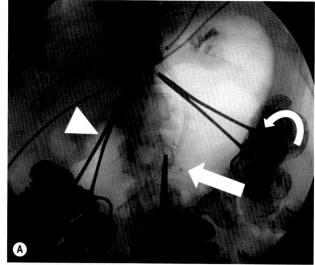

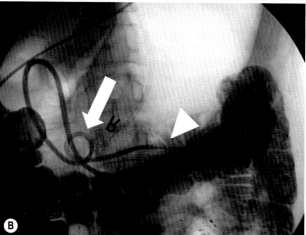

FIGURE 6-13 ■ **Gastrojejuenostomy tube insertion in a 68-year-old male.** (A) The stomach is inflated with air using a nasogastric tube. The colon contains barium administered the night before the procedure. Metal clamps have been placed to depict the left costal margin (curved arrow) and liver margin (arrowhead). There is a safe window to the stomach (arrow) and four 25G needles demarcate where gastropexy sutures will be placed. (B) Confirmation of tip within the small bowel (arrowhead) and locking loop in the stomach (arrow).

Peritoneum

Paracentesis is one of the most common image-guided procedures. Placement of a 7–8Fr catheter following normal preparation and local anaesthesia is generally sufficient. Portal hypertension and cirrhosis are common causes of voluminous ascites. These pathologies are associated with reduced plasma oncotic pressure. Induction of splanchnic vasodilation and an effective reduction of the circulating blood volume induces retention of water and sodium by the renin–angiotensin system and by antidiuretic hormone. Excess hepatic lymph exudes into the abdominal cavity to create ascites. Ascitic fluid should be tested for albumin content and for infection at least at the time of the first drainage. The serum albumin gradient (SAAG) is used to determine the cause of ascites. The serum-ascites albumin count on the day of paracentesis is subtracted from the ascitic albumin concentration. An

SAAG greater or equal to 1.1 g/dL indicates that ascites is due to portal hypertension with 97% accuracy.[41] Causes of a SAAG of less than 1.1 g/dL include carcinomatosis, nephrotic syndrome, pancreatitis and tuberculous peritonitis. The detection of a carcinoembryonic antigen (CEA) level greater than 5 ng/mL or an alkaline phosphatase level of 240 IU/L is suggestive of perforated bowel.[42] Administration of albumin is performed in selected patients with ascites who experience circulatory disturbance following large-volume paracentesis. The authors administer up to four 12.5 g bottles of 25% albumin in the peri-procedural period for these patients. For patients with intractable malignant ascites that requires frequent paracentesis despite medical therapy, implanted peritoneal catheters offer a safe and effective palliative measure.[43]

Infected peritoneal collections are a common indication for image-guided drainage. These include perforated appendicitis, Crohn's enteritis of colitis, diverticulitis and anastomotic leakage. Drainage in the setting of perforated viscous is reasonable in the absence of free perforation or signs of peritonism. Drainage is sometimes a temporising measure before surgery. However, percutaneous catheter drainage alone is deemed sufficient by the American College of Radiology Appropriateness guidelines for periappendiceal collections (Fig. 6-3). In patients with Crohn's disease, percutaneous abscess drainage is technically successful in 96% of cases. Drainage reduces the need for surgery by 50% within 60 days of presentation and reduces the overall need for surgery by 23%.[44] Approximately 16% of patients with Crohn's disease develop metachronous collections following drainage. Postoperative collections are more successfully treated by catheter drainage than primary collections. Treatment of postoperative collections of various causes by image-guided drainage and antibiotics often suffices and represents one of the most successful applications of these techniques. Drainage catheter placement is also often sufficient for treating an anastomotic leak, which can be difficult to treat surgically due to postoperative tissue inflammation and adhesions. Sometimes upstream diversion is necessary to promote healing. Previous administration of therapeutic radiation to the perianastomotic region, such as the presacral territory for rectal cancer treatment, is associated with fibrous stiff tissues, which are often slow to collapse, and require long-term drainage before catheter removal (Fig. 6-14).

Deep Pelvic Collections

Bowel, bladder, bone, blood vessels and nerves confined in a limited space constitute a recipe for challenging drainage in the deep pelvis. A pre-procedure CT should be carefully reviewed prior to draining a deep pelvic collection. Modern intracavitary ultrasound probes provide

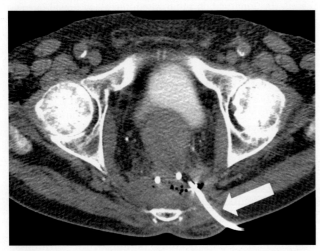

FIGURE 6-14 ■ **CT-guided drainage of presacral collection in an 89-year-old male following abdominoperioneal resection of rectal cancer.** Transgluteal catheter placement close to the sacrum (arrow) was performed using tandem-trochar technique under CT guidance.

high-resolution imaging through the rectum and vagina. Catheter placement through the vagina and rectum is often free-hand over a trochar although an improvised guide can be created using a peel-away introducer sheath. Either way, the catheter needs to be imaged throughout insertion. Care should be taken to apply gentle pressure on the probe during imaging in order to avoid compressing bowel or bladder, which can lead to inadvertent traversal. Transrectal drainage is favoured over transvaginal drainage where possible. Patients generally need to be placed in the decubitus position for intracavitary ultrasound probe insertion and image-guided drainage. Prone positioning is favoured for transgluteal drainage of deep pelvic collections, which are often performed using CT guidance. Optimal transgluteal drain insertion is at the level of the sacrospinous ligament inferior to the piriformis muscle and close to the sacrum in order to reduce pain and risk of blood vessel and nerve injury (Fig. 6-14). A CT drainage window to a high pelvic collection not accessible in an axial plane may be facilitated by tilting the CT gantry.

Organ Traversal

A collection deep to an organ should be approached with caution. Many organs should not be traversed in order to access a collection during image-guided drainage. These include blood vessels, the spleen, the gallbladder, the pancreas, the oesophagus, the large and small bowel, the bladder, the uterus and the ovaries (Fig. 6-15). Traversal of some organs during drain insertion may be necessary, especially in an ill patient with limited surgical options. Provided the coagulation profile is acceptable, it is feasible and often safe to traverse a minimal portion of liver, avoiding the hilar vessels and the gallbladder, in order to drain a collection. Care must be taken to ensure that all catheter sideholes are within the collection in order to avoid leakage back along the catheter into the liver. The stomach is frequently traversed in order to access retroperitoneal collections, especially those of pancreatic origin. Transrectal and transvaginal approaches are feasible for drainage of a deep pelvic collection under ultrasound guidance, although catheters in these locations have a notorious propensity to fall out.

Paediatric Patients

Image-guided drainage is performed in children for collections related to acute appendicitis, inflammatory bowel disease or in the postoperative setting (Fig. 6-3). Good paediatric care requires a different approach to that of an adult. Monitoring and resuscitation equipment are tailored to age, heat loss must be minimised and sedation requirements should be undertaken by an anaesthesiologist. Ultrasound imaging should be used where possible for guidance. CT parameters should be optimised to reduce dose by shielding the gonads, minimising the range and imaging time, reducing the kilovoltage and milliamperage, using automatic tube modulation and adaptive statistical iterative reconstruction. Once planning images are obtained, greater image noise is often acceptable for catheter check images. Post-procedure

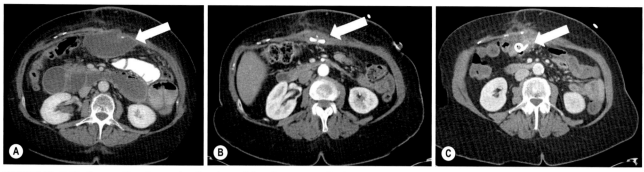

FIGURE 6-15 ■ **Drainage of peritoneal collection with subsequent displacement of drainage catheter into the colon in a 76-year-old female after midline laparotomy.** (A) Intra-abdominal collection present (arrow). (B) Drain placed into the collection with good decompression (arrow). (C) Interval CT demonstrated migration of the tip of the drainage catheter into the transverse colon (arrow). The catheter was withdrawn into the collection and left in place until the fistula closed.

imaging with CT should be performed sparingly and avoided altogether if possible, by relying more on clinical response, catheter outputs and ultrasound for decision making. Image-guided drainage is a safe and effective technique for treatment of appendicitis complicated by abscess formation.[45] Complications are reduced and interval appendectomy is often obviated if a perforated appendiceal abscess is treated successfully with catheter-directed drainage.

Complications

Many potential complications can occur after image-guided drainage. Some discomfort or scar formation at the site of insertion may be unavoidable. Involvement of the interventional radiologist in patient rounds is important for patient care, early detection of complications, exchange of information with referring physicians and continued learning. Although every effort is made to minimise the length of treatment, every patient is different, and catheter removal can sometimes take a long time.

There are many reasons why a collection may respond slowly to treatment, leading to prolonged drainage. Clear communication throughout the treatment process is vital to avoid misconceptions. It is important to stress from the outset what can be realistically expected. The presence of loculations, the development of a fistula and the presence of tumour can hamper catheter removal. Loculations can often be effectively treated by increasing the size of the drain or by repositioning it, or by tPA instillation as described earlier. Fistula development often results in long-term catheter placement. Diversion of upstream fluids (bile, urine, pancreatic juices, bowel content) by surgical or endoscopic means if necessary should be considered. Image-guided drainage of an infected tumour should be approached with extreme caution and should involve multidisciplinary discussion. Catheters placed into an infected tumour can rarely be removed, and often remain for life, or until surgical removal of the tumour.

Complications are uncommon following image-guided drainage of thoracic fluid collections; the National Patient Safety Agency in the United Kingdom reported 12

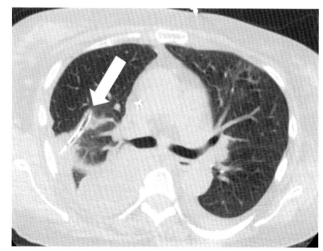

FIGURE 6-16 ■ **Intraparenchymal chest tube placement in a 54-year-old female.** CT demonstrates right-sided chest tube (arrow) with blood on both sides of the catheter. A new chest drain was placed and the catheter removed without further complication.

fatalities, and 15 instances of serious harm, caused by chest drain insertion.[46] Intraparenchymal chest tube placement, intercostal artery injury, iatrogenic infection and pneumothorax formation have been observed (Fig. 6-16). Transarterial embolisation for arterial injury, prophylactic antibiotics in some situations and aspiration of thoracentesis-related pneumothorax may be necessary (Fig. 6-17).[47] Catheter dislodgement is a frequent occurrence. It is important to adequately secure drainage catheters and educate patients regarding the risk of pulling on the catheter. The decision to reinsert a drainage catheter depends on the reason for insertion, the adequacy of treatment and need for further drainage. Long-term catheters such as a nephrostomy catheter, with an established tract, can generally be rescued within 24 h of catheter dislodgement. An established tract is formed approximately 2 to 4 weeks after catheter placement.

Bleeding is not uncommon after catheter placement. Bleeding from the skin site of catheter insertion may be due to the presence of altered blood in a postoperative

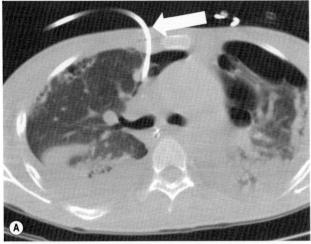

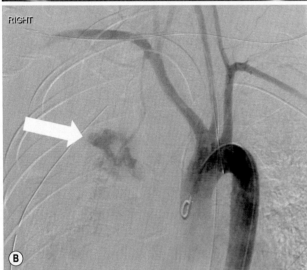

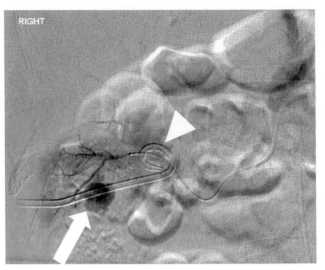

FIGURE 6-18 ■ Pseudoaneurysm in an 82-year-old male due to right percutaneous nephrostomy placement. Renal angiogram demonstrates pseudoaneurysm (arrow) over the nephrostomy catheter (arrowhead). The pseudoaneurysm was treated by coil embolisation.

FIGURE 6-17 ■ Bleed from intercostal artery following chest tube insertion in a 23-year-old male with chronic lung disease due to a mitochondrial disorder. (A) Chest tube (arrow) was placed into the right anterior chest adjacent to the sternum for treatment of pneumothorax. (B) The patient developed haemodynamic shock after removal of the chest tube. This was due to haemorrhage from the right internal mammary artery (arrow) and was successfully treated by coil placement.

collection and is often self-limiting. However, occasionally, it can be a sign of significant injury such as pseudoaneurysm formation (Fig. 6-18). In cases of concern, it is advisable to remove a catheter over a wire, so that the catheter can be replaced to tamponade significant bleeding as a temporary measure before definitive treatment by surgery or embolization.

CONCLUSION

Image-guided drainage can significantly contribute in a positive manner to patient management. Image-guided procedures continue to be widely used and to evolve. The principles of good image-guided drainage apply to many clinical situations. Careful patient preparation and catheter management are vital to safe practice.

REFERENCES

1. Duszak RL Jr, Levy JM, Akins EW, et al. Percutaneous catheter drainage of infected intra-abdominal fluid collections. American College of Radiology. ACR Appropriateness Criteria. Radiology 2000;215(Suppl):1067–75.
2. Harisinghani MG, Gervais DA, Hahn PF, et al. CT-guided transgluteal drainage of deep pelvic abscesses: indications, technique, procedure-related complications, and clinical outcome. Radiographics 2002;22(6):1353–67.
3. Gervais DA, Brown SD, Connolly SA, et al. Percutaneous imaging-guided abdominal and pelvic abscess drainage in children. Radiographics 2004;24(3):737–54.
4. Men S, Akhan O, Köroğlu M. Percutaneous drainage of abdominal abscess. Eur J Radiol 2002;43(3):204–18.
5. Levison MA. Percutaneous versus open operative drainage of intra-abdominal abscesses. Infect Dis Clin North Am 1992;6(3):525–44.
6. Solomkin JS, Mazuski J. Intra-abdominal sepsis: newer interventional and antimicrobial therapies. Infect Dis Clin North Am 2009;23(3):593–608.
7. Bradley MJ. An in-vitro study to understand successful free-hand ultrasound guided intervention. Clin Radiol 2001;56(6):495–8.
8. Carlson SK, Bender CE, Classic KL, et al. Benefits and safety of CT fluoroscopy in interventional radiologic procedures. Radiology 2001;219(2):515–20.
9. Maher MM, Gervais DA, Kalra MK, et al. The inaccessible or undrainable abscess: how to drain it. Radiographics 2004;24(3):717–35.
10. Miguel K, Hirsch JA, Sheridan RM. Team training: a safer future for neurointerventional practice. J Neurointerv Surg 2011;3(3):285–7.
11. Leonard MW, Frankel A. The path to safe and reliable healthcare. Patient Educ Couns 2010;80(3):288–92.
12. Goldberg MA, Mueller PR, Saini S, et al. Importance of daily rounds by the radiologist after interventional procedures of the abdomen and chest. Radiology 1991;180(3):767–70.
13. Harris A, O'Driscoll BR, Turkington PM. Survey of major complications of intercostal chest drain insertion in the UK. Postgrad Med J 2010;86(1012):68–72.
14. Romero S, Martinez A, Hernandez L, et al. Light's criteria revisited: consistency and comparison with new proposed alternative criteria for separating pleural transudates from exudates. Respiration 2000;67(1):18–23.

15. Heffner JE, Brown LK, Barbieri C, DeLeo JM. Pleural fluid chemical analysis in parapneumonic effusions. A meta-analysis. Am J Respir Crit Care Med 1995;151(6):1700–8.
16. Dewhurst C, O'Neill S, O'Regan K, Maher M. Demonstration of the course of the posterior intercostal artery on CT angiography: relevance to interventional radiology procedures in the chest. Diagn Interv Radiol 2012;18(2):221–4.
17. Boland GW, Gazelle GS, Girard MJ, Mueller PR. Asymptomatic hydropneumothorax after therapeutic thoracentesis for malignant pleural effusions. Am J Roentgenol 1998;170(4):943–6.
18. Gervais DA, Levis DA, Hahn PF, et al. Adjunctive intrapleural tissue plasminogen activator administered via chest tubes placed with imaging guidance: effectiveness and risk for hemorrhage. Radiology 2008;246(3):956–63.
19. Arellano RS, Gervais DA, Mueller PR. Computed tomography-guided drainage of mediastinal abscesses: clinical experience with 23 patients. J Vasc Interv Radiol 2011;22(5):673–7.
20. American College of Radiology Appropriateness Criteria. Radiologic Management of Infected Fluid Collections. http://www.acr.org/~/media/ACR/Documents/AppCriteria/Interventional/RadiologicManagementInfectedFluidCollections.pdf (Accessed 23 Oct 2013).
21. Tam A, Ensor JE, Snyder H, et al. Image-guided drainage of pericardial effusions in oncology patients. Cardiovasc Intervent Radiol 2009;32(6):1217–26.
22. Chou FF, Sheen-Chen SM, Chen YS, Chen MC. Single and multiple pyogenic liver abscesses: clinical course, etiology, and results of treatment. World J Surg 1997;21:384–9.
23. Pomerantz BJ. Biliary tract interventions. Tech Vasc Interv Radiol 2009;12:162–70.
24. Thoeni RF. The revised Atlanta classification of acute pancreatitis: its importance for the radiologist and its effect on treatment. Radiology 2012;262(3):751–64.
25. O'Connor OJ, Buckley JM, Maher MM. Imaging of the complications of acute pancreatitis. Am J Roentgenol 2011;197(3):W375–81.
26. Hirota M. Percutaneous transfistulous interventions for intractable pancreatic fistula. Radiol Res Pract 2011;109:259.
27. Saad WE, Wallace MJ, Wojak JC, et al. Quality improvement guidelines for percutaneous transhepatic cholangiography, biliary drainage, and percutaneous cholecystostomy. J Vasc Interv Radiol 2010;21(6):789–95.
28. Winbladh A, Gullstrand P, Svanvik J, Sandstrom P. Systematic review of cholecystostomy as a treatment option in acute cholecystitis. HPB (Oxford) 2009;11:183–93.
29. Joseph T, Unver K, Hwang GL, et al. Percutaneous cholecystostomy for acute cholecystitis: ten-year experience. J Vasc Interv Radiol 2012;23(1):83–8.
30. Ha JP, Tsui KK, Tang CN, et al. Cholecystectomy or not after percutaneous cholecystostomy for acute calculous cholecystitis in high-risk patients. Hepatogastroenterology 2008;55:1497–502.
31. Chung YH, Choi ER, Kim KM, et al. Can percutaneous cholecystostomy be a definitive management for acute acalculous cholecystitis? J Clin Gastroenterol 2012;46(3):216–19.
32. Zagoria RJ, Dyer RB. Do's and don't's of percutaneous nephrostomy. Acad Radiol 1999;6(6):370–7.
33. McInnes MD, Kielar AZ, Macdonald DB. Percutaneous image-guided biopsy of the spleen: systematic review and meta-analysis of the complication rate and diagnostic accuracy. Radiology 2011;260(3):699–708.
34. Robinette CD, Fraumeni JF Jr. Splenectomy and subsequent mortality in veterans of the 1939–45 war. Lancet 1977;16:127–9.
35. Lucey BC, Boland GW, Maher MM, et al. Percutaneous nonvascular splenic intervention: a 10-year review. Am J Roentgenol 2002;179(6):1591–6.
36. Singh AK, Shankar S, Gervais DA, et al. Image-guided percutaneous splenic interventions. Radiographics 2012;32(2):523–34.
37. Cantwell CP, Perumpillichira JJ, Maher MM, et al. Antibiotic prophylaxis for percutaneous radiologic gastrostomy and gastrojejunostomy insertion in outpatients with head and neck cancer. J Vasc Interv Radiol 2008;19:571–5.
38. Silas AM, Pearce LF, Lestina LS, et al. Percutaneous radiologic gastrostomy versus percutaneous endoscopic gastrostomy: a comparison of indications, complications and outcomes in 370 patients. Eur J Radiol 2005;56:84–90.
39. Wollman B, D'Agostino HB. Percutaneous radiologic and endoscopic gastrostomy: a 3-year institutional analysis of procedure performance. Am J Roentgenol 1997;169:1551–3.
40. Oyogoa S, Schein M, Gardezi S, Wise L. Surgical feeding gastrostomy: are we overdoing it? J Gastrointest Surg 1999;3(2):152–5.
41. Runyon BA, Montano AA, Akriviadis EA, et al. The serum-ascites albumin gradient is superior to the exudate-transudate concept in the differential diagnosis of ascites. Ann Intern Med 1992;117:215–20.
42. Wu SS, Lin OS, Chen YY, et al. Ascitic fluid carcinoembryonic antigen and alkaline phosphatase levels for the differentiation of primary from secondary bacterial peritonitis with intestinal perforation. J Hepatol 2001;34:215–21.
43. Mercadante S, Intravaia G, Ferrera P, et al. Peritoneal catheter for continuous drainage of ascites in advanced cancer patients. Support Care Cancer 2008;16(8):975–8.
44. Gervais DA, Hahn PF, O'Neill MJ, Mueller PR. Percutaneous abscess drainage in Crohn disease: technical success and short- and long-term outcomes during 14 years. Radiology 2002;222(3):645–51.
45. Simillis C, Symeonides P, Shorthouse AJ, Tekkis PP. A meta-analysis comparing conservative treatment versus acute appendectomy for complicated appendicitis (abscess or phlegmon). Surgery 2010;147(6):818–29.
46. National Patient Safety Agency. Risks of chest drain insertion. NPSA/2008/RRR003. 2008 May 15.
47. Matin TN, Gleeson FV. Interventional radiology of pleural diseases. Respirology 2011;16(3):419–29.

CHAPTER 7

HEPATOBILIARY INTERVENTION

Aoife N. Keeling • Bhaskar Ganai • Michael J. Lee

INTRODUCTION

Biliary intervention is not as prevalent as it was 20 years ago because of the advent of endoscopic retrograde cholangiopancreatography (ERCP). Skilled endoscopists can treat the vast majority of patients with biliary obstruction with stents, stone removal and/or sphincterotomy. In addition, the days of perfoming a diagnostic percutaneous transhepatic cholangiogram (PTC) are virtually over with the advent of magnetic resonance cholangiopancreatography (MRCP). PTC is now almost always performed before a therapeutic biliary drainage. Percutaneous biliary drainage remains an important technique for managing patients with biliary obstruction where ERCP fails or is not possible. Interventional radiology (IR) also plays a significant role in treating patients with benign biliary strictures and, particularly, patients with anastomotic strictures after hepatico-jejunostomy.

Careful patient preparation is essential before any biliary procedure to avoid potentially serious complications. All patients with obstructive jaundice should be commenced on intravenous fluids during and after biliary drainage. Patients with obstructive jaundice have usually fasted for a myriad of other tests before reaching IR and are often significantly dehydrated. Any significant choleresis after biliary drainage can place patients with long-standing obstructive jaundice and high serum bilirubin levels at risk of developing hepatorenal syndrome. Coagulation screening and a serum creatinine check should be performed before all biliary drainage procedures. Correction of any bleeding diathesis should be performed before any drainage. In addition, all patients should receive broad-spectrum antibiotic coverage within one hour of the drainage procedure, or indeed any further biliary procedure, including tube change or cholangiography, to protect against biliary sepsis. The authors prefer monotherapy with piperacillin/tazobactam which has broad Gram-negative and -positive coverage and achieves high concentrations in bile. Patient preparation also includes reviewing all imaging studies, including computed tomography (CT), ultrasound (US) and magnetic resonance (MR) cholangiography, so that a full picture of the biliary procedure can be discussed with the patient during the consent process.

MANAGEMENT OF BILIARY OBSTRUCTION

Background

Biliary obstruction can arise from both benign and malignant causes. Malignant causes are more common and include obstruction from pancreatic carcinoma, cholangiocarcinoma and metastatic disease. Ultrasound is the imaging modality of choice for determining the presence or absence of dilated bile ducts. Further investigation with CT or MRI/MRCP is used to determine the cause and level of biliary obstruction, and in cases of malignancy, for staging and assessment of surgical resectability. Most malignant tumours causing biliary obstruction are not surgically resectable at the time of diagnosis and these patients have a limited life expectancy. Malignancy should be confirmed with biopsy if possible. Cross-sectional imaging will also determine the level of biliary obstruction and any atrophy/compensatory hypertrophy in a liver lobe, which can impact the proposed biliary draiange.

Mid to lower biliary obstruction is now increasingly treated endoscopically in the first instance; lesions at the liver hilum are challenging to treat at ERCP and are best dealt with by percutaneous biliary drainage.

The goal of treatment is to relieve jaundice, treat or prevent sepsis and improve symptoms of pruritus.[1]

Percutaneous Transhepatic Cholangiography

Percutaneous transhepatic cholangiography is the first step in a range of biliary interventional procedures. This is usually performed under conscious sedation or general anaesthesia. Hilar lesions may cause atrophy or compensatory hypertrophy of a liver lobe which affects the decision on whether drainage of that lobe is indicated. MRCP is important in establishing the level of the hilar obstruction and the extent of involvement of the intrahepatic ducts. For example, if the anterior and posterior sectoral ducts on the right are both involved, it may be best to drain the left lobe only (if the size of the left lobe is sufficient to provide palliation of jaundice). Puncture of the ducts in the right lobe access can be performed under either fluoroscopic or ultrasound guidance, whilst left lobe punctures are usually performed under US guidance.

A coaxial introducer system employing a 21G Chiba needle and 0.018-inch guidewire which enables upsizing to a 0.035-inch guidewire reduces the risk of haemorrhage. If fluoroscopic guidance is used on the right side, the point of entry is the mid axillary line just above the tenth rib. A peripheral duct should be selected and, after aspiration of bile, a diagnostic cholangiogram is performed with iodinated contrast material. After cholangiography, the guidewire is passed into the central ducts to maintain access for further interventions.

Biliary Drainage: External, Internal–External

In most cases an external drain (tube is left above the level of obstruction) is a temporary measure and an internal–external biliary drain from the duodenum through the biliary system to the skin surface is preferred. In patients with biliary sepsis, the goal of treatment is rapid decompression and drainage with minimal catheter manipulation and contrast material injection. In cases where a stricture cannot be crossed in the first sitting an external drainage catheter can be placed. The stricture can be negotiated during a subsequent session.

An internal–external drainage catheter will have side holes both above and below the stricture and pass into the duodenum. It can be used after biliary stenting to preserve access to the biliary tree for a few days (a safety catheter) if the procedure has been difficult or there is blood in the biliary system limiting bile drainage and is usually followed by placement of a stent in patients with malignant obstruction.

Biliary Stenting: Metal, Plastic

Two main types of biliary stents are available: plastic or metallic. Plastic stents (e.g. Cotton-Leung stents; Cook

Medical, Bloomington, IN) offer lower patency rates due to encrustation of bile and often require a larger tract through the liver (10–12Fr), causing increased patient discomfort during insertion. They have the advantage that they are easily removed at endoscopy/surgery and can therefore be used preoperatively in patients who require drainage (e.g. for sepsis) before surgical resections.

Metallic stents offer better patency rates than their plastic counterparts.[2] These stents are inserted in a contracted state but when released, expand to a predefined diameter. This enables their placement though a smaller-calibre percutaneous tract (6–8Fr). Metallic stents elicit a marked fibrotic reaction; for this reason they should be avoided preoperatively and in benign disease. The larger-diameter lumen reduces the rate of occlusion from bile encrustation. Metallic stents occlude from either tumour growth through the interstices of the stent or, more frequently in hilar tumours, overgrowth at the ends of the stent. In lower common bile duct (CBD) strictures, stenting through the sphincter of Oddi may help provide better drainage with the theoretical risk of increased infection due to reflux of enteric contents.

Covered stents have been developed for the biliary system. These metallic stent grafts have a fabric covering which aims to prevent tumour ingrowth, but have the drawbacks of increased migration and coverage of side branches leading to cholecystitis or pancreatitis with cystic duct and pancreatic duct occlusions, respectively. Despite these drawbacks, early data are promising in both malignant[3] and benign[4] disease.

When stenting, the goal of treatment is to try and drain the largest volume of tumour-free liver. Careful review of pre-procedure imaging is mandatory to allow planning of the PTC approach for stent placement and the superior extent of obstruction. In a hilar obstruction, if both hepatic lobes require drainage then either a 'T' stenting configuration from a single percutaneous access site or a 'Y' configuration from bilateral access sites may be employed (Fig. 7-1). When the stent(s) have been placed, balloon dilatation can be performed to bring the stents up to nominal diameter (usually 8 mm in hepatic ducts, 10 mm in CBD), usually after administration of a further dose of analgesia as the dilatation can be very painful (Fig. 7-2).

Benign Disease

Benign strictures are often the result of iatrogenic ductal injury during laparoscopic cholecystectomy. Further causes include post-hepatic transplantation ischaemia, biliary atresia, choledochal cysts and sclerosing cholangitis.

Transhepatic drainage can be performed in benign strictures or stones to:

1. Drain an obstructed infected system not amenable to endoscopic drainage
2. Dilate benign strictures, often iatrogenic secondary to laparoscopic cholecystectomy, biliary-enteric anastomotic strictures (including post-hepatic transplant) or sclerosing cholangitis.
3. Treat intrahepatic or ductal calculi.

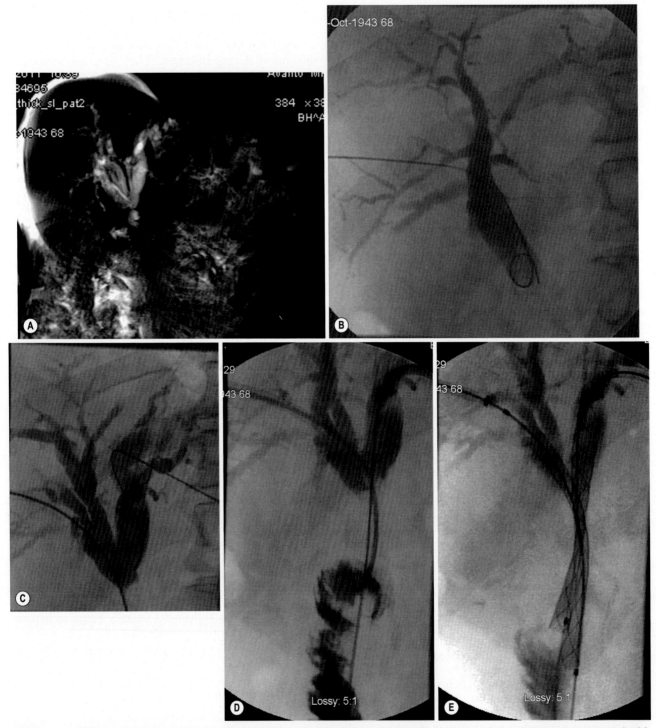

FIGURE 7-1 ■ **A 68-year-old female with a background of a prior Whipple's resection for a pancreatic head cancer re-presented with jaundice and weight loss.** MRCP demonstrated a tight stricture at the biliary-enteric anastomosis with a corresponding soft-tissue mass in keeping with local recurrence (A). A PTC was performed via the right side (B). The left side was then punctured (C) and the proximal tight stricture at the biliary-enteric anastomosis was elicited (D). It was elected to place metallic biliary stents from both the right and left sides in a Y configuration as the stricture was so high. Ten-millimetre metallic self-expanding stents were deployed simultaneously across the stricture (E).

Benign Strictures

PTC is performed as described above and a balloon dila-tation is performed with an 8- to 10-mm balloon. Following balloon dilatation, at least 2 weeks of biliary

drainage with the catheter crossing the stricture is required.

In cases of biliary-enteric anastomoses, the ERCP approach is less likely to be successful due to the forma-tion of a Roux loop or Billroth II gastric anastomosis.

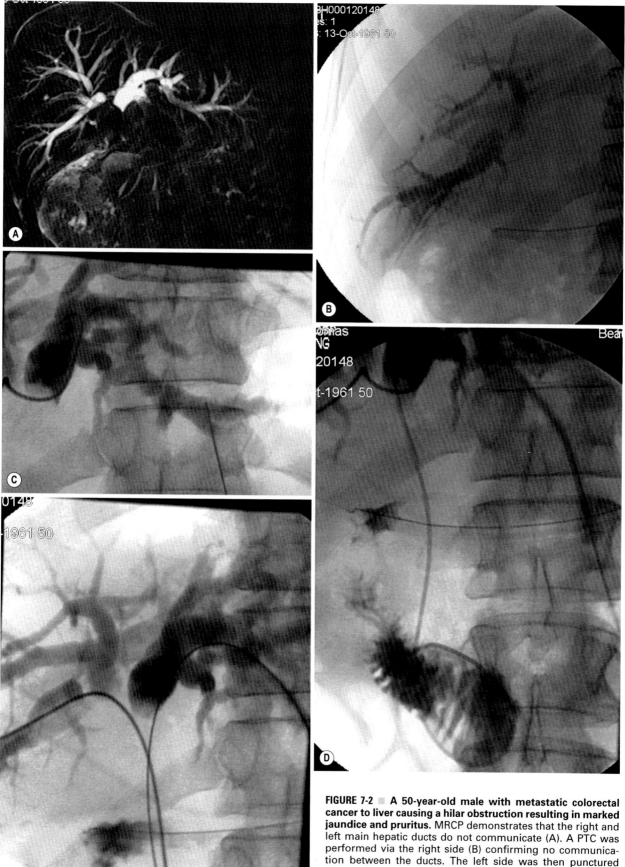

FIGURE 7-2 ■ **A 50-year-old male with metastatic colorectal cancer to liver causing a hilar obstruction resulting in marked jaundice and pruritus.** MRCP demonstrates that the right and left main hepatic ducts do not communicate (A). A PTC was performed via the right side (B) confirming no communication between the ducts. The left side was then punctured (C) and the long stricture within the hilum and common duct was elicited (D). Therefore it was elected to place metallic biliary stents from both the right and left sides in a Y configuration. Guidewires were placed through the stricture via both sides (E). *Continued on following page*

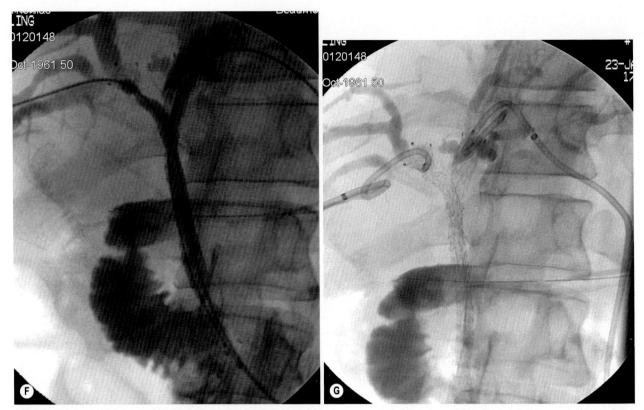

FIGURE 7-2, Continued ■ Ten-millimetre metallic self-expanding stents were deployed simultaneously across the stricture; note the tight stricture proximally within the right-sided stent which required balloon dilatation with an 8-mm balloon (F). Following balloon dilatation, the stents are widely patent, with safety external biliary drains placed for 24 hours (G).

Some surgeons advocate burying either the afferent or efferent Roux-en-Y loop during the biliary enteric anastomosis under the skin. The position of this loop is marked with surgical clips, enabling subsequent percutanous fluoroscopically guided access for stricture dilatation and stone extraction. This allows safe, well-tolerated access over many years.[5]

In patients with post-laparoscopic cholecystectomy bile duct injury or stricture, the goal is to cross the stricture or bile duct interruption and place a stent or stents to allow healing around the stent. It may be necessary to approach bile duct interruptions from both above and below so that a guidwire placed from one end can be snared in 'open space' from the other end to obtain through-and-through access.

Benign strictures should be dilated to approximately 10 mm. It is useful to leave a 4Fr acccss catheter in place for approximately 6 weeks, in order to facilitate redilatation if early recurrence occurs. If there is no significant restenosis, the catheter should be removed.

Percutaneous stents are not commonly used in benign strictures, as they will almost always become occluded after a few months.

Calculous Disease

Biliary obstruction secondary to distal CBD calculi is usually initially managed endoscopically. In cases where ERCP is unsuccessful or the calculi are intrahepatic, a percutaneous approach can be employed. A PTC is performed as described above and a guidewire manipulated past the calculus into the duodenum. A balloon catheter is placed over the guidewire and passed beyond the calculi and the sphincter of Oddi is dilated. The balloon is then deflated and placed above the calculus. The balloon is reinflated and then pushed forward to move the calculi into the duodenum.[6]

Post-cholecystectomy retained bile duct stones are usually removed endoscopically. If a T-tube has been placed at surgery, percutaneous removal can be performed. The T-tube tract is allowed to mature for 6 weeks and the T-tube is removed over a guidewire. A second safety guidewire is placed to maintain access and the calculi is then removed with a basket.

Percutaneous Biliary Intervention Complications

Percutaneous biliary drainage is relatively safe.[7] Procedure-related mortality is around 2% with 30-day patient mortality >10% in many series due to the underlying advanced malignant disease and co-morbid conditions.

Complications include localised pain, bile leak, bleeding including haemobilia and septicaemia. If the pleura

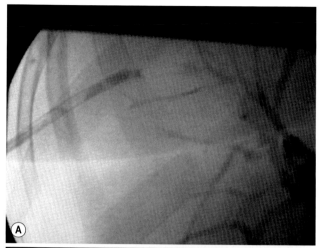

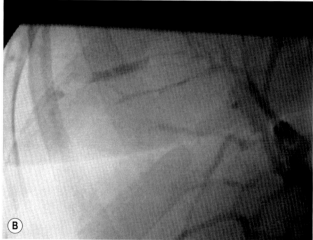

FIGURE 7-3 ■ **Patient in whom biliary stent was placed and track embolised with pledgets of Gelfoam.** (A) Peel-away sheath has been inserted into the hepatic track and contrast media injected to outline the track. One Gelfoam torpedo (air column in contrast-filled track) has been delivered and the second Gelfoam torpedo can be seen in the peel-away sheath. (B) Both Gelfoam torpedoes (torpedoes appear as air density tubular structures) have been delivered and the peel-away sheath removed.

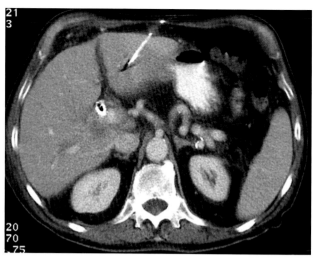

FIGURE 7-4 ■ **Patient in whom a biliary stent was placed from a left-sided approach.** CT was performed over the ensuing months. The CT shows the mixture of glue and lipiodol (1:1 mixture) in the percutaneous track in the left liver lobe. The glue is delivered using a fascial dilator.

is transgressed, there are additional risks or pneumothorax and haemothorax. External and internal–external drainage catheters can kink, become dislodged and exacerbate bilovenous fistulae.[8] Metallic stents can become blocked and 10–30% will require reintervention.

Track embolisation at the end of the procedure can also help to reduce the latter complications and reduce post-procedure pain. Track embolisation can be performed with pledgets of Gelfoam pushed into the peel-away sheath and left in the hepatic track as the peel-away sheath is withdrawn (Fig. 7-3). Alternatively, a 1:1 mixture of lipiodol:cyanoacrylate can be delivered with a dilator into the transhepatic track (Fig. 7-4).

VASCULAR INTERVENTIONAL TECHNIQUES IN THE LIVER

CHEMOEMBOLISATION

Background

Malignant tumours receive almost all their blood supply from the hepatic artery, whereas the normal liver parenchyma receives blood from both the portal vein and the hepatic artery. Transarterial chemoembolisation (TACE) aims to induce tumour ischaemic necrosis by occluding the blood supply to the tumour while preserving the blood flow to the normal liver parenchyma. Both hepatocellular carcinoma (HCC) and metastases may respond to TACE. Local delivery of chemotherapy directly into the tumour bed reduces systemic chemotherapy side effects.[9]

Indications

Patients with HCC with preserved liver function and Eastern Cooperative Oncology Group (ECOG)[10] performance status of 0–1 without extrahepatic disease are most suitable for chemoembolisation.[11,12] If the aim is to prolong life, patients with metastases should be treated if the disease is confined to the liver or if there is stable extrahepatic disease. In patients with neuroendocrine tumours, TACE can control symptoms such as flushing, sweating and palpitations.

TAE/TACE may be employed to reduce tumour bulk to allow an initially unresectable tumour to become resectable or to control or reduce tumour bulk in patients with HCC until a liver becomes available for transplantation.

TACE Contraindications

Poor outcomes occur in patients with little liver reserve and therefore chemoembolisation should be avoided in patients with more than 50–75% of liver parenchyma replaced by tumour, in patients with advanced cirrhosis and in those in liver failure. Advanced or progressive extrahepatic disease is also a contraindication. Relative contraindications include portal vein thrombus, Child-Pugh Class C, hepatic encephalopathy, active gastrointestinal (GI) bleeding, refractory ascites, transjugular intrahepatic portosystemic shunt and a serum bilirubin >5 mg/dL.[13] Patients with biliary-enteric anastomosis, prior sphincterotomy or CBD stents are at higher risk of infection and liver abscess formation due to reflux of enteric contents into the biliary system; thus antibiotic prophylaxis should be extended.

Pre-Procedure Medication/Sedation/Analgesia

Intravenous antibiotics and intravenous fluids are administered prior to chemoembolisation in most centres. Local analgesia and conscious sedation are given as per operator preference.

Performing the Procedure

Thorough good-quality digital subtraction angiography (DSA) is employed prior to embolisation to map out tumour arterial blood supply, identify anatomical variants, detect arteriovenous shunts, confirm portal vein patency and guide treatment strategy. Selective digital subtraction angiography is performed with microcatheters (Fig. 7-5). Dynamic CT can help to to map out tumour arterial feeders and recruitment of arterial feeders from unsuspected locations, i.e. dome lesions supplied from inferior phrenic arteries.

Chemoembolisation should be performed as superselectively as possible (Fig. 7-5). Various chemoembolisation agents are currently available. Slow controlled injections are necessary, watching closely under fluoroscopic guidance to avoid reflux or non-target embolisation. The end point is elimination of the tumour blush but not complete arterial stasis.

Post-Procedure Complications

Embolisation is often followed by the post-embolisation syndrome (PES), as a result of cell death and the release of various cytokines. It usually develops within 12 hours and manifests as nausea, vomiting, pain, fever and general malaise for a period of 2–7 days. PES may be prevented or ameliorated by the use of analgesia, antiemetics, antipyretics and intravenous fluids during and immediately after the procedure.

The overall complication rate of TACE is quoted at 4%[11] and includes hepatic failure due to infarction, abscess, biliary necrosis leading to biliary stricture, tumour rupture and non-target embolisation, especially of the gallbladder and the bowel wall.

Imaging Post-Chemoembolisation

Cross-sectional imaging with either CT or MRI can be utilised to assess tumour response following chemoembolisation and is usually performed 6 weeks after the

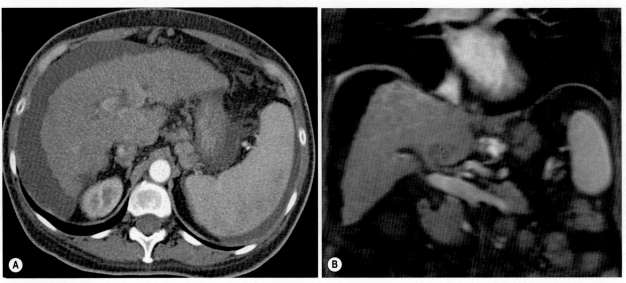

FIGURE 7-5 ■ A 59-year-old male with hepatitis C virus and long-standing cirrhosis with a raised AFP has both CT (A) and MRI (B; T1 fat-saturated post-contrast), demonstrating a caudate lobe mass lesion consistent with HCC. Note the irregular liver contour, ascites and splenomegaly.

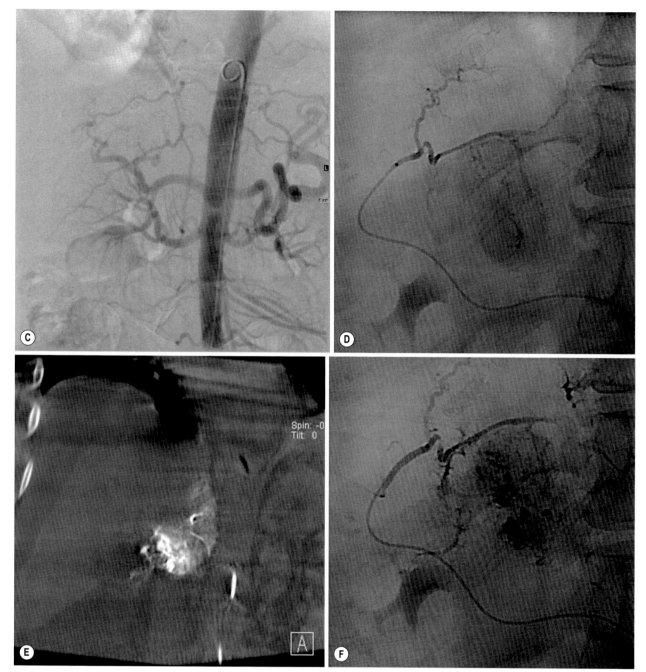

FIGURE 7-5, Continued ▪ Angiography demonstrates normal mesenteric anatomy (C) and tumour blush when the left hepatic artery is selectively catheterised with a microcatheter (D). Intense focal contrast opacification of the tumour with DynaCT (E) confirms that the microcatheter is perfusing all arterial tumour feeders. Chemoembolisation (TACE) was then performed with a cisplatin, doxorubicin, mitomycin combination regimen mixed with lipiodol, administered via the microcatheter (F).

procedure. Repeat embolisation can be considered if there is any viable residual tumour. Follow-up protocols are variable, with most centres performing further imaging at 3- or 6-monthly intervals.

The method of actual individual lesion size measurement and lesion number reporting is variable. The World Health Organisation (WHO) (bidimensional perpendicular measurements of the tumour) has published guidance on the anatomical assessment of tumour response to therapy.[14] As the measuring methods and

selection of target lesions are not clearly described in the WHO guidelines, assessment of tumour response is shown to be poorly reproducible between investigators.[15] In 2000 the Response Evaluation Criteria in Solid Tumours (RECIST) guidelines (unidimensional measurements of the tumour) were published.[16] The European Association for Study of the Liver (EASL) guidelines were published in 2001 and were based on the per cent change in the amount of enhancing tumoural tissue post-treatment.[17]

TACE Literature

There are two randomised controlled trials available, comparing chemoembolisation with conservative treatment for HCC and comparing bland embolisation against conservative treatment for HCC. Survival rates for patients with HCC following TACE at 1 and 2 years were 82 and 63% versus 63 and 27% for conservative treatment.[13] Survival rates for patients with HCC following TACE at 1, 2 and 3 years were 57, 31 and 26% versus 32, 11 and 3% for conservative treatment, respectively.[18] Survival rates for patients with HCC following TAE at 1 and 2 years were 75 and 50% versus 63 and 27% for conservative treatment, respectively.[13] A meta-analysis from Llovet's group demonstrated a significant 2-year survival benefit for patients with HCC treated with chemoembolisation versus conservative treatment alone.[19] There was no 2-year survival benefit for HCC patients treated with bland embolisation.[19] In the Precision V trial, Lammer et al. compared DC Bead chemoembolisation versus conventional TACE in patients with HCC and demonstrated higher rates of complete response, objective response and disease control in the DC Bead group than in the conventional TACE group (27 versus 22%, 52 versus 44% and 63 versus 52%, respectively).[20]

RADIOEMBOLISATION

Background

Also known as selective intra-arterial radiotherapy (SIRT) or selective intra-arterial brachytherapy, radioembolisation is a form of local radiotherapy. Micron-sized particles containing a radioisotope are given directly into the liver tumour via its feeding arteries in order to enable direct delivery of radiation. This technique delivers significantly higher radiation doses than external beam radiotherapy and minimises radiation dose to normal surrounding liver tissue.

Glass or resin particles impregnated with a β-emitting radio-isotope yttrium-90 (^{90}Y) are used to deliver the local tumour radiation. ^{90}Y is a pure β emitter with a half-life of 64.2 hours, which decays to stable zirconium-90. Despite the first clinical trials being conducted in the 1960s and its safety in human livers established in the 1980s, radioembolisation has only become readily available over the past decade. Two radioactive microsphere products are currently available on the market: a glass sphere known as TheraSphere (MDS Nordion, Canada) and a resin sphere known as SIR-Sphere (Sirtex Medical, Australia). TheraSphere gained FDA (Food and Drug Administration of America) approval in 1999 for use in the treatment of primary and/or metastatic HCC, with SIR-Sphere gaining FDA approval in 2002 for use in the treatment of colorectal cancer liver metastases.

Radioembolisation combines the advantages of embolisation and internal brachytherapy. It is necessary to perform detailed, pre-treatment angiography to map out tumour and liver arterial anatomy, to identify variant arterial anatomy, to delineate tumour arterial supply and to determine arterio-portal shunting.

Patient Selection

Patient selection for radioembolisation should be performed in a multidisciplinary team setting with both tumour characteristics and patient characteristics being highly important. Indications include an unresectable lesion, lack of fitness for transplantation, lesions unsuitable for thermal ablation and failed conventional chemotherapy. Patient characteristics include an ECOG performance status of 0–2 and an estimated life expectancy of greater than 12 weeks.[10]

Performing the Procedure: Planning

Pre-^{90}Y administration planning, diagnostic mesenteric angiography with meticulous technique is vital.[21] Diagnostic mesenteric angiography aims to determine hepatic arterial anatomy and variant anatomy, as 50% of the population will have aberrant hepatic arteries and 15% have aberrant arteries from the liver supplying the GI tract.[22] Salem et al. have provided an excellent description of the technique required to obtain good-quality angiography.[21] The use of a power injector pump to administer contrast, along with a base 5Fr catheter in the coeliac and superior mesenteric artery is mandatory.[21] Delayed venous imaging with the base catheter in the coeliac artery enables demonstration of a patent portal vein (Fig. 7-6).[21] A microcatheter, with an adjusted contrast flow rate on the power injector, is used to demonstrate the common, right, left and middle hepatic arteries, along with the gastroduodenal artery (GDA).[21] Dynamic CT or C-arm CT can be used to delineate tumour arterial supply via intra-arterial contrast administration during CT acquisition using a microcatheter at slow flow rates (Fig. 7-6).[21] This ensures the demontration of all arterial feeders to the lesion and avoids missing dual tumour supply, which is particularly important for dome lesions, which can parasitise flow from the inferior phrenic arteries.[22]

Non-target (normal tissue) embolisation is a greater problem with ^{90}Y than with chemoebolisation, as ^{90}Y not only causes ischaemia but also radiation injury to non-target tissue. The planning angiography procedure provides an opportunity to identify and deal with GI branches that could cause non-target ^{90}Y embolisation.[22] Coils may be used to embolise arteries to normal tissue, such as the GDA, left and right gastric artery, falciform artery and cystic artery in order to avoid non-target tissue damage, which may result in GI haemorrhage or pancreatitis. As there is a rich collateral arterial supply, proximal coils do not usually cause ischaemia and protect the bowel from ^{90}Y, thus allowing tumour-only delivery.

HCC is characterised by significant shunting, with lung shunting being of particular concern for treatment with ^{90}Y. The planning angiography procedure allows one to determine the lung shunt fraction (LSF) with a technetium ^{99m}Tc albumin aggregated (^{99m}Tc-MAA) shunt study.[22] LSF is calculated by injecting ^{99m}Tc-MAA into arteries to be treated with ^{90}Y and then imaging with a single photon emission computed tomography (SPECT) to detect shunting to pulmonary vasculature (Fig. 7-6). The size of the MAA particles is the same as the size of

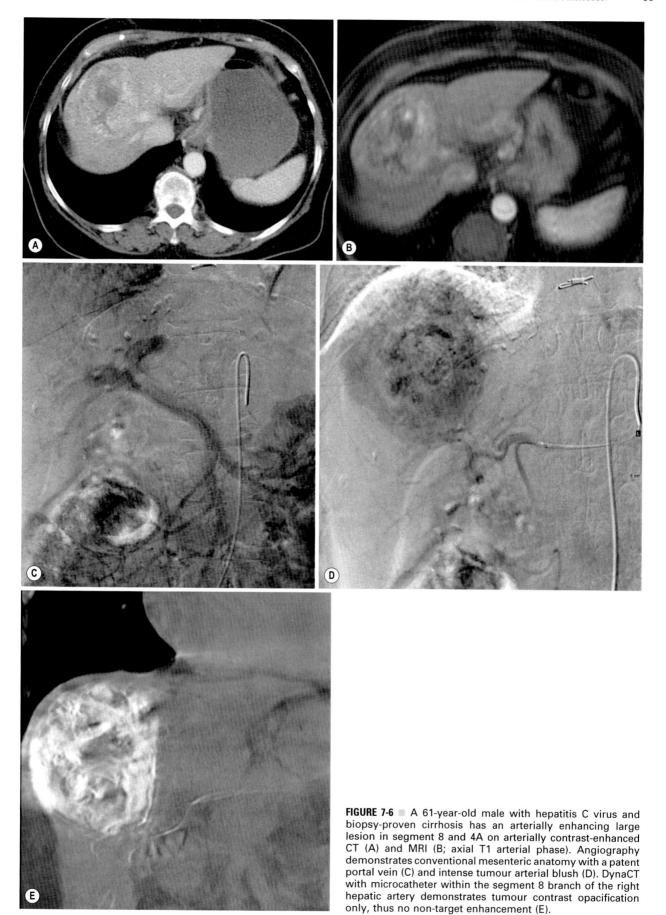

FIGURE 7-6 ■ A 61-year-old male with hepatitis C virus and biopsy-proven cirrhosis has an arterially enhancing large lesion in segment 8 and 4A on arterially contrast-enhanced CT (A) and MRI (B; axial T1 arterial phase). Angiography demonstrates conventional mesenteric anatomy with a patent portal vein (C) and intense tumour arterial blush (D). DynaCT with microcatheter within the segment 8 branch of the right hepatic artery demonstrates tumour contrast opacification only, thus no non-target enhancement (E).

Continued on following page

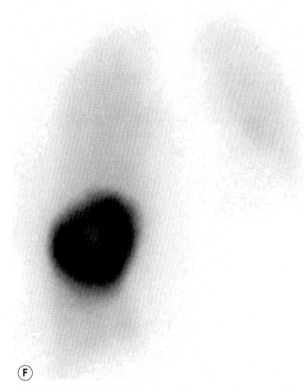

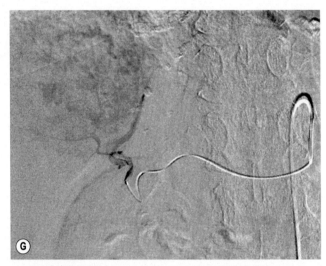

FIGURE 7-6, Continued ■ Radionuclide scan of segment 8 arterially injected MAA (F) demonstrates minimal lung shunting, thus confirming that it is safe to proceed with yttrium-90 radioembolisation. Microcatheter position for ^{90}Y injection (G).

[90]Y; thus, the MAA shunt study can be considered a test run for the [90]Y. If LSF exceeds 20%, radioembolisation is not considered a safe option.[23]

[90]Y Administration

One lobe is treated at any one time, with at least 4 weeks between lobar treatments. Repeat angiography should be performed prior to ^{90}Y administration to determine arterial flow characteristics, to detect failed coiling with reperfusion to non-target areas, thus enabling re-coiling if necessary. A slow, steady injection of ^{90}Y via a microcatheter with saline flushes and radiation monitoring should be performed (Fig. 7-6). Check angiography is performed on completion.

[90]Y Complications

Riaz et al. provided a concise review of complications following radioembolisation with [90]Y.[24] Post-radioembolisation syndrome, which is similar to the usual post-embolisation syndrome, can occur and is managed conservatively. Hepatic dysfunction, radiation cystitis/biliary stricture, portal hypertension, radiation pneumonitis, GI complications from non-target embolisation and hepatic arterial injury are the main potential complications following radioembolisation.[24]

Imaging Post-Radioembolisation

The assessment of response using imaging is similar to that following TACE. Riaz et al. demonstrated that the primary index lesion concept significantly correlates with disease progression and patient survival.[25]

Radioembolisation Results

Treatment of HCC with radioembolisation has demonstrated survival rates following ^{90}Y at 1, 2 and 3 years of 84, 54 and 27%, respectively.[26] Treatment of CRC metastases with radioembolisation with ^{90}Y have yielded survival rates at 1 and 2 years of 39.1 and 22.1%, respectively, with imaging response rates quoted from 23 to 74% across a number of studies.[27] [90]Y is better at HCC downstaging than TACE.[28] Colorectal cancer metastases treated with ^{90}Y in combination with irinotecan produced a median progression-free survival of 6.0 months, with a median survival of 12.2 months.[29] Randomised controlled trials (RCT)s of ^{90}Y versus TACE are currently ongoing.

HEPATIC ARTERIAL EMBOLISATION FOR HAEMORRHAGE

Liver arterial haemorrhage occurs following trauma, blunt or penetrating, spontaneously from tumour or cyst

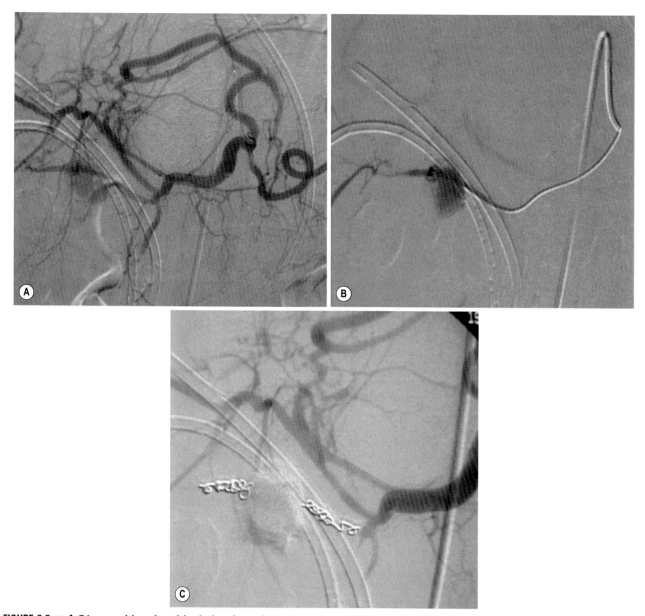

FIGURE 7-7 ■ **A 74-year-old male with cholangiocarcinoma causing obstructive jaundice recently had an internal–external biliary drain placed to enable biliary decompression prior to stenting.** He became hypotensive with bright red blood pouring out of his biliary drain. Digital subtraction angiography with a catheter in the coeliac artery demonstrated a large hepatic arterial pseudoaneurysm at the site of the internal–external biliary drain (A). Superselective catheterisation with a microcatheter eloquently identifies the pseudoaneurysm (B). Both the front door and the back door to the pseudoaneurysm were coil embolised to achieve haemostasis (C).

rupture or from iatrogenic causes such as following liver biopsy or biliary drainage (Fig. 7-7). Diagnosis can be made with triphasic liver CT. In the setting of an unstable patient with active arterial bleeding or a pseudoaneurysm, control of bleeding can be achieved by transcatheter embolisation. The pre-procedure planning and procedure technique is very similar to that employed for chemoembolisation or radioembolisation, with good-quality digital subtraction angiography with contrast pump injectors essential to delineate the arterial anatomy and the exact site of arterial injury. Embolisation can be performed with a variety of agents, depending on the configuration of the arterial injury: e.g. coils, particles or liquid embolic agents such as glue. The goal is to elicit a rapid diagnosis, clear demonstration of the anatomy and rapid haemorrhage control. Close liaison with surgical and anaesthetic colleagues is essential for optimum patient outcome.

TRANSJUGULAR INTRAHEPATIC PORTOSYSTEMIC SHUNT

Background

Transjugular intrahepatic portosystemic shunt (TIPSS) creates a transhepatic communication between a major intrahepatic portal vein branch (usually the right) and a hepatic vein using a needle system from the jugular vein. The transhepatic tract patency is maintained with a metallic covered stent. The creation of the shunt reduces the portal venous pressure. Accepted indications for TIPSS include variceal bleeding, both acute and refractory to endoscopic therapy,[30] refractory ascites[31] and hepatic hydrothorax. Further indications include Budd–Chiari syndrome[32] and hepatorenal/hepatopulmonary syndromes.

Imaging

Preoperative imaging is geared towards delineating hepatic vascular anatomy and confirming patency of the portal vein. Cardiovascular status should be assessed with cardiac failure contraindicating TIPSS due to the haemodynamic changes associated with the creation of a portosystemic shunt. Sepsis and biliary obstruction are further contraindications and coagulopathy should be corrected.

Pre-Procedure Evaluation

Various preoperative scoring systems are available, with the model for end-stage liver disease (MELD) scoring system developed for those undergoing elective TIPSS.[33] The prognosis according to MELD score is as follows:[34]

  MELD <17: 3-month mortality: 16%
  MELD >18: 3-month mortality: 35%
  MELD >24: 3-month mortality: 65%.

Performing the Procedure

The procedure is generally performed under general anaesthesia. The right internal jugular vein is accessed and a vascular sheath is placed to the right atrium and the right hepatic vein is catheterised. The portal vein is delineated by various methods: percutaneous placement of portal vein guidewire before the procedure; aortoportography with delayed imaging after contrast injection from the SMA; or wedged CO_2 portography from the hepatic vein. A transhepatic trocar is advanced from the hepatic vein to the region of the portal vein, the needle withdrawn and the catheter is aspirated as it is withdrawn. Once blood is aspirated, a small amount of contrast material is injected to confirm portal venous position (Fig. 7-8). A guidewire is passed to the portal vein and pressure measurements are obtained in the portal vein and right atrium. The tract is measured with a calibated catheter from the portal vein to the confluence of the hepatic vein with the inferior vena cava (Fig. 7-8). The tract is dilated with an angioplasty balloon and a covered stent (e.g. Viatorr; Gore Medical, Flagstaff, AZ) is placed. The stent is balloon dilated. Pressure measurements are performed to ensure that adequate shunting has been established (pressure <12 mmHg or halving the portosystemic gradient). Angiography is performed at the end of the procedure. If there is continued opacification of varices, these should be embolised, if the patient has had a significant variceal bleed (Fig. 7-8).

Post-Procedure

The haemodynamic changes can lead to cardiac failure and diuretics may help reduce central venous pressure. The risk of encephalopathy ranges from 5 to 35%.[35] Periprocedural lactulose and rifaximin are effective in reducing gut flora.

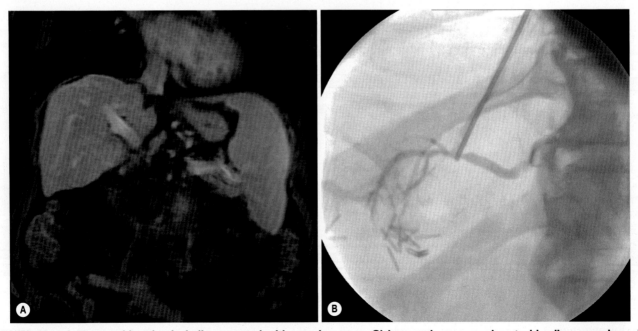

FIGURE 7-8 ■ A 55-year-old male alcoholic presented with massive upper GI haemorrhage secondary to bleeding oesophageal varices, with a MELD of 11. MRI demonstrated a patent portal vein, cirrhosis and splenomegaly (A). Due to the massive variceal bleeding it was elected to perform a TIPSS. A right hepatic vein to right portal vein approach was taken (B).

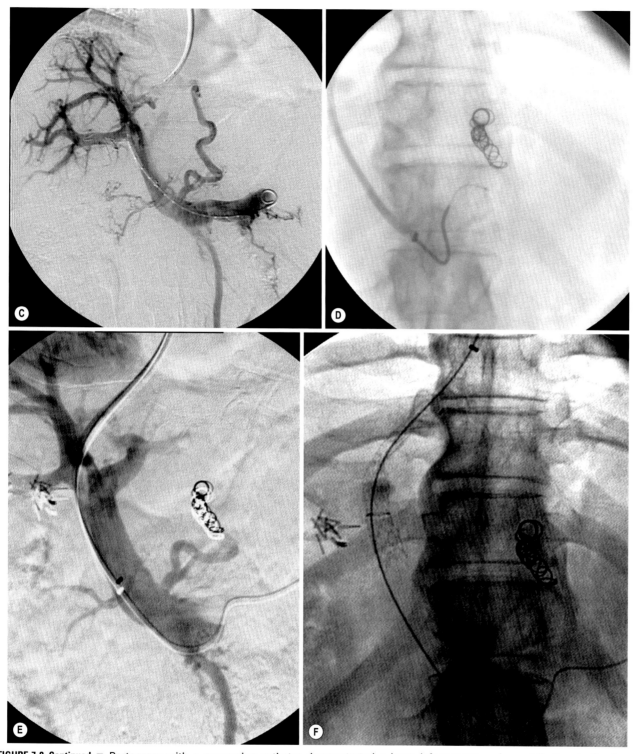

FIGURE 7-8, Continued ■ Portogram with a measuring catheter demonstrated a large left coronary vein contributing to the large oesophageal varices (C). The coronary vein was coil embolised (D). Repeat portogram demonstrated no flow within the left coronary vein following embolisation (E). A Viatorr 10 mm × 8 cm TIPSS was placed, which demonstrated some stenosis initially (F).

Continued on following page

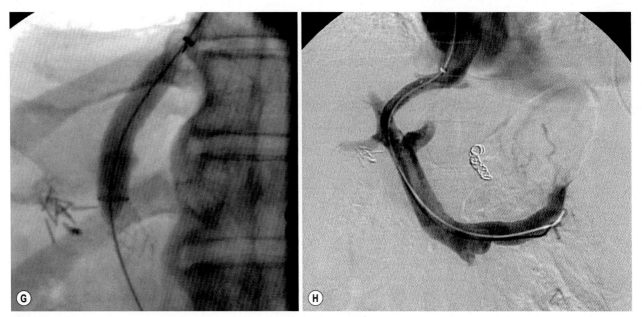

FIGURE 7-8, Continued ■ The stent was ballooned to 8 mm (G). Completion venography demonstrates a widely patent TIPSS with no variceal flow (H).

Complications

Direct procedural-related mortality is lower than 2%[35] and relates to hepatic arterial injury, capsular perforation or direct puncture of the extrahepatic portal vein with intraperitoneal haemorrhage. Right atrial perforation may occur from misplaced stents. Bile duct injury with haemobilia and intraparenchymal haematoma may occur at the time of the procedure. Further complications include heart failure and encephalopathy due to shunting. Stent occlusion and subsequent sepsis have been reduced with the advent of covered stents but remain problematic.

PORTAL VEIN EMBOLISATION

Background

Preoperative portal vein embolisation is performed in patients undergoing liver resection for localised metastases to the liver or primary hepatocellular carcinoma. It is used in cases where the future liver remnant (usually left lobe) will not provide sufficient function, and exploits the ability of the liver to regenerate. Volumetric analysis from CT is undertaken to calculate the functional liver volume required, which is related to body surface area. If the future liver remnant is less than 25% in a normal liver, or less than 40% in a cirrhotic liver, then portal vein embolisation should be considered.[36] In addition, systemic disease with diabetes mellitus may limit the degree of hypertrophy.[37] The portal vein embolisation is performed 4–6 weeks before surgical resection, and the section of liver to be resected is embolised to divert portal venous blood flow to the remaining liver to allow hypertrophy.

Performing the Procedure

US-guided percutaneous access is gained to the portal vein with a coaxial microaccess set (e.g. Neff Set (Cook)). A sheath is placed and portal venography is performed to delineate the anatomy. An angiographic catheter is placed to the branch portal vein supplying the tumour. Embolisation is performed with glue, coils, plugs or a combination of these. Specific complications of portal vein embolisation include main portal vein thrombosis, which would preclude surgery and portal hypertension resulting in variceal haemorrhage.[37]

HEPATIC VENOUS INTERVENTIONS: BUDD–CHIARI SYNDROME

Background

Budd–Chiari syndrome is a heterogeneous group of disorders characterised by hepatic venous outflow obstruction at the level of the hepatic veins, the inferior vena cava (IVC) or the right atrium.[38] Budd–Chiari syndrome is not a primary condition of the liver parenchyma; it is due to partial or complete obstruction of hepatic venous outflow. This obstruction subsequently leads to progressive sinusoidal congestion, centrilobular necrosis, fibrosis and nodular regeneration. Percutaneous therapies performed in properly selected patients can help improve liver function and arrest hepatic destruction.[39]

Diagnosis

Clinically, patients usually present with tender hepatomegaly and ascites. However, they may present in fulminant hepatic failure and rarely present with chronic liver impairment. Doppler ultrasound may demonstrate lack of flow in the hepatic veins, hepatic venous thrombus or intrahcpatic venous collaterals. Flow reversal in the distal hepatic veins, a caval web, caval stenosis or occlusion may also be demonstrated. Cross-sectional imaging with CT or MRI can confirm the ultrasound findings.

Treatment

The aim is to restore normal hepatic venous drainage from the liver. In acute thrombus, direct catheter-based thrombolysis with tissue plasminogen activator (tPA) is employed. A hepatic venous or caval stenosis can then be unmasked with clot dissolution, enabling venoplasty and/ or stenting. However, restenosis is common. TIPSS creation is an alternative option to maintain venous outflow drainage from the liver in Budd–Chiari. Close post-TIPSS surveillance is needed in this patient group to detect shunt restenosis and enable balloon dilatation. Liver transplantation may be necessary in some patients.

REFERENCES

1. George C, Byass OR, Cast JE. Interventional radiology in the management of malignant biliary obstruction. World J Gastrointest Oncol 2010;2:146–50.
2. Lammer J, Hausegger KA, Fluckiger F, et al. Common bile duct obstruction due to malignancy: treatment with plastic versus metal stents. Radiology 1996;201:167–72.
3. Krokidis M, Fanelli F, Orgera G, et al. Percutaneous palliation of pancreatic head cancer: randomized comparison of ePTFE/FEP-covered versus uncovered nitinol biliary stents. Cardiovasc Intervent Radiol 2011;34:352–61.
4. Gwon DI, Shim HJ, Kwak BK. Retrievable biliary stent-graft in the treatment of benign biliary strictures. J Vasc Interv Radiol 2008;19:1328–35.
5. McPherson SJ, Gibson RN, Collier NA, et al. Percutaneous trans-jejunal biliary intervention: 10-year experience with access via Roux-en-Y loops. Radiology 1998;206:665–72.
6. Ozcan N, Kahriman G, Mavili E. Percutaneous transhepatic removal of bile duct stones: results of 261 patients. Cardiovasc Intervent Radiol 2012;35:890–7.
7. van Delden OM, Lameris JS. Percutaneous drainage and stenting for palliation of malignant bile duct obstruction. Eur Radiol 2008;18:448–56.
8. Inal M, Aksungur E, Akgul E, et al. Percutaneous placement of metallic stents in malignant biliary obstruction: one-stage or two-stage procedure? Pre-dilate or not? Cardiovasc Intervent Radiol 2003;26:40–5.
9. Soulen MC. Chemoembolization of hepatic malignancies. Oncology (Williston Park) 1994;8:77–84; discussion, 9–90 passim.
10. Oken MM, Creech RH, Tormey DC, et al. Toxicity and response criteria of the Eastern Cooperative Oncology Group. Am J Clin Oncol 1982;5:649–55.
11. Llovet JM, Burroughs A, Bruix J. Hepatocellular carcinoma. Lancet 2003;362:1907–17.
12. Bruix J, Sala M, Llovet JM. Chemoembolization for hepatocellular carcinoma. Gastroenterology 2004;127:S179–88.
13. Llovet JM, Real MI, Montana X, et al. Arterial embolisation or chemoembolisation versus symptomatic treatment in patients with unresectable hepatocellular carcinoma: a randomised controlled trial. Lancet 2002;359:1734–9.
14. Miller AB, Hoogstraten B, Staquet M, Winkler A. Reporting results of cancer treatment. Cancer 1981;47:207–14.
15. Therasse P. Measuring the clinical response. What does it mean? Eur J Cancer 2002;38:1817–23.
16. Therasse P, Arbuck SG, Eisenhauer EA, et al. New guidelines to evaluate the response to treatment in solid tumors. European Organization for Research and Treatment of Cancer, National Cancer Institute of the United States, National Cancer Institute of Canada. J Natl Cancer Inst 2000;92:205–16.
17. Bruix J, Sherman M, Llovet JM, et al. Clinical management of hepatocellular carcinoma. Conclusions of the Barcelona-2000 EASL conference. European Association for the Study of the Liver. J Hepatol 2001;35:421–30.
18. Lo CM, Ngan H, Tso WK, et al. Randomized controlled trial of transarterial lipiodol chemoembolization for unresectable hepato-cellular carcinoma. Hepatology 2002;35:1164–71.
19. Llovet JM, Bruix J. Systematic review of randomized trials for unresectable hepatocellular carcinoma: Chemoembolization improves survival. Hepatology 2003;37:429–42.
20. Lammer J, Malagari K, Vogl T, et al. Prospective randomized study of doxorubicin-eluting-bead embolization in the treatment of hepatocellular carcinoma: results of the PRECISION V study. Cardiovasc Intervent Radiol 2010;33:41–52.
21. Salem R, Thurston KG. Radioembolization with 90Yttrium micro-spheres: a state-of-the-art brachytherapy treatment for primary and secondary liver malignancies. Part 1: Technical and methodologic considerations. J Vasc Interv Radiol 2006;17:1251–78.
22. Covey AM, Brody LA, Maluccio MA, et al. Variant hepatic arterial anatomy revisited: digital subtraction angiography performed in 600 patients. Radiology 2002;224:542–7.
23. Lewandowski RJ, Sato KT, Atassi B, et al. Radioembolization with ^{90}Y microspheres: angiographic and technical considerations. Cardiovasc Intervent Radiol 2007;30:571–92.
24. Riaz A, Lewandowski RJ, Kulik LM, et al. Complications following radioembolization with yttrium-90 microspheres: a comprehensive literature review. J Vasc Interv Radiol 2009;20:1121–30; quiz 1131.
25. Riaz A, Miller FH, Kulik LM, et al. Imaging response in the primary index lesion and clinical outcomes following transarterial locoregional therapy for hepatocellular carcinoma. JAMA 2010;303:1062–9.
26. Kulik LM, Atassi B, van Holsbeeck L, et al. Yttrium-90 micro-spheres (TheraSphere) treatment of unresectable hepatocellular carcinoma: downstaging to resection, RFA and bridge to transplan-tation. J Surg Oncol 2006;94:572–86.
27. Salem R, Thurston KG. Radioembolization with yttrium-90 microspheres: a state-of-the-art brachytherapy treatment for primary and secondary liver malignancies: part 3: comprehensive literature review and future direction. J Vasc Interv Radiol 2006;17:1571–93.
28. Lewandowski RJ, Kulik LM, Riaz A, et al. A comparative analysis of transarterial downstaging for hepatocellular carcinoma: chem-oembolization versus radioembolization. Am J Transplant 2009;9:1920–8.
29. van Hazel GA, Pavlakis N, Goldstein D, et al. Treatment of fluorouracil-refractory patients with liver metastases from colorec-tal cancer by using yttrium-90 resin microspheres plus concomitant systemic irinotecan chemotherapy. J Clin Oncol 2009;27:4089–95.
30. Garcia-Pagan JC, Caca K, Bureau C, et al. Early use of TIPS in patients with cirrhosis and variceal bleeding. N Engl J Med 2010;362:2370–9.
31. Saab S, Nieto JM, Lewis SK, Runyon BA. TIPS versus paracentesis for cirrhotic patients with refractory ascites. Cochrane Database Syst Rev 2006;CD004889.
32. Garcia-Pagan JC, Heydtmann M, Raffa S, et al. TIPS for Budd-Chiari syndrome: long-term results and prognostics factors in 124 patients. Gastroenterology 2008;135:808–15.
33. Malinchoc M, Kamath PS, Gordon FD, et al. A model to predict poor survival in patients undergoing transjugular intrahepatic por-tosystemic shunts. Hepatology 2000;31:864–71.
34. Ferral H, Gamboa P, Postoak DW, et al. Survival after elective transjugular intrahepatic portosystemic shunt creation: prediction with model for end-stage liver disease score. Radiology 2004;231:231–6.
35. Freedman AM, Sanyal AJ, Tisnado J, et al. Complications of trans-jugular intrahepatic portosystemic shunt: a comprehensive review. Radiographics 1993;13:1185–210.
36. Abdalla EK, Hicks ME, Vauthey JN. Portal vein embolization: rationale, technique and future prospects. Br J Surg 2001;88:165–75.
37. Madoff DC, Hicks ME, Vauthey JN, et al. Transhepatic portal vein embolization: anatomy, indications, and technical considerations. Radiographics 2002;22:1063–76.
38. Ludwig J, Hashimoto E, McGill DB, van Heerden JA. Classifica-tion of hepatic venous outflow obstruction: ambiguous terminology of the Budd-Chiari syndrome. Mayo Clin Proc 1990;65:51–5.
39. Cura M, Haskal Z, Lopera J. Diagnostic and interventional radiol-ogy for Budd-Chiari syndrome. Radiographics 2009;29:669–81.

CHAPTER 8

VASCULAR GENITOURINARY TRACT INTERVENTION

Jonathan G. Moss • Reddi Prasad Yadavali

CHAPTER OUTLINE

KIDNEY

Renal Artery Stenosis

Background

Stenosis of the renal artery (RAS), which is usually focal, can cause a cascade of ischaemic-driven events in the kidney plus other potential insults such as cholesterol embolisation. This can lead to clinical consequences, which include secondary hypertension, impaired renal function and fluid retention (flash pulmonary oedema). Much interest has focused on correcting the anatomical abnormality, initially with angioplasty and latterly with stents in an attempt to reverse or halt the clinical manifestations.

Aetiology and Pathology

In Western populations, atherosclerosis is the leading cause in over 90% of cases. However, in younger age group, the non-atheromatous arteritides should be considered (Table 8-1) particularly in the non-Caucasian individual.

Diagnosis of RAS

Once suspected clinically, the optimal imaging modality is contrast-enhanced magnetic resonance angiography (MRA) (Fig. 8-1). However, due to a small number of reported cases of nephrogenic systemic fibrosis linked to gadolinium contrast media exposure, guidelines suggest caution if the e GFR is <30 mL/min and is contraindicated when <15 mL/min. Other imaging options include computed tomographic angiography (CTA) and newer MRI sequences, avoiding contrast media altogether. Although Doppler ultrasound and functional nuclear medicine scans can be used, they have largely fallen out of favour in recent years. Despite this, they may still play a limited role specific circumstances, however, they similarly selective renal vein sampling is seldom used nowadays.

Atheromatous Renovascular Disease (ARVD)

ARVD is by far the commonest cause of RAS and usually develops as part of a systemic inflammatory atheromatous syndrome with disease in other vascular beds (coronary, peripheral). There is a strong correlation with both smoking and type 2 diabetes. Anatomically over 90% of ARVD involves the renal ostium as a result of encroaching aortic plaques.

Clinical Presentation of ARVD. Many patients are asymptomatic and the condition is often detected whilst investigating other symptoms, e.g. lower limb ischaemia. Others present with hypertension, impaired renal function or 'flash pulmonary oedema'. The latter is a poorly understood condition where there are recurrent attacks of fluid overload with normal or near normal cardiac function but the kidney's ability to excrete fluid is impaired.

Treatment of ARVD. Treatment of the global atherosclerotic burden should be addressed with smoking cessation, aspirin, statins and optimising blood pressure control. Although intuitively contraindicated, ACE inhibitors should be given with careful monitoring of renal function. There is some evidence that this 'package of medical treatment' can stabilise atheromatous plaque and even induce regression.

Revascularisation of the stenotic artery has evolved over the years. Initially performed by open surgical repair, percutaneous transluminal angioplasty (PTA) gained rapid acceptance in the 1980s. However, high restenosis rates due to elastic recoil from the aortic plaques led to

TABLE 8-1 Non-Atheromatous Arteritides

- Fibromuscular disease
- Neurofibromatosis
- Takayasu arteritis
- Williams syndrome

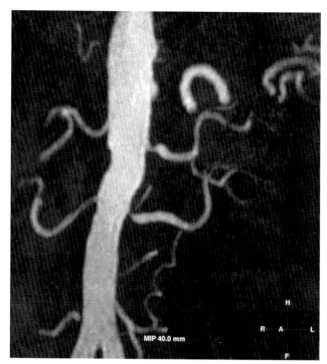

FIGURE 8-1 ■ Renal artery stenosis. Coronal MIP MRA shows osteal stenoses of superior and inferior left renal arteries.

disappointing anatomical and clinical results.[1] The introduction of metallic stents in the early 1990s led to a resurgence in endovascular activity and the mechanical limitations of renal PTA were overcome with a significant reduction in restenosis.[2] Almost overnight renal stenting became the dominant strategy for ARVD.

However, although stenting clearly led to improved patency it was often difficult to clearly link this with clinical benefit, e.g. blood pressure reduction or improvement in renal function. It was often said that the 'rule of thirds' applied with one-third showing some improvement, another third static and the final third deteriorating. This continuing uncertainty triggered several randomised trials which spanned both the PTA and stenting era.

Renal Revascularisation Trials. The early trials[3–5] predated stents and focussed on blood pressure outcomes. The later trials used stents exclusively and focussed on renal function.[6,7] None of these trials with meta-analyses of over 1000 patients have been able to prove any clear benefit of either PTA or stenting over medical treatment alone.[8,9] These trials, including the largest (ASTRAL $n = 806$), have all been criticised and the debate continues. A large ultrasound (US) trial (CORAL) is due to report in 2014 and may provide more information.[10]

Routine renal stenting for hypertension or impaired renal function is therefore difficult to justify in view of the lack of evidence. However, not all patients entered these trials and possible but unproven indications for renal stenting may include the following:

- Intractable hypertension on maximum medical treatment;
- Rapidly deteriorating renal function;
- A single kidney with a critical stenosis (>90%);
- Flash pulmonary oedema; and
- Acute renal failure with preserved renal size (>8 cm).

Careful individualised patient evaluation is necessary as complications can occur in 5–10% of procedures. These are mostly minor, e.g. groin haematoma, but can include damage to the renal artery, cholesterol embolisation and occasional loss of the kidney. Very rarely a patient will present with acute renal failure and an occluded single renal artery; stenting in these circumstances is worthwhile and can restore renal function with little to lose (Fig. 8-2).

Technique for Renal Angioplasty and Stenting

Renal Angioplasty. The angle from which the renal artery leaves the aorta will help decide between a femoral and an arm (brachial or radial) approach. Over 90% are approachable from the femoral artery. Similarly the angle at which the renal artery ostium lies in the coronal plane will determine the correct angle to place the 'C-arm', in order to project the origin of the renal artery clear of the aorta. Careful perusal of the baseline imaging is essential. Advances in guidewire and catheter technology have meant most operators now use the so-called 'low platform' systems, which use a 3–4F catheter with 0.014–0.018 guidewires. Delivered through a 6–7F guiding catheter, they are less traumatic than the old 0.035 guidewire systems. Having accessed the renal artery ostium and placed a guide catheter, the lesion is crossed and angioplastied with an appropriate sized balloon. Intraoperative heparin and a proprietary antispasmodic should be given. When dealing with non-atheromatous lesions angioplasty is usually sufficient (Fig. 8-3) but atheromatous lesions are almost always stented to overcome elastic recoil.

Renal Stenting. The procedure is similar to PTA and again uses a 'low platform' stent. The lesion is crossed as above and the stenosis pre-dilated to 3 mm and then the stent placed. Accurate C-arm positioning is critical to ensure accurate stent placement with 2–3 mm protruding out into the aorta. Most operators use balloon-expandable rather than self-expanding stents because they are easier to place accurately at the renal artery ostium (Fig. 8-4).

Fibromuscular Disease. In the West, fibromuscular disease accounts for 10% of all cases of RAS. Although it is most frequently found in the renal arteries (60%) other major vessels such as the carotid, visceral and coronaries can be involved. There are at least five different pathological types but the most common is medial fibroplasia where there are alternating areas of stenosis

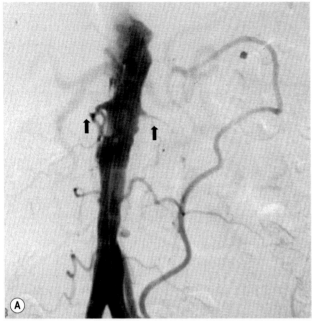

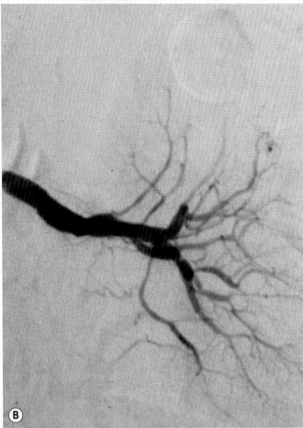

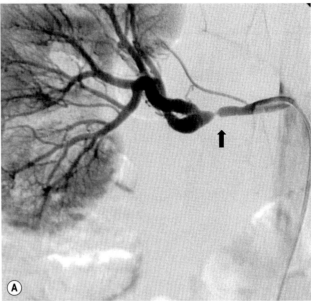

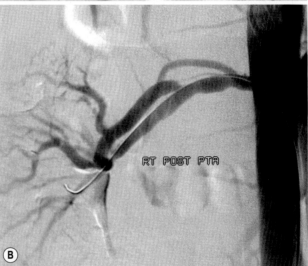

FIGURE 8-2 ■ (A) Patient presenting with acute kidney injury. Angiogram showing bilateral renal artery occlusions. (B) Selective left renal angiogram following successful recanalistion and stenting of the renal artery. Satisfactory renal function was re-established with a massive diuresis.

FIGURE 8-3 ■ **Female patient aged 23 years with severe hypertension.** (A) Selective right renal angiogram showing a tight focal stricture due to fibromuscular disease. (B) Aortogram showing good post angioplasty result. There was a dramatic drop in blood pressure, necessitating cessation of all antihypertensive medications.

and aneurysmal dilation leading to the classical 'string of beads' appearance (Fig. 8-5). A much rarer type leads predominantly to aneurysm formation (Fig. 8-6) and requires a different management strategy. The typical presentation is a young person, commonly female, with new onset hypertension. Renal function is usually normal and although the lesion may progress, complete vessel occlusion is rare. Although initial management with drugs is usual there is a strong case for angioplasty as the lesions respond well and there is often a good chance of 'cure' or significant improvement in blood pressure control.[11]

Takayasu Arteritis. The epidemiology of RAS is different in the Indian subcontinent and the Far East, with vasculitis, including Takayasu arteritis, said to be responsible for up to 60% of RAS cases. Although PTA can be used, this inflammatory condition can be resistant to dilation. Steroids are often successfully used to suppress the inflammatory component.

Neurofibromatosis. This rare congenital condition is known to cause a myriad of symptoms and signs. Less well recognised is the involvement of vessels, commonly the renal arteries. The pathology is usually one of stenosis and aneurysmal dilatation. Although PTA can be utilized, the lesions are often resistant to dilatation and in this young patient group surgical reconstruction of the vessel may be a better option.

Williams Syndrome. This rare congenital condition presents in childhood. Although the renal arteries are commonly involved there is almost always aortic hypoplasia and the extent to which angioplasty and stenting can help is very limited.

Renal Denervation (RDN)

Background

Essential hypertension is extremely common in Western societies where approximately one-third of adults have high blood pressure. With an ageing population, Westernisation and increasing obesity and diabetes, the prevalence of hypertension will only increase. In the USA in 2011, 69% of first heart attacks, 77% of first strokes and 74% with congestive cardiac failure had a blood pressure higher than 140/99 mmHg.[12] The costs to the global

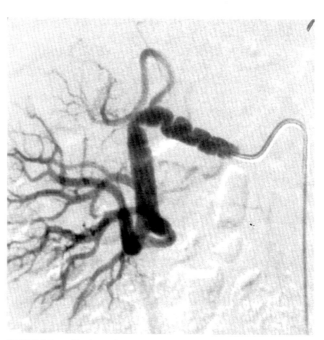

FIGURE 8-5 ■ **'String of beads'.** Right renal angiogram showing multifocal stenosis secondary to fibromuscular disease.

FIGURE 8-4 ■ **Renal artery stent.** Balloon-expandable stent in the proximal left renal artery for atheromatous osteal stenosis.

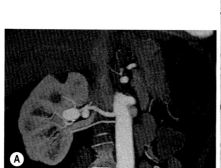
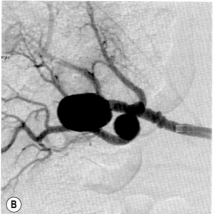
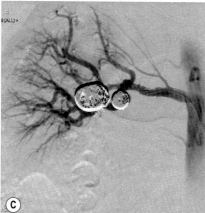

FIGURE 8-6 ■ **Renal artery aneurysms.** (A) CT MIP image showing two renal artery aneurysms. Both are complex with no neck and arising from branch divisions. (B) Right renal angiogram showing additional irregularity of the proximal renal artery thought to represent fibromuscular disease. (C) Completion right renal angiogram afer second embolisation. Three solitaire detachable stents were used in a stent through stent configuration to preserve blood flow to the kidney and then coils placed through the stents to gain aneurysm thrombosis. A complex case like this can take several hours and cost £15–20,000 in disposable equipment alone.

healthcare system are huge. There is a direct correlation between high blood pressure and cardiovascular risk. Although many patients can be controlled with antihypertensive drugs there is a cohort who do not achieve good control despite multiple medications. This group is estimated to be as high as 30% although in specialist centres, with drug optimisation and having excluded poor compliance and secondary causes, the figure is more likely to be 5%. In this significant minority, until very recently, there was little to offer that was effective.

History of Sympathectomy

The idea of renal denervation is not a new one. Since the 1920s open radical surgical sympathectomy had been practised mainly for malignant hypertension. Although a very invasive procedure it clearly reduced blood pressure and observation studies of over 2000 patients have been reported.[13] Carried out into the 1960s the introduction of modern antihypertensives such as beta-blockers ultimately relegated the procedure to the history books. It was not until the 1990s that interest was renewed with initially rhizotomy in rats and then selective renal denervation using an endovascular approach in pigs. The first reports of successful renal denervation in humans appeared in 2009 with a multicentre 'proof of principle' study.[14]

Pathophysiology

The kidneys receive an efferent sympathetic supply from preganglionic brain fibres via the thoracic and lumbar sympathetic trunks, which run through the major visceral ganglia before providing postganglionic supply to the kidneys. Efferent stimulation of the kidneys results in activation of the renin–angiotensin–aldosterone system and leads to water and sodium retention and reduced renal blood flow. In addition, the kidneys have an afferent sympathetic output from both mechanoreceptors and chemoreceptors responding to stretch and ischaemia, respectively. Via the dorsal root ganglia these afferent fibres travel to the cardiovascular centres in the brain (Fig. 8-7). Afferent activation leads to antidiuretic hormone and oxytocin secretion and also plays a role in modulation of systemic vascular resistance. Surrogate markers such as noradrenaline spillover and microneurography have demonstrated sympathetic overactivitiy in essential hypertension and this has a myriad of effects described above, all of which ultimately increase blood pressure.

Both the afferent and efferent sympathetic fibres run within the adventitia of the renal arteries and this is where they are targeted by the RDN procedure.

Technique

This technology is evolving rapidly and at the time of writing only one device is CE marked for clinical use. However, at least another six devices are at various stages of development and will be soon arriving on the market. The current device (Medtronic Inc, USA) uses a small steerable radiofrequency probe placed into the lumen of

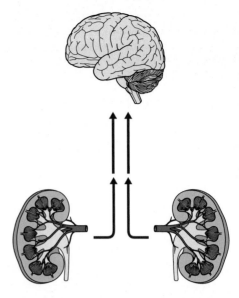

Renal nerves and the SNNS

Afferent renal sympathetics

(A) The kidney is a source of central sympathetic drive in hypertension, heart failure, chronic kidney disease and ESRD

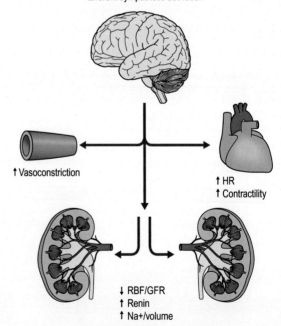

Renal nerves and the SNNS

Efferent sympathetic activation

↑ Vasoconstriction

↑ HR
↑ Contractility

↓ RBF/GFR
↑ Renin
↑ Na+/volume

(B) Patients cannot develop and/or maintain elevated BP without renal involvement

FIGURE 8-7 ■ Afferent and efferent sympathetic innervations of the kidney. (Redrawn from Papademetriou V, Doumas M, Tsioufis K 2011 Renal sympathetic denervation for the treatment of difficult-to-control or resistant hypertension. Int J Hypertens 2011: 196518, Fig. 6.)

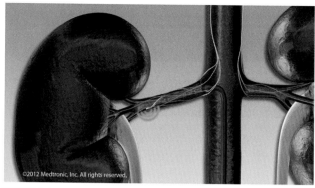

FIGURE 8-8 ■ **RDN procedure showing the sympathetic nerves in the adventitia of the renal arteries being ablated with the Ardian device.** (Reproduced with permission from Medtronic Inc.)

the renal artery through a guiding catheter from a trans-femoral approach (Fig. 8-8). Several pulses (5–7) of energy deployed in a spiral fashion are used to heat up and destroy both the afferent and efferent renal sympathetic nerves lying in the adventitial layer. The procedure is repeated in both kidneys.

Although performed under local anaesthesia the procedure is relatively painful and an analgesic protocol is required. A regimen similar to that needed for fibroid embolisation is suggested. The procedure is commonly carried out as a day case admission.

Indications

The precise indications for RDN are not yet fully developed. The reader is directed to the recent guidance issued by the Joint UK Societies Consensus Statement and NICE in 2012.[15]

Broadly speaking, patients should have a sustained blood pressure of ≥ 160 mmHg (≥ 150 mmHg in type 2 diabetes) on three or more medications. Ambulatory blood pressure measurements should be used. As the procedure is evolving other potentially beneficial effects are being reported. These include reduced insulin resistance, and improved renal and cardiac function. Further research is ongoing in these patient groups.

Results

The early results have been very promising and a randomised controlled trial (Symplicity HTN-2) reported in 2010 showed a mean reduction in blood pressure of 32/12 mmHg in the active group compared to 1/0 mmHg in the control group.[16] This was a highly significant difference $p < 0.0001$. There were no serious procedure-related or device-related complications and occurrence of adverse events did not differ between groups. At the time of writing, further trials are underway (Symplicity HTN-3) and longer term follow-up on both safety and efficacy is needed. NICE have produced guidance for the UK, stating the procedure can be undertaken with 'special arrangements for clinical governance, consent and audit or research'.

Renal Tumours

Intervention for renal tumours is essentially limited to the control of haemorrhage. Preoperative embolisation to facilitate surgical excision although popular in the past is rarely undertaken nowadays with improvements in surgical management.

Benign

Benign renal tumours are rare. Oncocytomas are often indistinguishable from malignant tumours when small and even differentiation at pathology can be challenging. Bleeding is rare but there are case reports in the literature of embolisation being used. Angiomyolipomas are much more common and present a challenge to the interventional radiologist. Although the majority are isolated there is a well-known link with tuberous sclerosis where they are said to be the commonest cause of death. It is in this syndrome and when lesions are > 4 cm in size that the risk of bleeding increases significantly. Spontaneous bleeding occurs in 50–60% when > 4 cm and up to a third of patients present with shock.[17]

Embolisation is the procedure of choice and controls bleeding in over 90% (Fig. 8-9). Embolic agents include particles, alcohol and coils, often in combination. Although there is a potential risk of loss of renal function, this is rare or minimal. Re-bleeding is reasonably common but can be treated with repeat embolisation. Complications are uncommon but include aneurysmal rupture. The angiomyogenic component of the tumour is more sensitive to embolisation than the lipomatous elements and it is the former that is thought to bleed.[18]

Malignant

This group essentially consists of renal cell carcinoma. Spontaneous haemorrhage is not uncommon and indeed may be the initial presentation often with a history of trivial trauma. Usually hypervascular (85%) these tumours are very amenable to embolisation. Provided the other kidney is normal, embolisation of the entire kidney is the simplest approach. Although placing coils in the main proximal renal artery is tempting and easy, a more distal embolisation should be performed as parasitic supply from other vessels, e.g. lumbar arteries, is common and these in turn may need to be embolised. A careful eye should be kept for connections with other vessels such as colic arteries, particularly if liquid embolic agents are contemplated. The choice of embolic agent includes particulate matter (e.g. polyvinyl alcohol), liquids (e.g. alcohol), histoacryl glue or Onyx. When using alcohol, temporary balloon occlusion of the main renal artery will considerably reduce the peri-procedural pain.

Renal Arteriovenous Malformation (AVM)

Renal arteriovenous malformations are abnormal connections between the intrarenal arteries and veins. They are either congenital or acquired (often iatrogenic). Acquired lesions are often termed A-V fistula and are

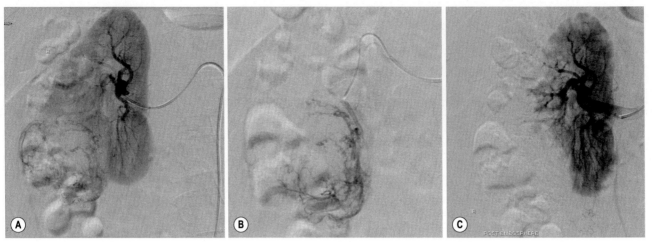

FIGURE 8-9 ■ **Renal embolization—angiomyolipoma presenting with acute loin pain and haematuria.** (A) Right renal angiogram showing abnormal mass of tissue at the lower pole. (B) Super selective angiogram showing multiple abnormal vessels supplying the angiomyolipomatous tissue. (C) Image taken following embolisation with particulate matter showing complete de-vascularisation of the AML.

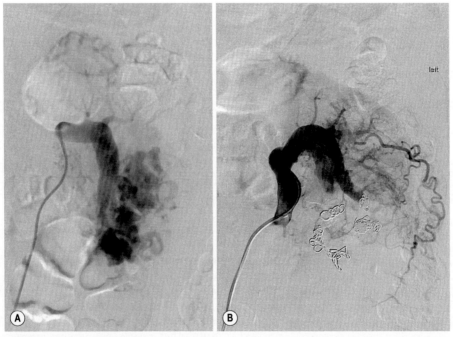

FIGURE 8-10 ■ **Renal arteriovenous malformation.** (A) Left renal angiogram showing massively enlarged left renal artery with a complex AVM involving the middle and lower pole of the kidney. A small upper pole branch is not involved. Patient presented in high output cardiac failure. (B) Renal AVM embolisation. Left renal angiogram following embolisation of the AVM with a combination of coils, alcohol and histoacryl glue.

dealt with in the section 'Trauma Embolisation'. AVMs are either detected coincidentally or present with haematuria and a renal mass. Patients are commonly hypertensive and occasionally there may be so much shunting that high output cardiac failure ensues (Fig. 8-10A). The more common cirsoid lesion has multiple feeding arteries and draining veins with a definite mass. The less common cavernous type consists of a single artery feeding a dilated chamber draining through a single vein. Embolisation has almost completely replaced surgery for these lesions and the results are good with cure being a realistic expectation. However, embolisation of any AVM is always complex and should only be undertaken by those with adequate experience and training. Referral to a tertiary centre is frequent. Embolisation is almost always from the arterial side and it may be necessary to use temporary occlusion balloons to reduce blood flow to control the embolisation process (Fig. 8-10B). Alcohol, histoacryl glue, Onyx and particles have all been used and each has their advocates.

Renal Artery Aneurysms

Visceral artery aneurysms are rare but renal aneurysms make up 22% of the group. The main aetiologies are atherosclerosis, fibromuscular disease (Fig. 8-6) and the other rarer arteritides. Usually asymptomatic and detected incidentally, they can present with hypertension, haematuria or flank or abdominal pain. Indications for treatment are size > 2 cm, symptoms and women who wish to become pregnant. Pseudoaneurysms are usually a result of trauma and dealt with in the section 'Trauma Embolisation'.

Technique

Although there may be the occasional argument for open surgical repair, advances in endovascular technology have led to embolisation being employed in the vast majority of cases. However, embolisation of these aneurysms can be technically very demanding and should be undertaken only by experienced operators. Every attempt should be made to preserve renal tissue and the only excuse for simple embolisation (closing off the vessel distal to the aneurysm) is in small intra-renal lesions where functional loss would be minimal. Loss of renal tissue or even ischaemic renal tissue may lead to troublesome post embolisation hypertension.

Treatment options include coil or liquid embolisation with either an adhesive agent, e.g. histoacryl or a non-adhesive agent such as Onyx. Although these can be used as stand alone therapy some form of protection for the distal renal vessel is often required. Examples include using an angioplasty balloon to prevent reflux of liquid Onyx or stents to 'jail in' coils. New neuroradiology systems with electrolytic released stents (Solitaire EV3, UK) allow complex branches to be preserved by stenting through stents and then using retrievable coils placed through the stent lattices. Although very expensive this technology lends itself to challenging anatomy (Fig. 8-6). There is a case for some form of continued imaging surveillance on an annual basis and smaller aneurysms not treated should also be kept under review.

TRAUMA EMBOLISATION

Haemorrhage control has recently become a major focus for interventional radiology (IR) service provision with increased recognition of its benefits over more invasive open surgery. There is reasonable evidence (although no trials) to show that embolisation can halt traumatic arterial haemorrhage with the advantage over surgery of offering a minimally invasive approach with minimal tissue or organ loss. It can often be carried out under local anaesthesia.

Kidney

Although both blunt and penetrating trauma, e.g. stabbing, is well recognised the majority of cases are iatrogenic in origin from either percutaneous nephrostomy or renal biopsy. Imaging studies have shown a high prevalence (1–10%) of traumatic pseudoaneurysm or A-V fistula following renal biopsy. The majority of these settle with simple observation and embolisation should only be considered if there is expansion of the pseudoaneurysm, persistent pain or frank haemorrhage. If treatment is deemed necessary then embolisation using coils is the procedure of choice. Care should be taken to use a superselective technique with coaxial catheters to ensure a distal embolization, minimising any loss of renal tissue (Fig. 8-11).

Occasionally following major blunt abdominal trauma the main renal artery may be either avulsed or occluded. Usually the kidney will have suffered irreversible ischaemia but on occasion it may be worth considering an

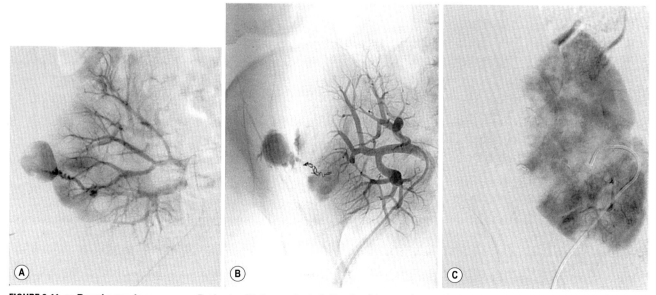

FIGURE 8-11 ■ **Renal pseudoaneurysm. Patient with haematuria following biopsy of a renal transplant.** (A) Angiogram shows a large pseudoaneurysm. (B) Angiogram following coil occlusion of feeding branch. (C) Late nephrogeic phase showing minimal loss of renal tissue.

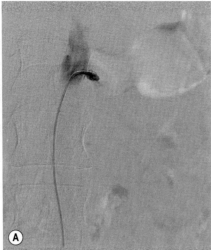

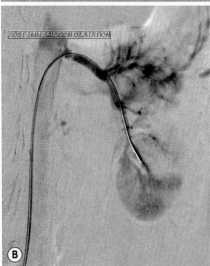

POST 5MM BALLOON DILATATION

FIGURE 8-12 ■ **Renal artery traumatic occlusion.** (A) Angiogram shows occluded left renal artery with a short stump at origin. (B) Successful recanalistion and angioplasty. (Reproduced by kind permission of Dr A. Todd Raigmore Hospital Inverness.)

attempt to recanalise the vessel using angioplasty or stenting (Fig. 8-12).

Ureter

Ureteric trauma is rare and almost always iatrogenic. Rarely a fistula between the ureter and the adjacent iliac artery can develop and present with massive haematuria. The aetiology is usually related to a ureteric stent eroding through the ureter or direct invasion by cancer. Treatment involves placing an appropriate sized stent graft in the iliac artery.[19]

Bladder

Vascular damage to the bladder or prostate causing intractable haemorrhage is very rare but there are case reports of prostatic embolisation being used after prostatic surgery. Rarely chemotherapy (e.g.

cyclophosphamide) can cause a severe haemorrhagic cystitis requiring embolisation.[20]

PROSTATIC ARTERY EMBOLISATION

Symptomatic benign prostatic hyperplasia (BPH) is a common condition typically presenting in the sixth and seventh decades. Over 40% of males will be symptomatic usually presenting with lower urinary tract symptoms (LUTS) such as hesitancy, frequency and urgency. Extreme cases present as an emergency with acute urinary retention. Standard treatment is usually with drugs such as 5-alpha reductase inhibitors and selective alpha-blockers. When these fail, the classical surgical procedure is transurethral resection of the prostate (TURP), although recently other options such as laser and microwave ablation have been under evaluation.

Prostatic artery embolisation is not new and has been used sporadically for haemorrhage since 1976. However, its potential use in controlling the symptoms of BPH has only recently been reported.[21]

Rather similar to fibroid embolisation it relies on occluding the blood supply to the prostate gland, thereby reducing the volume of the gland and its pressure on the urethra (Fig. 8-13). The procedure involves catheterising the prostatic arteries and embolising with a propriety embolic agent, e.g. PVA particles. Early experience to date (2012) is limited to two centres (in Brazil and Portugal) who have collectively treated about 90 patients. The procedure is technically demanding due to the size of the vessels, tortuosity and anatomical variation and failure rates of up to 30% are reported. Complications have included bladder wall ischaemia, rectal bleeding and urethral pain. Mean reduction in prostatic volume appears to be around 30% with an improvement in both quality of life and objective urinary symptom scores. Several patients using long-term catheters have been able to re-establish normal micturition. Advantages over surgery may include lack of incontinence and preserved sexual function.

Clearly an exciting new procedure, the long term outcomes and durability are unknown. Prostatic embolisation is currently undergoing assessment by NICE (2012) in the UK.

FIBROID EMBOLISATION

Uterine Artery Embolisation (UAE)

Uterine fibroids are the commonest tumour found in women of reproductive age and the prevalence increases up to the menopause where it can be as high as 80% in some ethnic groups (Afrocarribean). At least half of women with fibroids are asymptomatic and need no active treatment. Symptoms include menorrhagia, pain and pressure; the pressure symptoms commonly involve the bladder and occasionally the bowel. A further group either has problems conceiving or suffers early pregnancy loss. The pathophysiology behind all these symptoms is not clear and in particular the link between fibroids and infertility is tenuous and may only apply to submucosal locations. Women with fibroid-related menorrhagia often have more severe menstrual loss than those with dysfunctional uterine bleeding and are more resistant to standard medical care.

Treatment Options

Medical management includes drugs such as non-steroidal anti-inflammatories, anti-fibrinolytics and hormonal manipulation. Second-line treatment includes the progesterone intrauterine device (Mirena coil) and endometrial ablation. These second-line measures are only technically feasible if the uterine cavity is less than 12 cm in length and not distorted by the fibroids. Third-line management is either surgical (myomectomy or hysterectomy) or uterine artery embolisation (UAE). Current guidance states that all treatment options should be discussed with patients so that they can make an informed choice.

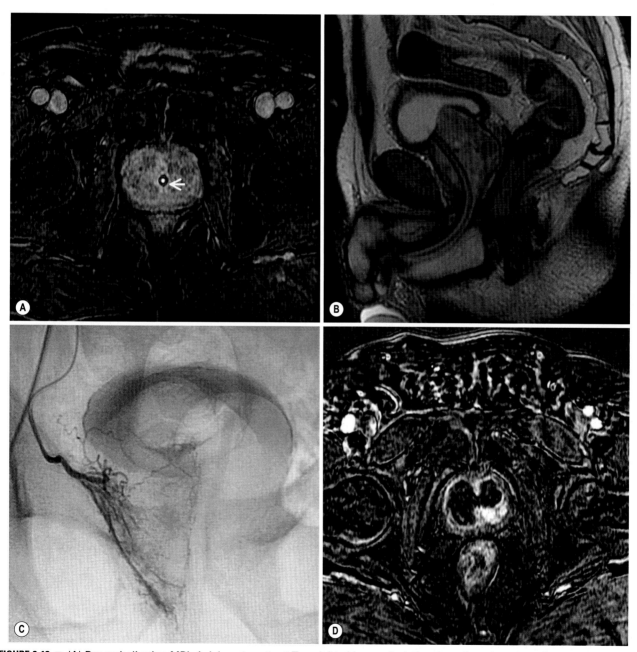

FIGURE 8-13 ■ (A) Pre-embolization MRI. Axial post-contrast T_1-weighted image depicting the enlarged prostate due to central gland nodules. Note the presence of the urethral catheter (white arrow). (B) MRI pre-embolization. Sagittal T_2-weighted image depicting an enlarged prostate due to central gland nodules protruding into the bladder neck. Note the presence of the urethral catheter. (C) Arteriogram after superselective catheterization of the right inferior vesical artery showing the right prostate arteries—urethral arteries (black arrow) and the capsular arteries (white arrow). (D) One-month post-embolization MRI. Axial post-contrast T1-weighted image depicting bilateral avascular areas (mainly on the right side) in the central gland (white arrows), and reduction of the prostate size.

Continued on following page

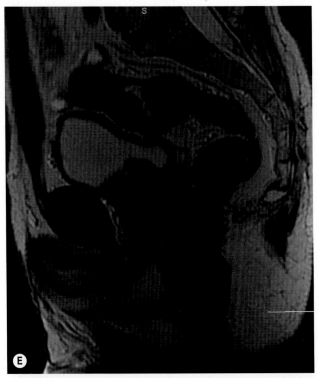

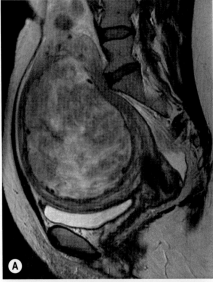

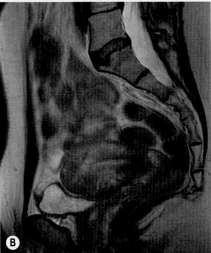

FIGURE 8-13, Continued ■ (E) MRI post-embolization. Sagittal T$_2$-weighted image showing a reduction of the central gland size. (Reproduced with kind permission from Dr FC Carnevale, MD. PhD, Professor and Chief of Interventional Radiology, University of Sao Paulo, Brazil.)

FIGURE 8-14 ■ **Fibroid uterus.** (A) Sagittal T$_2$-weighted image showing a large intramural fibroid. (B) Sagittal T$_2$-weighted image following uterine artery embolisation shows complete resolution of fibroid.

Imaging

Some form of baseline imaging is essential prior to embarking on UAE. This is to firmly establish the diagnosis, exclude other pathologies and assess the number of fibroids and their location. Although ultrasound is inexpensive, it lacks the precision of MRI and suffers from operator expertise and poor assessment of vascularity. The general availability of MRI should make this the imaging modality of choice (Fig. 8-14A) and contrast enhancement should be used routinely. Occasionally a non-enhancing fibroid which would not be suitable for UAE is seen. Adenomyosis is a not-infrequent concomitant finding and can cause identical symptoms to fibroids. It is not a contraindication to embolisation but the outcomes are less robust than with fibroids alone. Although almost any fibroid can be embolised there are situations where surgery may be more effective, examples include a submucosal fibroid on a stalk where hysteroscopic resection is simple and effective. More controversy surrounds pedunculated subserosal fibroids and very large lesions but increasingly these are being safely embolised. Clearly UAE is not appropriate if the diagnosis of fibroids is in any doubt and it should be remembered that neither MRI nor any other imaging modality can reliably detect the very rare coincidental leiomyosarcoma unless there are signs of extrauterine spread.

It is increasingly common practice and reassuring to repeat the MR imaging at around 6 months to confirm infarction and tumour shrinkage (Fig. 8-14B).

Technique

Preoperative preparation is essential for this procedure. The patient will usually be admitted on the day of the procedure and expect to be staying for one night. This is purely to manage the post embolisation pain, which if improperly controlled can be very severe. An analgesic protocol should be in place ideally agreed in liaison with the anaesthetic department. Analgesia should be administered on the ward prior to UAE, during and after the procedure. Opioid drugs are required with antiemetics and can be given using a patient-controlled pump if desired. Patients will be discharged on oral analgesia.

The procedure itself is relatively straightforward and not painful. Prophylactic antibiotics are often administered. Access is from the right common femoral artery and using a 4–5F cobra-shaped catheter the aortic bifurcation is crossed and the contralateral anterior division of the internal iliac artery selected. It is common practice

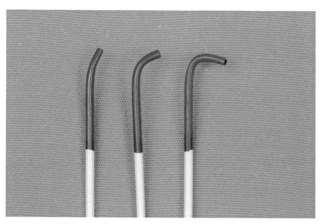

FIGURE 8-15 ■ **Catheters.** The various types and shapes of Vanschie catheter tips (Cook, UK) used for selective uterine artery catheterisation.

at this stage to use a coaxial catheter to select the uterine artery. This minimises the risk of spasm, allowing free flow embolisation. The choice of embolic agent is often one of operator preference and there is no evidence that any of the newer more expensive agents are superior to standard non-spherical PVA. Particle size ranges between 300 and 700 μm and a frequently used embolic end-point is complete stasis in the uterine artery. The catheter is then withdrawn and the ipsilateral internal iliac and uterine artery selected and embolised. Occasionally the anatomy can be challenging and other catheter shapes such as a reverse curve or Vanschie (Cook, Europe) are required (Fig. 8-15). A minority of operators use a bilateral femoral artery approach claiming a reduction in radiation burden.

Safety and Efficacy

NICE has recently (2011) updated its guidance on UAE, stating it can be carried out using 'normal arrangements'.[22] Complications are usually minor and include the post embolisation syndrome (pain, fever, raised inflammatory markers), vaginal discharge and infection. Major complications are less frequent and include severe infection, fibroid expulsion and premature ovarian failure. When compared with surgical options the incidence of complications is very similar, albeit the complications are different.

Long-term follow-up from several randomised trials,[23–25] a Cochrane review[26] and a meta-analysis[27] has shown a similar improvement in quality of life and patient satisfaction compared with surgery but there is a need for re-intervention in a significant minority (20–30%) after UAE due to either complications or recurrent/persistent symptoms. The advantage of UAE over surgery is a significantly faster recovery time with more rapid return to normal activities and uterine preservation. Re-intervention does not always mean hysterectomy and if there is incomplete fibroid infarction, repeat UAE can be offered and is often successful.

Questions still remain, particularly the role of UAE in women wishing to preserve their fertility. A small trial

has suggested superior pregnancy outcomes with myomectomy[28] but a much larger trial (FEMME; <http://www.hta.ac.uk/project/2378.asp>) is now underway in the UK.

OBSTETRIC HAEMORRHAGE

The World Health Organisation estimates that severe bleeding complicates 10% of all live births and accounts for 24% of all maternal deaths annually.[29] However, in the developed world there has been a dramatic reduction in maternal death due to haemorrhage. Advances in blood transfusion, surgical techniques and critical care have all made major contributions. However, major obstetric haemorrhage (MOH) remains a major cause of maternal morbidity and is the leading cause in Scotland (4.3/1000 live births).[30] A wide range of clinical interventions is now available and has been proposed in the management of MOH, including:

- Pharmacological agents (recombinant activated factor VII);
- Intrauterine balloons;
- Uterine compressive suture (B Lynch suture);
- Supportive interventions (cell salvage); and
- Interventional radiological techniques (embolisation and balloon occlusion).

In 2006 the Royal College of Obstetricians and Gynaecologists recommended the early involvement of interventional radiology in the management of post partum haemorrhage (PPH).[31] One challenge for IR is to provide a deliverable 24/7 service (which is still patchy in some countries, e.g. the UK) before obstetricians will fully accept its role.

Post Partum Haemorrhage

The definition of PPH depends on the timing and blood loss. Primary PPH occurs within the first 24 hr of delivery and involves a blood loss of at least 500 cc. Secondary PPH occurs after 24 hr and is usually linked to either retained parts and/or infection.

Causes of PPH

- Uterine atony—the commonest cause > 50%
- Genital tract lacerations
- Abnormal placentation
- Post caesarean section or hysterectomy
- Rare causes, e.g. uterine AVM

Management of PPH

Embolisation is never the first-line treatment but should also not be used as a last resort. Units should develop their own agreed algorithm but a generic strategy would include standard use of uterotonics, and removal of any retained parts. If this fails then an intrauterine balloon is a simple and effective next step with reported success rates as high as 91%.[32] If the abdomen is already open then a uterine compression suture, e.g. B-Lynch, can be placed. If these measures are ineffective then embolisation should be used with the primary aim of stopping bleeding and preserving the uterus. Avoidance of maternal mortality is critical. Obstetric units can measure the effectiveness of their PPH algorithm by auditing the peri-partum hysterectomy rate.

Technique

Although CT angiography is now used routinely prior to embolisation in the gut or following trauma, it is infrequently deployed in PPH, as it is usually obvious on clinical grounds whether haemorrhage is occurring. However, it may have a role in recurrent bleeding or post hysterectomy. The embolisation technique is fairly standard and very similar to that used for fibroids. Access, however, is best from a bilateral common femoral artery approach with catheterisation of the anterior divisions of the internal iliacs and embolisation of the offending bleeding point (usually the uterine artery) with Gelfoam. A negative angiogram should prompt a search for other vessels particularly if post-caesarean section or hysterectomy (Fig. 8-16). However, a negative angiogram is not uncommon particularly with uterine atony. It has become accepted practice to carry out 'empirical embolisation' in these circumstances although there is little high quality evidence to support this strategy. Almost always bilateral embolisation will be required as there is such a good cross flow collateral circulation in the pelvis. Failure to control PPH by embolisation is rare but more likely to occur with abnormal placentation (see section below). Continued haemorrhage requires good clinical judgement and a hysterectomy may be unavoidable. Recurrent bleeding can usually be re-embolised.

Abnormal Placentation

Abnormal placentation occurs when a defect within the decidua basalis allows invasion of the chorionic villi into the myometrium. There are three types (Fig. 8-17) with the least invasive (accreta) being the most prevalent (84%). Placenta accreta refers to a placenta invading the myometrium. Placenta increta (13%) occurs when the serosa is reached and percreta (3%) when invasion occurs beyond the serosa into adjacent structures such as the bladder. Maternal morbidity is clearly related to the degree of invasion. Abnormal placentation has increased in incidence by a factor of 10 over the past 50 years and the most important risk factors are the combination of previous caesarean sections and placenta previa. Ideally this condition should be suspected and confirmed prenatally to allow a management plan. Imaging modalities include US and increasingly MRI but the sensitivities vary from 33 to 95%. The more severe case with bladder invasion is easier to detect. This condition is the leading cause of a peri-partum hysterectomy and carries a maternal mortality of up to 7%.

Management of Abnormal Placentation. If confirmed or suspected pre-natally an organised pre-delivery strategy should be put in place involving an interventional

radiologist. The plan must include the location of delivery, e.g. interventional or obstetric theatre, availability of cell salvage for blood transfusion and a decision whether to try to preserve the uterus, possibly leaving the placenta in situ or a planned caesarean hysterectomy. Whatever is decided these are complex procedures and fully informed consent should be obtained by both the obstetrician and interventional radiologist. The patient's view on caesarean hysterectomy is important and should be respected if possible. Bilateral common femoral artery access should be established. Some suggest that after establishing access, the IR should wait and see how the caesarean section progresses. If the bleeding can be controlled by surgical means no embolization may be required. However, many would be more pro-active and place at least guidewires and possibly occlusion balloons in the common iliac, internal iliacs or uterine arteries and inflate these just prior to incising the uterus or placenta. Care should be taken to correctly size the balloons and particular care taken if the uterine arteries are catheterised prior to delivery (Fig. 8-18). There are anecdotal reports of anoxia in the child where balloons have been inflated in the uterine arteries, which are sensitive to spasm. There are reports of parasitic supply to the uterus from branches arising from the common femoral artery and others and the author's preference is to use common iliac balloons, which will cater for most extrauterine supply. On occasion an aortic occlusion balloon may be useful as a last-resort life-saving manoeuvre. If balloon inflation controls the haemorrhage, and the obstetrician can suture satisfactorily, embolisation may not be needed. However, if on deflating the balloons bleeding returns then embolisation will be required. Depending on the balloon position, this may require further selective catheterisation. Embolisation should always be as targeted as possible. Gelfoam is the usual embolic agent although almost all other particle types have been reported. If the decision has been made to leave the uterus and placenta in situ, embolisation of the uterus may facilitate subsequent placental involution.

Complications of Embolisation and Balloon Occlusion

In experienced hands the complications rates should be low and this is supported by the literature. Most complications are minor and puncture site-related. However, major complications can occur and include buttock and lower limb ischaemia, small bowel, uterine, vaginal, cervical and bladder wall necrosis.[33] Neurological damage involving the sciatic and femoral nerves has occurred. Control of PPH can be challenging for the interventional radiologist; sometimes the imaging equipment is suboptimal, e.g. a mobile C-arm, plus the added pressure of needing to work quickly in an already overcrowded obstetric theatre environment.

Results of Haemorrhage Control for PPH

There is little doubt that embolisation for PPH works: a meta-analysis of nonsurgical management found a

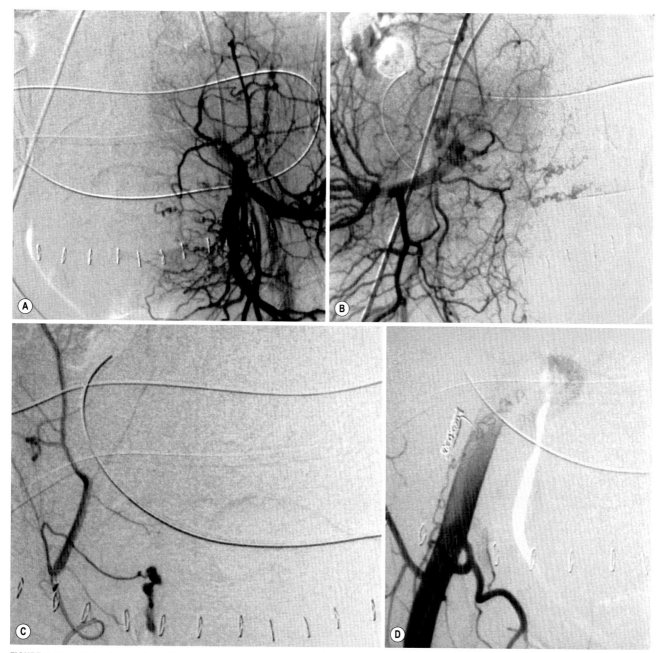

FIGURE 8-16 ■ **Patient bleeding after emergency caesarean section.** (A) Selective left and (B) right internal iliac artery angiograms show no evidence of uterine bleeding. (C) A selective angiogram of the right inferior epigastric artery shows frank extravasation of contrast from a muscular branch of the rectus muscle. (D) Initial occlusion of the distal inferior epigastric prior to particulate embolisation of the small branch.

cumulative success rate of 91%.[34] A recent national cohort study carried out in the UK (226 maternity units) identified 272 women who were treated with one or more second-line treatments, representing an estimated rate of 2.2 cases per 10,000 women delivering.[35] The success rates of the first second-line therapy were as follows: uterine compression sutures 75%, pelvic vessel ligation 36%, embolisation 86% and rFVII 31%. The overall peri-partum hysterectomy rate was 26%.

Outcomes for abnormal placentation are less clear and the literature produces conflicting results. It is likely that an invasive placenta is a predictor for embolisation failure and the more invasive the placenta, e.g. percreta, the

worse the outcome. This probably reflects the aggressive blood supply from both uterine and non-uterine arteries. Clear benefit to mother and child requires further research and study.

Ectopic Pregnancy and Spontaneous Abortion

Cervical ectopic pregnancy is very rare (0.15% of all ectopics) but carries a significant haemorrhagic risk. Embolisation has been reported for both active bleeding and prior to dilation and curettage.[36] Re-bleeding is relatively frequent (25%) and may require further embolisation or a more radical surgical solution. Post abortion haemorrhage can usually be controlled medically but there are sporadic case reports of successful embolisation in the literature.[37]

PELVIC CONGESTION SYNDROME

Chronic pelvic pain is a common problem affecting women aged between 18 and 50 years. Pelvic congestion syndrome (PCS) is one of the many possible causes of

this condition. Dull pelvic ache is thought to be secondary to ovarian and pelvic varicosities. Incompetent venous valves, multiple pregnancies, effect of oestrogen, retro-aortic left renal vein, compression of left ovarian and renal veins by superior mesenteric artery and compression of left common iliac vein by right common iliac artery are proposed predisposing factors.[38] By the time of referral to an interventional radiologist patients will usually have already undergone extensive investigation and imaging often including laparoscopy. Cystic ovaries are seen in more than half of these women. Vulval or leg varicosities may also be present. MRI with MR venography (Figs. 8-19, 8-20) is a valuable

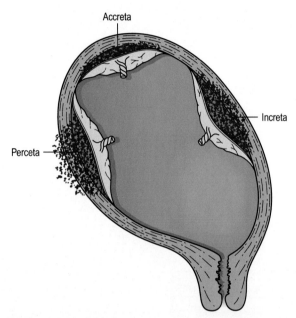

FIGURE 8-17 ■ **Classification of invasive placenta.** Image showing different degrees of placental invasion into the uterine wall.

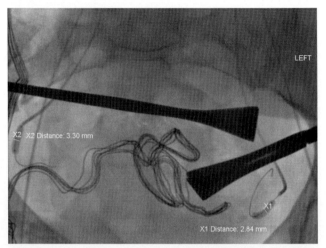

FIGURE 8-18 ■ **Uterine artery balloon occlusion.** Patient with an invasive placenta undergoing prophylactic balloon occlusion of both uterine arteries to minimise blood loss during caesarean section.

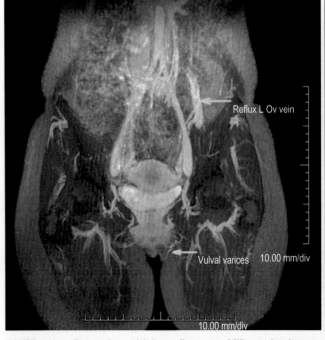
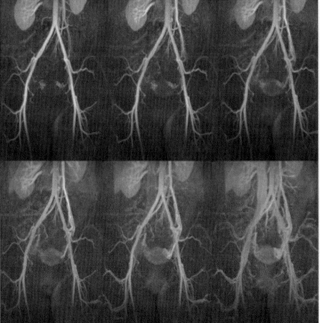

FIGURE 8-19 ■ **Dynamic multiphase first-pass MIPs and subsequent steady-state phase slab MIP of contrast-enhanced MRA/V of abdominopelvic veins.** Patient with vulval varicosities demonstrating rapid early reflux in incompetent left ovarian vein. (Reproduced with permission from Giles Roditi, Magnetic Resonance Venography in Clinical Blood Pool MR Imaging 2008, pp 115–130. Fig 10.16A.)

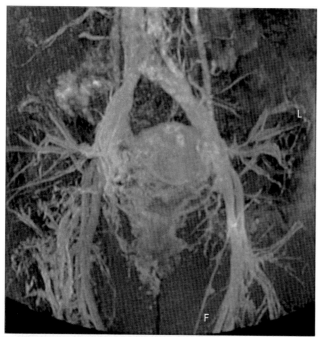

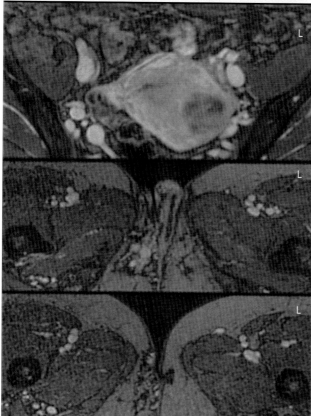

FIGURE 8-20 ■ Coronal MIP of pelvis in steady state in patient with vulval varicosities demonstrating ipsilateral deep venous varicosities in right thigh draining to internal iliac pelvic venous varicosities (incidental uterine fibroid). (Reproduced with permission from Giles Roditi, Magnetic Resonance Venography in Clinical Blood Pool MR Imaging 2008, pp 115–130.)

TABLE 8-2	Diagnostic Criteria for PCS on Venography

- 5 mm or greater diameter of ovarian vein
- Retrograde flow in ovarian or pelvic veins
- Presence of tortuous collateral veins in pelvis crossing the midline
- Delayed clearance of contrast from pelvic veins

non-invasive imaging tool. However, all non-invasive imaging suffers from potential venous collapse in the supine position and many will still perform conventional catheter ovarian vein venography with the table tilted head up to fully assess gonadal vein incompetence. Generally agreed diagnostic criteria for PCS[39] are listed in Table 8-2.

Treatment

Ovarian vein embolisation (Fig. 8-21) is usually straightforward and performed through either a right common femoral vein or increasingly a right internal jugular vein approach. This is a day case procedure and embolisation has been reported using a wide variety of embolic agents including liquids, sclerosants, gelfoam, coils and vascular plugs. It is often necessary to embolise both ovarian veins. Technical success rates are high and some have reported clinical improvement in 83% of patients.[40] Clinical failures may be due to additional incompetent internal iliac venous collaterals and more aggressive workers also target these claiming good results. Complications are rare and include venous perforation, non-target embolisation and thrombophlebitis.

Vulval varices can cause labial hypertrophy affecting one or both side. If troublesome these can be treated by direct injection sclerotherapy using sodium tetradecyl sulphate (STD). It is important in these cases always to exclude and treat any ovarian venous incompetence first.

VARICOCOELE

The male equivalent of PCS, a varicocoele, is an abnormal dilatation of the pampiniform plexus of veins draining the testes resulting from an incompetent testicular vein. A common condition said to afflict up to 10% of males it is usually asymptomatic, requiring simple reassurance. When symptomatic the discomfort is described as a dragging sensation usually in the left testicle often worse during strenuous activity. In 10–15% of cases they can be bilateral. Patients with unilateral right-sided varicocoele should be evaluated for pathology such as renal tumours, retroperitoneal lymphadenopathy and anatomical variants such as situs inversus. Ultrasound has a very high sensitivity and specificity and tortuous veins greater than 3 mm are considered diagnostic.[41] Typically, on palpation they are described as a 'bag of worms'.

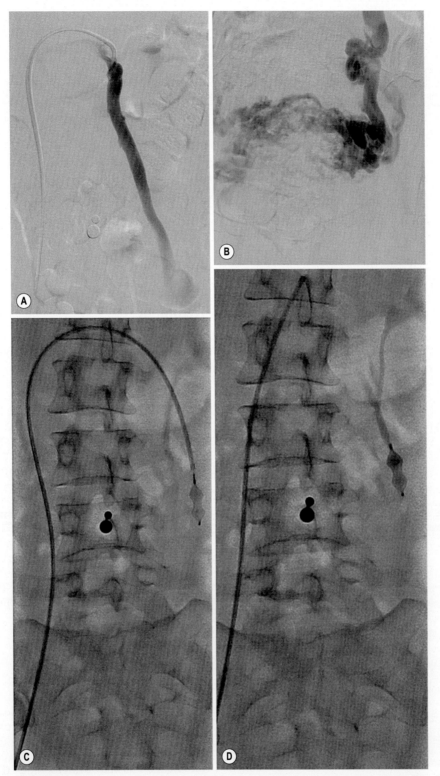

FIGURE 8-21 ■ Ovarian vein embolisation. (A) Left renal venogram shows reflux into the left ovarian vein. (B) Venogram shows enlarged left ovarian vein and tortuous pelvic veins crossing midline. (C, D) Deployment of Amplatzer vascular plug in the left ovarian vein from right femoral vein approach.

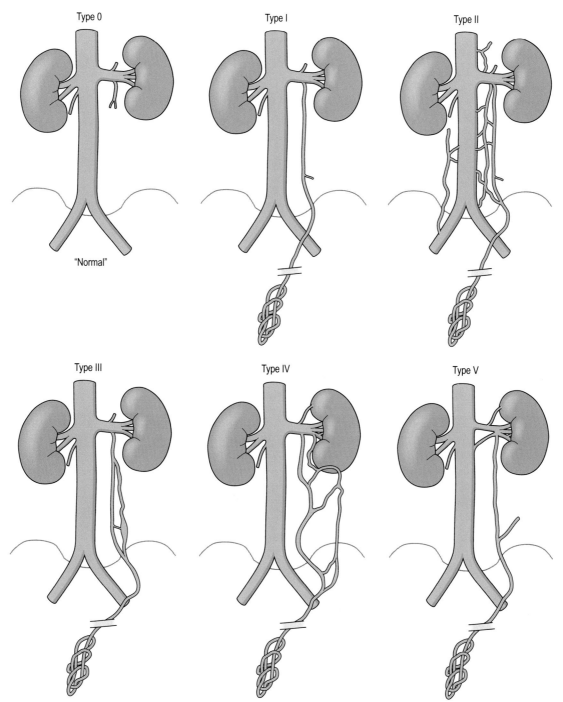

FIGURE 8-22 ▪ **Line diagram showing anatomical variants of testicular venous drainage.** (Redrawn from Sigmund G, Bahren W, Gall H, et al 1987 Idiopathic varicoceles: feasibility of percutaneous sclerotherapy. Radiology 164(1):161–168.)

Varicocoeles are sometimes discovered during investigations for male infertility but although improvement in sperm density, motility, morphology and testicular volume after treatment have been reported, NICE guidelines currently state, 'Men should not be offered surgery for varicocoeles as a form of fertility treatment because it does not improve pregnancy rates.'[42]

There is a lot of anatomical variation in testicular venous drainage. A recognised description is presented as shown in Fig. 8-22. See also Table 8-3.

Treatment

Although the gonadal vein can be ligated in the inguinal canal or from a pre-peritoneal laparoscopic approach,

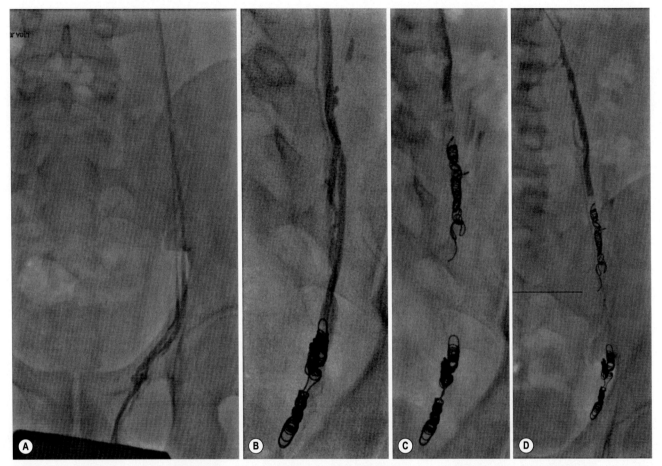

FIGURE 8-23 ■ **Left varicocoele embolisation.** (A) Venogram of left spermatic vein and (B–D) images showing embolisation with multiple coils.

TABLE 8-3   **Classification of Gonadal Vein Anatomy**

Type 0	Normal
Type I	Single testicular vein without valves
Type II	Afferent collateral medial retroperitoneal vessels to the ascending lumbar or retroperitoneal veins
(IIa	No valve)
(IIb	Valve present at entry into renal vein)
Type III	Duplicated testicular vein/internal spermatic vein
Type IV	Collateral flow from lateral renal vein and peri-renal veins to testicular vein
(IVa	No valve)
(IVb	Valve present and bypassed by insufficient collaterals)
Type V	Bifurcated renal vein with a retroaortic component

embolisation (Fig. 8-23) has become the mainstay of modern minimally invasive treatment. A simple day case procedure undertaken from either a common femoral but increasingly right jugular vein approach, the left renal vein and the left testicular vein are selectively catheterised. Venography is performed to confirm reflux and delineate the anatomy. The right testicular vein usually arises from the IVC directly around the level of the right renal vein and is more difficult to select. Almost every embolic agent manufactured has been reported in this procedure but the majority of operators will choose to use simple embolisation coils, placing these fairly distal at the level of the inguinal ligament. Embolisation is performed from distal to proximal. Complications related to the procedure include venous spasm, perforation and non-target embolisation and thrombophlebitis post procedure. Care is taken to minimise the radiation dose to the testes by using a gonadal shield.

Although the technical success rate is close to 100% the clinical results are lower at around 85%. It should be appreciated there are other causes of scrotal pain and the varicocoele may simply be coincidental.

REFERENCES

1. Textor SC. Revascularization in atherosclerotic renal artery disease. Kidney Int 1998;53:799–811.
2. Van de ven PJG, Kaatee R, Beutler JJ, et al. Arterial stenting and balloon angioplasty in ostial atherosclerotic renovascular disease: a randomised trial. Lancet 1999;353:282–6.
3. Plouin PF, Chatellier G, Darne B, Raynaud A. Blood pressure outcome of angioplasty in atherosclerotic renal artery stenosis: a randomized trial. Hypertension 1998;31:823–9.
4. Webster J, Marshall F, Abdalla M, et al. Randomised comparison of percutaneous angioplasty vs continued medical therapy for hypertensive patients with atheromatous renal artery stenosis. J Hum Hypertens 1998;12:329–35.
5. Van Jaarsveld BC, Krijnen P, Pieterman H, et al. The effect of balloon angioplasty on hypertension in atherosclerotic renal artery stenosis. N Engl J Med 2000;342:1007–14.
6. Bax L, Woittiez AJ, Kouwenberg HJ, et al. Stent placement in patients with atherosclerotic renal artery stenosis and impaired renal function: a randomized trial. Ann Intern Med 2009;150(12):840–8, W150–1.
7. Wheatley K, Ives N, Gray R, et al. Revascularization versus medical therapy for renal-artery stenosis. N Engl J Med 2009;361(20):1953–62.
8. Shetty R, Biondi-Zoccai GG, Abbate A, et al. Percutaneous renal artery intervention versus medical therapy in patients with renal artery stenosis: a meta-analysis. EuroIntervention 2011;7(7):844–51.
9. Kumbhani DJ, Bavry AA, Harvey JE, et al. Clinical outcomes after percutaneous revascularization versus medical management in patients with significant renal artery stenosis: a meta-analysis of randomized controlled trials. Am Heart J 2011;161:622–30.
10. Cooper CJ, Murphy TP, Matsumoto A, et al. Stent revascularization for the prevention of cardiovascular and renal events among patients with renal artery stenosis and systolic hypertension: rationale and design of the CORAL trial. Am Heart J 2006;152:59–66.
11. Tegtmeyer CJ, Matsumoto AH, Angle JF. Percutaneous transluminal angioplasty in fibrous dysplasia and children. In: Novick A, Scoble J, Hamilton G, editors. Renal Vascular Disease. 1st ed. London: WB Saunders; 1995. p. 363–83.
12. Statistical fact sheet 2012 Update | American Heart Association. Available from: http://www.heart.org/idc/groups/heart-public/@wcm/@sop/@smd/documents/downloadable/ucm_319587.pdf. Accessed 1 July 2012.
13. Smithwick RH. Hypertensive vascular disease: results of and indications for splanchnicectomy. J Chronic Dis 1955;1:477–96.
14. Krum H, Schlaich M, Whitbourn R, et al. Catheter-based renal sympathetic denervation for resistant hypertension: a multicentre safety and proof-of-principle cohort study. Lancet 2009;373:1275–81.
15. NICE | Interventional procedure guidance 418. Percutaneous transluminal radiofrequency sympathetic denervation of the renal artery for resistant hypertension. Available from: http://www.nice.org.uk/nicemedia/live/13340/57923/57923.pdf. Accessed 1 July 2012.
16. Esler MD, Krum H, Sobotka PA, et al. Renal sympathetic denervation in patients with treatment-resistant hypertension (The Symplicity HTN-2 trial): a randomised controlled trial. Lancet 2010;376:1903–9.
17. Soulen MC, Faykus MH Jr, Shlansky-Goldberg RD, et al. Elective Embolization for Prevention of Hemorrhage from Renal Angiomyolipomas. J Vasc Interv Radiol 1994;5(4):587–91.
18. Ewalt DH, Dimond N, Rees C, et al. Long-term outcome of transcatheter embolization of renal angiomyolipomas due to tuberous sclerosis complex. J Urol 2005;174(5):1764–6.
19. Yamasaki T, Yagihashi Y, Shirahase T, et al. [Endovascular stent graft for management of ureteroarterial fistula: a case report.] Hinyokika Kiyo 2004;50(9):641–4.
20. Cho CL, Lai MH, So HS, et al. Superselective embolisation of bilateral superior vesical arteries for management of haemorrhagic cystitis. Hong Kong Med J 2008;14(6):485–1488.
21. Carnevale FC, Antunes AA, Motta-Leal-Filho JM, et al. Prostatic artery embolization as a primary treatment for benign prostatic hyperplasia: preliminary results in two patients. Cardiovasc Intervent Radiol 2010;33(2):355–61.
22. NICE | Interventional procedure guidance 94. Uterine artery embolisation for fibroids. Available from: http://www.nice.org.uk/nicemedia/live/11025/51706/51706.pdf.
23. Edwards R, Moss J, Lumsden M, et al. Uterine-artery embolization versus surgery for symptomatic uterine fibroids. N Engl J Med 2007;356:360–70.
24. Van der Kooij SM, Hehenkamp WJ, Volkers NA, et al. Uterine artery embolization vs hysterectomy in the treatment of symptomatic uterine fibroids: 5-year outcome from the randomized EMMY trial. Am J ObstetGynecol 2010;203:105.e1–13.
25. Moss J, Cooper K, Khaund A, et al. Randomised comparison of uterine artery embolisation (UAE) with surgical treatment in patients with symptomatic uterine fibroids (REST trial): 5-year results. BJOG 2011;118:936–44.
26. Gupta JK, Sinha A, Lumsden MA, Hickey M. Uterine artery embolisation for symptomatic uterine fibroids. Cochrane Database Syst Rev 2012;(5):CD005073.
27. Van der Kooij SM, Bipat S, Hehenkamp WJK, et al. Uterine artery embolization versus surgery in the treatment of symptomatic fibroids: a systematic review and metaanalysis. Am J Obstet Gynecol 2011;205:317.e1–18.
28. Mara M, Maskova J, Fucikova Z, et al. Midterm clinical and first reproductive results of a randomized controlled trial comparing uterine fibroid embolization and myomectomy. Cardiovasc Intervent Radiol 2008;31:73–85.
29. World Health Organization (WHO) Department of Reproductive Health and Research. Maternal mortality in 2000: estimates developed by WHO, UNICEF, and UNFPA. WHO, Geneva; 2004.
30. Lennox C, Marr L. Scottish Audit of Severe Maternal Morbidity 7th Annual Report, Healthcare Improvement Scotland. Available at: http://www.healthcareimprovementscotland.org/his/idoc.ashx?docid=7c8fc48a-dd38-45d7-be00-05a0ec1be61a&version=-1. 2011.
31. Royal College of Obstetricians and Gynaecologists. The role of emergency and elective interventional radiology in postpartum hemorrhage. Royal College of Obstetricians and Gynaecologists Good Practice Guideline No. 6. Royal College of Obstetricians and Gynaecologists, London. Available at: http://www.rcog.org.uk/womens-health/clinical-guidance/role-emergency-and-electiveinterventional-radiology-postpartum-haem; 2007.
32. Georgiou C. Intraluminal pressure readings during the establishment of a positive 'tamponade test' in the management of postpartum haemorrhage. BJOG 2010;117:295–303.
33. Tixier H, Loffroy R, Guiu B, et al. Complications and failure of uterine artery embolisation for intractable postpartum haemorrhage. BJOG 2009;116:55–61.
34. Doumouchtsis SK, Papageorghiou AT, Arulkumaran A. Systematic review of conservative management of postpartum hemorrhage: what to do when medical treatment fails. Obstetr Gynecol Surv 2007;62:540–7.
35. Kayem G, Kurinczuk JJ, Alfirevic Z, et al. Specific second-line therapies for postpartum haemorrhage: a national cohort study. BJOG 2011;118:856–64.
36. Yu B, Douglas NC, Guarnaccia MM, et al. Uterine artery embolization as an adjunctive measure to decrease blood loss prior to evacuating a cervical pregnancy. Arch Gynecol Obstet 2009;279:721–4.
37. Steinauer JE, Diedrich JT, Wilson MW, et al. Uterine artery embolization in postabortion hemorrhage. Obstet Gynecol 2008;111:881–9.
38. Ignacio EA, Dua R, Sarin S, et al. Pelvic congestion syndrome: diagnosis and treatment. Semin Intervent Radiol 2008;25(4):361–8.
39. Kies DD, Kim HS. Pelvic congestion syndrome: a review of current diagnostic and minimally invasive treatment modalities. Phlebology 2012;27(Suppl 1):52–7.
40. Kim HS, Malhotra AD, Rowe PC, et al. Embolotherapy for pelvic congestion syndrome: long-term results. J Vasc Interv Radiol 2006;17:289–97.
41. Bittles MA, Hoffer EK. Gonadal vein embolization: treatment of varicocele and pelvic congestion syndrome. Semin Intervent Radiol 2008;25(3):261–70.
42. NICE | Clinical Guideline 11. Fertility: assessment and treatment for people with fertility problems. Available from: http://www.nice.org.uk/nicemedia/live/10936/29267/29267.pdf.

CHAPTER 9

NON-VASCULAR GENITOURINARY TRACT INTERVENTION

Uday Patel • Lakshmi Ratnam

INTRODUCTION

The genitourinary (GU) tract is especially prone to anatomical and morphological variations and successful intervention relies on careful anatomical appreciation and planning. This chapter describes the various interventional procedures currently used in the GU tract, but commences with a review of the anatomy relevant to renal access, as this is the cornerstone of most GU interventions.

PERCUTANEOUS RENAL ACCESS—IMPORTANT ANATOMICAL FACTORS

Renal Position

The kidneys lie in the perinephric space at the level of T12 to L2/3 vertebral bodies. The upper pole is more medial than the lower, with a coronal axis tilt of about 15°. The upper pole is also more posterior facing than the lower. In the short axis the renal pelvis points anteromedially. Anatomical disposition in the 3 planes is illustrated in Fig. 9-1.

Relations of the Kidney

The important relations regarding renal access are those adjacent structures that may be inadvertently injured—the liver, spleen, diaphragm, pleura/lung and the colon.

Variant anatomy should also be remembered: for example, the splenic flexure of the descending colon may be abnormally high and posterior (said to be more common in obese women). Pre-procedure ultrasound (US) will identify these hazards.

Pelvicalyceal Anatomy of the Kidney

The adult kidney has approximately 8–9 calyces. Typically, the upper and lower pole calyces are fused; and therefore larger and easier to access. Calyces will also vary in orientation, facing either relatively anterior or posterior. The posterior calyx is ideal for access, being closer to the skin surface. Posterior calyces also allow better intrarenal navigation; e.g. the route from a posterior to an adjacent anterior calyx or the renal pelvis is more or less in a straight line forward. However, access to the pelviureteric junction (PUJ) and ureter is easier from an interpolar or upper pole calyx. These points are illustrated in Fig. 9-2.

Renal Vascular Anatomy

The main renal artery divides into a (larger) anterior division and smaller posterior division, and each division further separates into segmental and lobar divisions (Fig. 9-3). Peripherally, the lobar and arcuate arteries skirt around the calyx. Thus, the safest place to puncture a calyx is its middle.[1,2] Puncture into the infundibulum or renal pelvis may lacerate larger arterial branches. A

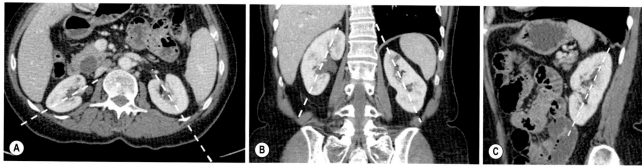

FIGURE 9-1 ■ **CT images of the renal axis and disposition.** CT images of the renal axis and disposition in the axial (A), coronal (B) and sagittal (C) planes. Note that the pelvis faces anteromedially and the upper pole is more medial and posterior.

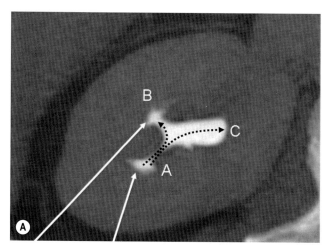

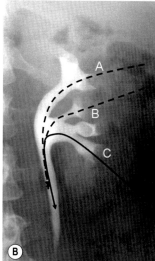

FIGURE 9-2 ■ **Calyceal selection for renal access.** These two images illustrate the importance of choosing the right calyx for renal access. (A) Axial CT image showing entry into a posterior-facing calyx A allows easy navigation into the anterior calyx B as well as towards the infundibulum and the renal pelvis C. Entry into an anterior calyx B would be poor for intrarenal navigation. (B) Coronal fluoroscopic image demonstrating that upper pole A or interpolar entry B is better for ureteric access. Lower pole entry C is less favourable.

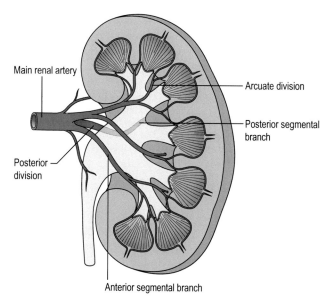

FIGURE 9-3 ■ **Normal renal arterial anatomy as seen from the front.** Note that the posterior division of the main renal artery lies behind the collecting system, and is vulnerable during percutaneous renal access in the prone position, especially if a more medial puncture is made.

further potential hazard is the posterior division, which is the only major renal arterial division that lies *posterior* to the collecting system. Typically it lies behind the upper renal pelvis but occasionally it is behind the upper pole infundibulum, where it may be injured if entry is misdirected towards the infundibulum rather than the upper pole calyx. Normally there is a single renal artery and vein, but up to 25% of kidneys have more than one renal artery and variant renal veins are seen in 3–17%. These do not influence access, but may explain the occasional vascular injury that occurs despite adherence to safe anatomical principles.

Other Anatomical Factors Important for Renal Access

Part of either kidney will lie above the eleventh/twelfth rib, especially the left kidney, and upper pole access may require an intercostal entry, placing the intercostal artery or pleura at risk. The intercostal artery runs in a groove

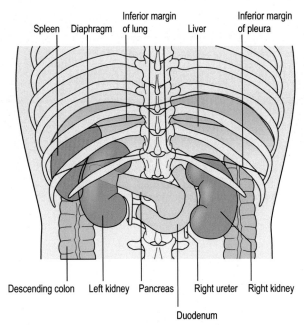

FIGURE 9-4 ■ Posterior view of the kidneys and their immediate anatomical relationships. The pleura can reach down to the twelfth rib, but veers away from the ribs laterally. Therefore, if renal access is performed above the twelfth rib, it should be laterally placed. However, too lateral a puncture may injure the liver or spleen.

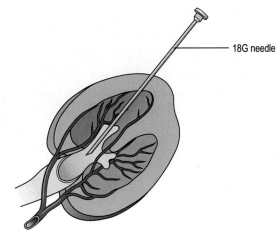

FIGURE 9-5 ■ The safest place to puncture a calyx. The safest place to puncture a calyx is its middle, (see text).

underneath the rib and is vulnerable with angled cephalad needle puncture. The posterior reflection of the parietal pleura is horizontal and reflected off the lateral portions of the ribs, and puncture through the latter half of the intercostal space is theoretically safer (Fig. 9-4).

Renal Anatomy and Percutaneous Entry

From this discussion, it can be appreciated that there are numerous factors to consider when planning safe, effective percutaneous renal access. The important considerations are summarised in Table 9-1. The safest point for calyceal puncture is the centre of the calyx, approached through the relatively avascular plane (Brödel's line) between the branches of the anterior and posterior divisions of the renal artery. Puncturing the centre of the calyx avoids injury to the arcuate divisions that course around the infundibulum. This is the ideal, and is illustrated in Fig. 9-5.

GENERAL EQUIPMENT FOR RENAL ACCESS

Personal preference may determine choice of equipment, but some general principles can help guide selection.

Access Needle

The two broad choices are a one-part 21G needle system (sometimes known as a micropuncture access system) or a one-part 18G/4Fr sheath system. With the former, the

TABLE 9-1	**Anatomical Considerations That Influence Renal Access in a Normally Sited Kidney**

1. The Lie of the Kidney
   a. The upper pole is more posterior.
   b. The short axis lies posterolaterally.
2. The Calyces
   a. The calyces lie either anterior or posterior.
   b. Upper or lower calyces are often compound or fused and so bigger.
3. Vascular
   a. There is a theoretically 'avascular' line along the lateral margin of the kidney.
   b. The lobar branches course in a curvilinear fashion around the calyx and papilla.
   c. The posterior segmental division may lie *behind* the upper pole infundibulum.
4. Adjacent Structures
   a. Pleura lies above the 12th and 11th ribs laterally.
   b. Intercostal artery lies underneath the rib.
   c. Liver, spleen and (left) colon may overlie the upper pole.
To summarise: A lower pole, posterolateral puncture of the centre of the calyx is theoretically the safest. The upper pole is more posterior and allows for easier navigation but must be approached with due care.

puncture is with a 21G needle, through which a 0.018-inch. platinum-tipped wire is inserted, followed by a 4Fr dilator and finally a 0.035-inch. working guidewire. A one-part system is an 18G diamond point needle, over which is a 4Fr sheath and the whole is inserted as a single unit. The puncture size is smaller with the two-part system (21 G vs 18G or 0.032 inch vs 0.048 inch diameter) and should be safer, but this has not been proven.[3]

Guidewires

The ideal puncture site is the centre of a calyx, but the calyx is a small structure with a usually even smaller outlet. Thus to navigate out of the calyx, a soft flexible wire with good torque is important, whereas rigidity is less vital. We favour either a straight-tipped Bentson wire or an angled-tipped hydrophilic wire. With the former wire, the floppy tip should not be too long. Once the guidewire has been manipulated out of the calyx (ideally down into the ureter, or at least into the renal pelvis), rigidity becomes more important, and a stiffer Amplatz-type wire is useful, especially if the track is being dilated for PCNL or a stent is being inserted through a malignant stricture. A stiff shaft hydrophilic wire has particular merits, being both rigid and kink resistant, whereas the other guidewires can kink. Kinks impede catheter advancement and lead to rupture of the renal pelvis.[4] The standard diameter is 0.035 inch, but thinner wires, especially with stiff inner cores, e.g. nitinol core, can be useful with tight ureteric strictures.

Catheters

Used for either navigation or drainage. For the former, a short angled-tip (e.g. Kumpe) or Cobra shape, high-torque catheter is best. Hydrophilic catheters are useful for bypassing tight ureteric strictures. For drainage, a pigtail catheter with large holes along the inner surface of the pigtail is chosen, as these are less likely to obstruct once the system decompresses. Any size > 6Fr should suffice, but the pigtail may not easily form in a small renal pelvis. The location and size of the drainage holes in the pigtail ensures good drainage. The pigtail should assist anchorage, especially with a locking system, but they do still fall out, and we routinely also further secure them in place (see below). Drainage catheters less frequently used are straight catheters or those with a Malecot-type tip, both useful with the small renal pelvis.

PERCUTANEOUS NEPHROSTOMY (PCN)

Percutaneous nephrostomy insertion is a commonly performed interventional procedure, most frequently for the relief of renal obstruction, with or without associated infection, and some further indications are listed in Table 9-2.

Ideally, a nephrostomy should be performed within working hours, on a stable, well-resuscitated and monitored patient. However, it is also important not to unnecessarily delay renal decompression, especially in those

with suspected pyonephrosis or infected hydronephrosis, as these patients can rapidly deteriorate.[4] Our practice is to only perform out-of-hours nephrostomy in infected obstructed kidneys and obstructed single or transplant kidneys, but this is an area of debate and department policies differ. Discussion between the urology and radiology department is important, and an agreement reached depending on local skill sets and resources. The only two published randomised studies comparing nephrostomy and ureteric stents showed them to be equally effective.[5,6] The technical success rate for PCN is quoted as 98–99% of patients, but it is possible that previous series may have under-represented non-dilated kidneys as the success rate is reduced in patients with non-dilated collecting systems, complex stone disease or staghorn calculi.[7-9] Available practice guidelines quote a success rate of 98% for dilated systems and transplants and 85% for non-dilated systems and staghorn calculi.[10]

There are no absolute contraindications to performing a PCN. Severe coagulopathy is a relative contraindication but this can be corrected. In patients with a limited life expectancy, a nephrostomy should be inserted only if this would lead to improved quality of life and survival. In all cases a multidisciplinary approach and close liaison with referring clinicians is essential.

Techniques

Patient Preparation and Procedure

Written consent should be obtained for all PCNs. Acceptable thresholds for complications are listed in Table 9-3. Where local complication rates are known, these should inform the consent process. Intravenous access and adequate hydration should be established; metabolic acidosis and hyperkalaemia should be corrected. A normal coagulation profile, with an INR <1.3 and platelet count of >80,000/dL, should be ensured. Antibiotic prophylaxis should be given,[11] especially if there is clinical evidence of infection. A single dose of a wide-spectrum agent is sufficient for low-risk patients. In high-risk cases, (elderly, diabetic, indwelling urinary catheter, bacteriuria, ureteroenteric conduit), antibiotics may have to be continued and modified appropriately once urine culture results are known.

TABLE 9-2 Indications for Insertion of PCN

1. Urinary tract obstruction from internal or external causes: stones, malignancy, sloughed papillae, crossing vessels, retroperitoneal fibrosis, iatrogenic causes (operative damage to ureter producing oedema/stricture)
2. Pyonephrosis or infected hydronephrosis
3. Urinary leakage or fistulas
4. Access for interventional or endoscopic procedures: ureteric stenting, PCNL, delivery of chemotherapy/medication (stone dissolution, antibiotic therapy for fungal infection), foreign body retrieval, biopsy
5. Urinary diversion for haemorrhagic cystitis

TABLE 9-3 Accepted Thresholds for Major Complications for PCN

Complication	Incidence (%)
Septic shock requiring major increase in level of care	4
Septic shock (in setting of pyonephrosis)	10
Haemorrhage requiring transfusion	4
Vascular injury (requiring embolisation or nephrectomy)	1
Bowel transgression	<1
Pleural complications	<1
Complications resulting in unexpected transfer to an intensive care unit, emergency surgery or delayed discharge	5

From ref 10.

Insertion is usually performed in the prone or prone oblique position. A true lateral or supine/oblique position is feasible; however, this increases the technical difficulty, with a greater risk of trauma to the liver, spleen or bowel. CT guidance may help if there is concern about variant anatomy. The procedure is usually performed under monitored sedo-analgesia. In addition, a local anaesthetic agent is infiltrated down to the renal capsule. Occasionally, when dealing with a confused or restless patient it may be safer to perform the procedure with the assistance of an anaesthetist, who can maintain a deeper level of sedation with safety, whilst the interventionist focuses on performing the procedure.

Following puncture of an appropriate calyx, a small amount of urine is aspirated to confirm the position of the needle. If the urine is clear, and the patient does not demonstrate any signs of sepsis, a small volume of iodinated contrast medium (approximately 10 mL) is injected into the collecting system. Over-distension should be avoided as this greatly increases the risk of bacteraemia. If the puncture site is acceptable, a wire is inserted and the track dilated for catheter insertion (single puncture PCN—Fig. 9-6). If the puncture site is revealed to be unsuitable (i.e. entry is into an infundibulum or the renal pelvis) then a second puncture should be performed into a more suitable calyx (double puncture PCN—see below).

Single Puncture Ultrasound-Guided PCN

On ultrasound, the posterior calyces are the most superficial and medial with the patient lying prone. With advances in ultrasound equipment and technique, primary puncture of a target calyx has become more common and is usually uneventful in a dilated system,[7] allowing for a single puncture PCN.

Single Puncture Fluoroscopically Guided PCN

Intravenous iodinated contrast medium can be used to opacify and select a suitable calyx. On fluoroscopy of an opacified collecting system, the calyces that demonstrate the largest range of movement when viewed on continuous screening (with tube below couch) from +30 to −30 oblique positions are the most posterior calyces. Being non-dependent, posterior calyces will be also be the least densely opacified in a prone position. Double contrast pyelography can also be used to highlight the posterior calyces as any gas (air or CO_2), being buoyant, will preferentially gravitate into the non-dependent parts of the collecting system. Not more than 20 mL of gas should be injected slowly and under continuous fluoroscopy. Care should be taken to avoid gaseous extravasation into the surrounding tissues, vessels or the retroperitoneum. Once a suitable calyx is identified, the needle is inserted under fluoroscopic guidance (Fig. 9-7).

Double Puncture Combined Ultrasound and Fluoroscopy-Guided PCN

The collecting system is initially punctured under ultrasound guidance. Ideally the definitive calyx for PCN

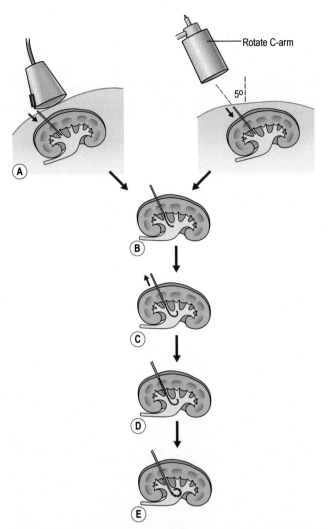

FIGURE 9-6 ■ **Single puncture PCN.** (A) Needle is inserted into the kidney either under ultrasound or fluoroscopic guidance. (B) Guidewire is passed through the needle (C) Needle is removed over the wire. (D) The nephrostomy is inserted over the wire. (E) The final position of the nephrostomy.

should be punctured and subsequent tract dilatation and catheter insertion carried out under fluoroscopic guidance. However, if definitive calyceal entry is not feasible (e.g. when the calyces are small), then any part of the collecting system visualised on ultrasound is entered with a 22G needle, a single or double contrast pyelogram performed and the pyelographic information used to select a target calyx. The chosen calyx is then punctured under fluoroscopic guidance, the tract dilated and a catheter inserted.

CT-Guided Nephrostomy

This technique is useful and safer when variant renal anatomy is suspected: e.g. horseshoe kidney, pelvic kidney or suspected retrorenal colon. A planning pyelographic phase CT is performed in the prone or supine/oblique position. The procedure can be performed under sole CT guidance or as a combined CT/fluoroscopy method. Needle access is gained under CT guidance and a guidewire inserted. Subsequent tract dilatation and

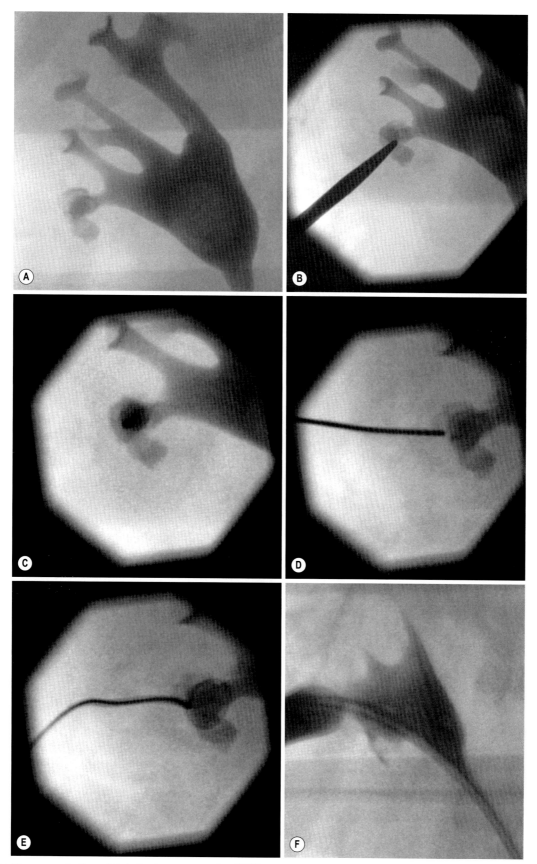

FIGURE 9-7 ■ **Fluoroscopically guided single puncture for PCNL access.** (A) Collecting system opacified with IV contrast medium demonstrating large stone in renal pelvis and smaller stone in lower pole calyx. (B) Tip of forceps over calyceal target used to centre image. (C) The needle centred over the target calyx 'like a dart'. (D) Angled screening once the needle is seen to move with the kidney in order to advance it to the calyx. (E) The wire coiled within the calyx. (F) Wire through calyx and into ureter with PCNL sheath in place.

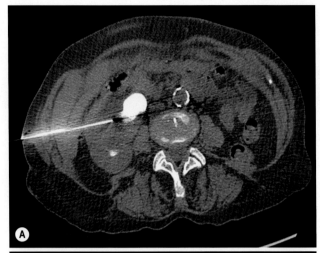

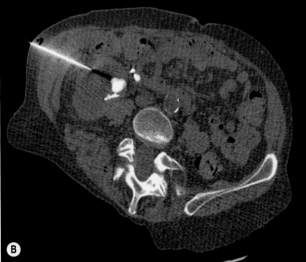

FIGURE 9-8 ■ CT-guided nephrostomy. (A) The procedure being performed in the supine position. (B) Puncture in the supine/oblique position. Either position is suitable, as is prone insertion. The procedure can be carried out solely under CT guidance or as a combined CT–fluoroscopic procedure (see text for details).

catheter insertion is done under fluoroscopic control. For the latter, care should be taken to ensure the access is secure before transferring the patient to the interventional suite[12] (Fig. 9-8).

Catheter Fixation and Removal

Displacement of a nephrostomy catheter is a constant hazard, particularly with long-term drainage. Definitive management (e.g. ureteric stenting) should not be delayed. The catheter should also be meticulously secured. Most nephrostomy tubes have a self-retaining suture, which once pulled forms a 'locked' pigtail within the collecting system. However, anchorage is not guaranteed and we further secure the tube to the skin (Fig. 9-9). A single anchoring suture through skin should be made close to the tube entry site. A small piece of tape is secured around the tube. The suture is then wrapped around the tube in a 'roman sandal' configuration with

knots at every turn going away from the skin entry site. The suture should be firmly tightened against the catheter but not so tightly as to kink the tube. Once the top of the tape is reached, the suture is returned towards the skin entry site, as a reversed 'roman sandal' pattern. In addition we also apply a standard 'drain-fix' dressing.

Removal of a nephrostomy tube should be performed under fluoroscopic control and, using a guidewire. The pigtail should be unlocked and, if this fails, the nephrostomy tube can be cut at the hub; however, this increases the likelihood of the suture being caught in the soft tissues on withdrawal of the nephrostomy tube, leaving a fragment behind. A retained suture acts as a foreign body and a nidus for stone formation.[13] Therefore, it is preferable to unlock the catheter whenever possible and not to cut the suture.[13]

Difficult or Complicated Nephrostomy

Non-dilated Kidneys

Non-dilated calyces are not visualised on ultrasound examination and, being small, they are difficult to puncture. Also the space is too restricted for wire/catheter manipulation. The double contrast technique can be used in these cases. If the renal pelvis can be seen on US then this can be punctured with a 22G needle and a double contrast pyelogram performed to identify and distend the posterior calyces. If no part of the collecting system can be seen on US, then intravenous contrast medium is used to opacify the system and a posterior calyx selected and punctured. Using this technique, a success rate of up to 96% can be achieved in the non-dilated system.[14]

Horseshoe Kidney

Because of its anatomical disposition, the horseshoe kidney is prone to impaired drainage, infection and stone formation but the orientation of the calyces and vessels are such that percutaneous access is relatively safe. As horseshoe kidneys are located more inferiorly, the upper poles are usually well below the ribs. The lower pole and pelvis are usually more anterior facing and a lower pole lateral entry may damage large anterior division arteries or accessory branches from the iliac artery. Thus a medial lying, upper pole calyx entry should be chosen for PCN (Fig. 9-10).

Transplant Kidney

Ultrasound-guided PCN is usually relatively straightforward in a transplant kidney as it is superficial and good views can be obtained.[15] The procedure is performed with the patient supine. A lateral, upper pole entry is preferred to avoid puncturing the peritoneum. An upper pole or interpolar anterior-facing calyx is ideal as this allows more favourable access to the PUJ and ureter for subsequent ureteric stenting. Careful ultrasound technique helps reduce the risk of bowel injury or puncture of the inferior epigastric artery. Often, there is marked capsular fibrosis around the transplant and this can make dilation and catheter insertion difficult. Over-dilation of the tract by 2Fr will facilitate catheter passage.

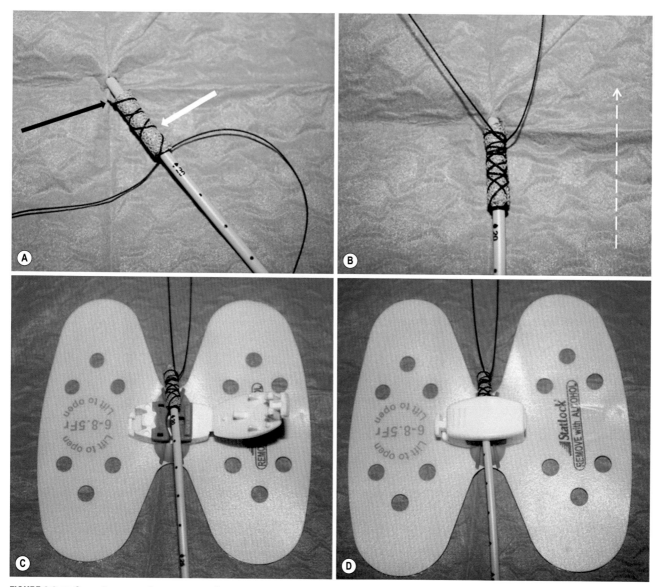

FIGURE 9-9 ■ **Securing a nephrostomy catheter.** (A) Small piece of tape secured onto nephrostomy tube. Anchoring suture (black arrow) is made through the skin; the suture is then wrapped around the tape in a 'roman sandal' configuration (white arrow) going away from the skin entry site. (B) 'Reversed roman sandal' knot along the tape in the direction of the dashed arrow. (C) The sutured tube is placed within a drain-fix dressing. (D) The top of the drain-fix dressing is locked in place to further secure the tube.

Paediatric Nephrostomy

Percutaneous nephrostomy in children should be performed under general anaesthesia. Ultrasound-guided PCN is technically straightforward as the collecting system is well seen, as it is superficial and usually generously dilated. However, in children the collecting system can rapidly decompress on needle entry and access may be lost. Decompression may occur because the system is under high pressure or because it is non-compliant. Therefore, the catheter must be inserted as swiftly as feasible. In straightforward cases with a dilated collecting system, initial puncture is performed with a sheathed needle, a stiff 0.035-inch. guidewire is inserted and the nephrostomy catheter advanced directly over this, as previous dilatation is not necessary. Special neonatal nephrostomy catheters (5Fr) are available; however, a standard 6Fr pigtail system works well. Care should be taken to minimise radiation dose to the patient by using low-dose techniques, good collimation and fluoroscopic image capture with minimal screening.[16]

Pregnancy

Urolithiasis is the common cause of true ureteric obstruction in pregnancy and will usually resolve with conservative measures. If this fails, nephrostomy may be required and an ultrasound-guided procedure should be performed. Fluoroscopy should be used sparingly and only if necessary. A lateral or supine/oblique approach may be used and intravenous opiates alone utilised to minimise fetal respiratory depression.

When fluoroscopy is used, radiation exposure should be minimised by lead shielding of the mother's abdomen

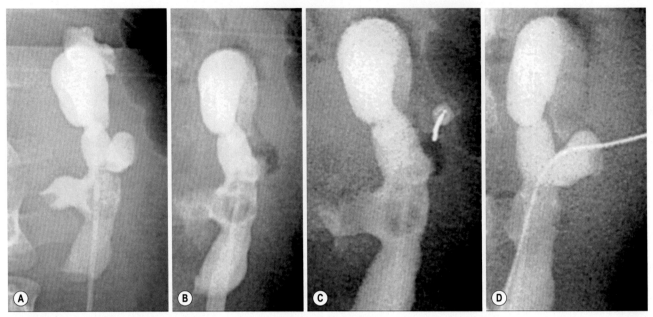

FIGURE 9-10 ■ Fluoroscopically guided PCN of a horseshoe kidney. (A) Ureteric catheter in situ used to perform a double contrast pyelogram. (B) The posterior-facing, non-dependent calyx is seen outlined by the introduced gas. (C, D) Percutaneous access achieved.

and by using similar safeguards as those recommended for paediatric cases.[17]

Complications of PCN and Management

The commonest serious complications following PCN insertion are sepsis and haemorrhage—Table 9-3. Patients at risk of pyonephrosis should receive pre-procedural antibiotics and nephrostomy insertion should not be delayed. Over-distension and manipulation of the collecting system should be avoided as these increase the risk of bacteraemia. In the well-dilated system, the entire procedure can be performed under ultrasound guidance, without any contrast pyelography. Performing a diagnostic nephrostogram should be delayed until the patient has recovered from the septic episode.

Haematuria, with or without clots, for a few days is not uncommon and usually resolves spontaneously but occasionally may require bladder catheterisation and washout. Major haemorrhage requires blood transfusion and/or further intervention. If the bleeding is venous in origin, continued drainage via the nephrostomy, catheter tamponade and blood transfusion, as necessary, can usually deal with the problem. Arterial bleeding can sometimes be managed in this way but more prolonged catheter tamponade, sometimes for several weeks, may be necessary. If this fails or the bleeding is not controllable with catheter tamponade, then renal angiography and embolisation should be undertaken.[18] Angiography should be performed with the catheter initially in situ and, if no bleeding point is seen, then the catheter should be withdrawn over a wire, whilst maintaining access, and repeat angiographic images are acquired in order to unmask an occult bleeding point.

Renal or pelvic injury is usually due to poor technique. Overzealous tract dilatation can rupture the pelvis. Care should be taken when inserting dilators and when advancing peel-away sheaths, particularly towards the renal pelvis and ureter. Avoidance of kinked guidewires will reduce dilator or sheath injuries. Most of these injuries are self-limiting and are treated with prolonged internal or external drainage.[19]

Bowel injuries are rare. If recognised during the procedure, the guidewire should be withdrawn out of the kidney and a drain left in the colon. A separate, second nephrostomy should be performed for renal drainage. Adequate renal drainage either via a PCN or a stent helps prevent renal-enteric fistulation. After a few days, a nephrostogram should be performed to exclude a renocolic fistula. If this is excluded, the colonic catheter can be removed. Theoretically, a mature track should minimise colonic spillage. If the patient develops signs of peritonitis, surgical intervention is required. Pleural complications include pneumothorax, empyema, hydrothorax and haemothorax. These are rare (0.1–0.2%) and are generally avoided by not performing punctures above the twelfth rib[19] and treated expectantly.

PERCUTANEOUS NEPHROLITHOTOMY (PCNL)

The indications for percutaneous endoscopic surgery are renal pelvic stones >2 cm, staghorn calculi, lower pole stones > 1 cm or stones in kidneys with poor drainage (e.g. stones in calyceal diverticula, horseshoe kidneys etc.). Hard stones (CT density > 1000 HU) and cysteine content are relative indications.[20] Less common indications are resection of transitional cell carcinoma of the renal pelvis, balloon dilatation or incision of PUJ obstruction and retrieval of foreign bodies. All these procedures require large-bore (30Fr) tract dilatation and sheath insertion.

Technique of PCNL

Leaving aside stone fragmentation, the key steps are access and tract dilatation. Regarding access, in addition to the sound anatomical principles discussed above in relation to renal puncture, the key consideration is that the entry should be well planned, in order to facilitate good intrarenal navigation and enable all/most stones to be removed.

Tract Planning

Appreciation of the intrarenal anatomy and the precise location of the stone are crucial and a good-quality IVU or 3D CT pyelogram will provide this key information (Fig. 9-11).[21] If complete stone clearance is not achievable, at the least the renal pelvis should be cleared in order to de-obstruct the kidney. If possible, the lower pole calyces should be cleared as fragments here may not drain naturally. The underlying principles regarding tract planning are summarised in Fig. 9-12.

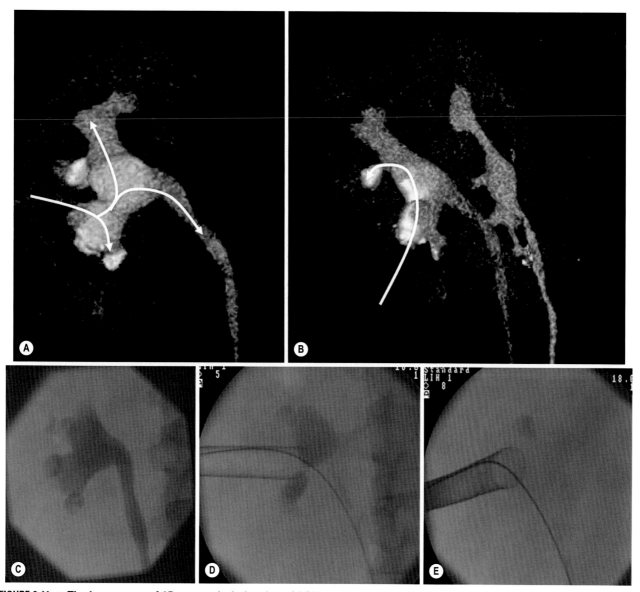

FIGURE 9-11 ■ **The importance of 3D anatomical planning of PCNL tracts.** The 3D CT pyelograms demonstrate a staghorn calculus with calyceal extension into the lower pole calyx and also a fragment in an interpolar calyx. As planned, a single tract will allow navigation into the lower pole calyces, pelvis and upper pole (arrow), as well as the ureter (A). However, the posterior-facing interpolar calyx presents an excessively acute angle from this access (arrow) (B). The three intraoperative images (C–E) confirm the accuracy of the pre-operative navigational map, as at the end of procedure the interpolar calyceal calculus was not retrievable. This was later treated with extracorporeal lithotripsy.

Tract Dilatation

The tract can be any size from 16Fr to 32Fr, but 30Fr is usual. Ideally, two guidewires should be inserted: a stiff wire for dilatation and a safety wire. There are three systems available for dilatation—a balloon mounted sheath system, serial plastic dilators or concentric/ telescopic metal dilators. Balloons are quick, serial plastic dilators are easy to use and the metal dilators are reusable. The latter are especially useful when dilating onto a calyceal diverticulum. In a recent study,[22] bleeding and operating times were higher after balloon dilatation, but there were many uncontrollable variables in the study and other studies disagree.[23]

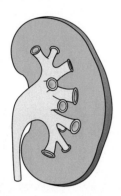

Principles of PCNL access
Aims
1. Aim for complete stone clearance
2. If complete clearance is not possible:
   • Clear renal pelvis to improve renal drainage.
   • Clear lower pole calyces as these may not respond to ESWL.
   • Residual stones in the upper/interpolar calyces can later be treated with ESWL.

Renal access
1. Posterior calyces allow access to anterior calyces.
2. Anterior calyceal entry poorer for intrarenal navigation.
3. Upper pole entry allows deep access of the PUJ/upper ureter:
   • May puncture posterior division artery.
   • May puncture pleura
4. Some interpolar calyces may be difficult with either lower or upper entry.

 A

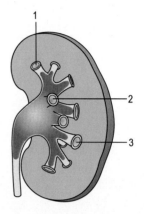

Complete staghorn
Stone clearance may be impossible with a single puncture.

1. Route 1 or 2 may be preferred—with Route 3 PUJ/ureteric clearance may be difficult.
2. With either routes some interpolar calyces may be difficult.

 B

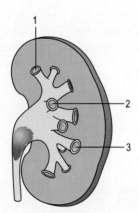

Stone in renal pelvis
Stone removed with minimal fragmentation. Ureteric fragments may be difficult to chase. Access planned according to PUJ anatomy.

1. Routes 1 and 2 are preferred with straight navigation to PUJ.
2. Route 3 may be difficult if the infundibulo-pelvic angle is acute and distal stone may be beyond reach.

 C

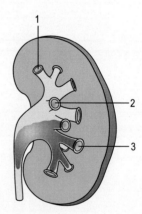

Stone in pelvis and lower calyces
Complete clearance is important (see under Principles/Aims).

1. Route 1 is often best.
2. Poor views of the interpolar calyx.
3. Poor views of upper ureter

 D

FIGURE 9-12 ■ **(A–F) The principles of tract planning for PCNL.** A well-planned tract should allow for maximal/all stone removal and easy intrarenal navigation, such that most/all calyces should be endoscopically accessible.

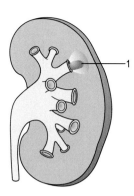

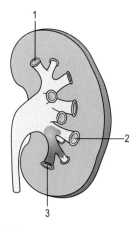

Stone in calyceal diverticulum with tight neck
Complete clearance is ideal. To decrease chances of recurrence, the neck should be dilated (thereby improving drainage) or the diverticulum should be obliterated. Direct puncture onto stone (1). Hydrophilic wire and good distension (with air/CO_2) help in searching for neck.

Lower-pole branched calculus
Stones in anterior and posterior parallel calyces. Complete clearance as ESWL may not work.
1. Route 1 preferred as both parallel calyces can be seen.
2. Route 2 (posterior calyx) better than 3 (anterior calyx) as navigation easier.

FIGURE 9-12, Continued

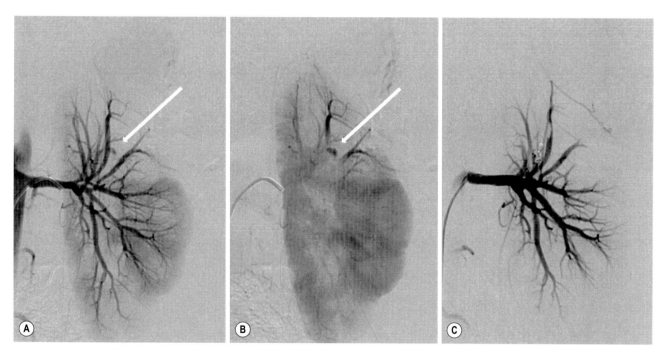

FIGURE 9-13 ■ **Embolisation of pseudoaneurysm (PSA).** (A) Upper pole PSA (white arrow) in early phase of contrast medium injection. (B) More prominent filling of the PSA in later stage of contrast medium injection (white arrow). (C) Post-embolisation image with coils in place. PSA is no longer seen to fill.

Complications of PCNL and Management

In a large international study, significant complications were bleeding (7.8%), renal pelvic injury (3.4%) and pleural effusion (1.8%). Bowel and visceral injury are less frequent. The principles of management are similar to those detailed under post-nephrostomy complications.

Embolisation is necessary in < 1% of cases. Pneumothorax and pleural effusions should be treated on their merits. Bowel injury should be treated expectantly to let the tract mature, but may require operative correction. Delayed complications include late pseudoaneurysm, haemorrhage (Fig. 9-13) and ischaemic stricture of the collecting system (Fig. 9-14), which can occur weeks or months after the procedure.

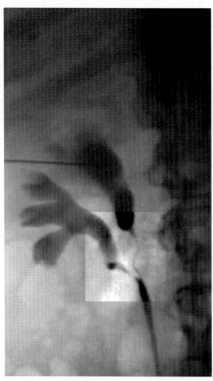

FIGURE 9-14 ■ **Post-PCNL ischaemic stricture.** Stricture of the renal pelvis extending into both infundibula post-PCNL. This was successfully balloon dilated.

ANTEGRADE URETERIC STENTS

A stent functions both as a splint and a conduit for natural flow. In the urinary tract, it is an alternative to a nephrostomy and although a stent is free of the complications of an external drain (external bag, leakage, skin irritation, accidental removal and infection) and better for home care, it has disadvantages.[24] The urinary tract does not tolerate artificial materials well. Stents can irritate the bladder or become infected. All stents, irrespective of their design or material of construction, will eventually become occluded, necessitating replacement.

Indications for Ureteric Stents

The common indications are relief of ureteric obstruction or leakage, and splinting of the ureter after balloon dilatation of ureteric strictures or after ureteric surgery. Stenting prior to stone therapy is now a relative indication.[25]

Ureteric Stents versus Percutaneous Nephrostomy

There are only two randomised studies comparing stents with nephrostomy (also referred to above under PCN). Both were in the setting of acute urolithiasis.[5,6] One reported no clinical difference and the other found a higher technical failure with retrograde stenting, but the numbers were small in both series. In a separate survey,[26]

respondents (radiologists and urologists) favoured antegrade approaches with pelvic malignancy, and retrograde in those with uncomplicated benign disease or coagulopathy. Regarding quality of life, the two methods were rated equal in one study.[27]

Types of Ureteric Stents

Plastic Stents

The standard design is a hollow tube with a double pigtail (or double J) stent which covers the full length of the ureter. There are drainage holes in both pigtails and, in some designs, along the shafts. The earliest stents, which were made of polyethylene or polyurethane, had a high encrustation and fracture rate. Polymers are now used because of their better biocompatibility. However, these stents require regular exchange. Novel designs include a softer, narrow bladder tail, to reduce bladder irritation. A metal braided double pigtail stent is more rigid and durable and may have a role in malignant strictures.

Metal Stents

Unlike double J stents, metal ureteric stents become permanently incorporated into the wall by epithelialisation. Many metallic designs have been tried[28–30] but only one, the Memokath 051, has been specifically designed for the urinary tract.[31] Unlike the others, the Memokath does not epithelialise and can be removed even after several years. Covered metal stents have been used but they also become occluded as a result of urothelial overgrowth.

Pathological and Functional Changes after Stenting

All stents, including modern polymer stents, lead to reactive urothelial hyperplasia, thickened mucosa and periureteral inflammation.[32] In both animals and humans,[24] reduced and ineffective peristalsis is seen with stents in situ and early drainage is passive, and dependent on the renal-bladder pressure gradient. In one study, peristalsis was rarely seen before 2 months and in other studies intrapelvic pressures rose after stenting.[24,33,34] Plastic stents also develop a biofilm and eventually become encrusted and blocked. Open mesh metal stents are also not well tolerated, exciting a profuse inflammatory response with urothelial hyperplasia.[35] Stent incorporation into ureteric mucosa is also unpredictable and eventually stents will obstruct due to malignant ingrowth or overgrowth, or as a result of encrustation.

Clinical Efficacy of Current Stents

Technical success varies from 77 to 95%.[24,36–39] However, in one study, 30% were blocked at 3 months.[40] Stent material and infection all have a bearing on encrustation. Dysuria or urinary frequency affects up to one half of all patients. Stent reflux can lead to infection and loin pain.

Practical Aspects of Antegrade Stenting

Antegrade ureteric stenting may be performed either as a primary stenting procedure [36] or as a second procedure following several days of external drainage. The technical success rate for the former is around 85% and near 100% for the latter.[24] Primary stenting is contraindicated with infected obstructed systems.

Technique of Antegrade Stenting

Interpolar or upper pole renal access is better but lower pole entry can be used, though with some difficulty. A nephrostogram will confirm the level and completeness of the stricture. The stricture can be negotiated with a curved tip hydrophilic wire combined with an angled tip, high torque catheter for stricture cannulation; or with a straight tip guidewire combined with a Cobra shape catheter. Once the stricture is crossed, the catheter is advanced into the bladder and the wire exchanged for a stiff guidewire to support stent insertion. A long peel-away sheath may be used to support stent insertion, especially if the perinephric track is long and/or with lower pole access. The tract is dilated to one size larger, or to 1Fr or 2Fr larger than the chosen stent.

Stent Lumen Size

A lumen >5Fr can accommodate a flow rate of up to 10 mL/min with minimal rise of the intrapelvic pressure. The nature of the obstruction may influence choice. Stents for bypassing obstructing ureteric stones are used for relatively short periods. Benign strictures also allow drainage around the stent as the ureter dilates (so-called peri-stent drainage), whereas malignant tissue does not permit such dilatation. We tend to use 8Fr stents for malignant or ischaemic/post-surgical strictures; and 6Fr to bypass ureteric calculi or inflammatory strictures. There is no consensus regarding metal stents, but 6- to 8-mm diameter stents have been used.

Stent Length

Direct ureteric length measurement can be used: the wire tip is advanced to the ureterovesical junction and a clip placed on the wire at the skin exit site. Then the wire is withdrawn until the wire tip is just in the renal pelvis and a second clip is placed. The inter-clip distance is the length of the ureter. However, this method can be inaccurate, particularly if the ureter is tortuous. An alternative is to use the patient's height. One formula suggests <175 cm height = 22-cm-long stent; 175–195 cm = 24 cm; and >195 cm = 26 cm.[41] This is a reliable method of calculating the length of the ureter, unless there is an anatomical anomaly or the two fixed points (the PUJ and VUJ) have changed position, e.g. because of a large bladder tumour or after renal pelvic surgery. In such cases a longer stent is selected. Patients with a urostomy usually require a 22-cm stent or shorter. A 12-cm length is generally sufficient for transplant ureters. The ureteric length in children should be judged according to their height.

Type of Stent

Polymer stents offer the best combination of rigidity, lumen flow and durability but no material is of proven superiority. Hydrophilic coatings allow easier passage but are expensive. The release method is a matter of individual preference. The presence of an internal stiffener, positioning thread loops and visible markers may benefit the novice. Occasionally the stiffener and the thread loops can create their own difficulties and the simplest design has no stiffener or thread lops, and uses only a pusher. Extra care is needed with this simple design, as there is no scope for repositioning.

Insertion of a Plastic Stent

The site of obstruction can be pre-dilated with either long dilators or with a 4- to 6-mm-diameter balloon catheter. High pressures may be necessary, especially with benign strictures. The stent is advanced with short, firm thrusts over the stiff guidewire, until the distal tip lies in the bladder and the proximal tip is in the renal pelvis. If it has been advanced too far, reposition by pulling on the stent assembly—and also the thread loops, if present. The distal tip should be within the bladder, but an excessively long bladder loop increases stent-related dysuria.

The stent is released by withdrawing the guidewire (and internal stiffener if one is being used). The thread loops can then be removed under fluoroscopic control, in order to avoid pulling the proximal pigtail into the renal parenchyma. The guidewire can then be re-advanced to regain renal access, a catheter is inserted and a check nephrostogram performed (Fig. 91-15). If stent patency is confirmed and there is no substantial clot in the renal pelvis, then all access can be removed. However, if flow is poor and/or there is marked clot, then a covering nephrostomy should be inserted and left on external drainage. This can be removed after 24–48 hours if the clot has cleared and the stent is functioning normally.

Insertion of a Metal Ureteric Stent

The length and position of the stricture are carefully documented. A stent longer than the stricture is used. Overlapping stents should be avoided, as this increases the risk of encrustation. No stent is of proven superiority. The Memokath stent is made of a coiled nickel–titanium shape memory alloy, which expands to its full diameter (9Fr shaft and 17Fr proximal flange) when the ureter is flushed with water at 50°C. When flushed with cold water, it returns to its smaller size even months/years after insertion, and can be fully retrieved. With all metal stents, immediate drainage can be unreliable, perhaps because of mucosal oedema over the ends and a covering nephrostomy may be necessary. This can be removed after a 24-h trial of nephrostomy clamping.

Further Issues about Ureteric Stents
Retroperitoneal Looping of Stent/Wire

This can occur as a result of a long retroperitoneal tract or an extrarenal cavity such as an urinoma. The tract

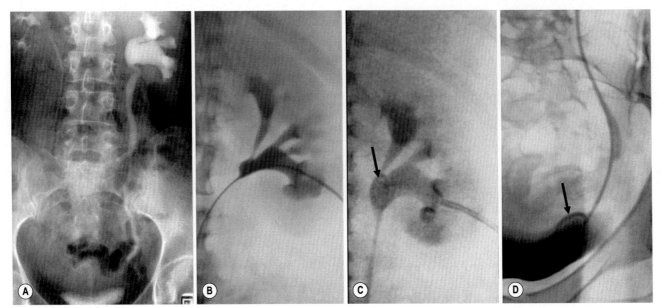

FIGURE 9-15 ■ **Ureteric stent insertion.** (A) Complete obstruction of the lower third of the ureter. (B) Renal access through a posterior-facing lower calyx. A wire was manipulated across the stricture (not shown) and a double pigtail stent was inserted. (C, D) The stent length was ideal as the upper pigtail (C) is coiled in the renal pelvis (arrow) and the lower pigtail (D) is just beyond the vesicoureteric junction (arrow) and not too long. We find the patient's height the most reliable method for choosing stent length, but there are other methods (see text).

needs to be supported using a stiff wire and a peel-away sheath. Some advocate the routine use of a sheath. We use it selectively, but the sheath should be one French size larger than the stent.

False Passage Created during Stricture Cannulation

If this complication occurs, it is best to stop, commence antibiotics and insert a protective nephrostomy catheter. Stenting can be reattempted after 3–7 days of external drainage.

Stenting of Ureteroileal or Ureterocolic Anastomosis

This can be performed by the standard antegrade route, or retrogradely under fluoroscopic guidance if the ureter can be demonstrated on loopography. Shorter stents are necessary but mucus can obstruct the stent. Use at least an 8Fr lumen stent and irrigation of the stoma may be necessary. A separate problem is the pressures generated by small bowel peristalsis. This will result in stent reflux and the urine may preferentially drain through the covering nephrostomy and stent blockage may be incorrectly assumed. A covering Foley catheter can be inserted into the urostomy or bladder to assist stent drainage. Both mucus and pressure problems can be overcome by using an extra-long stent with the distal pigtail externalised into the stoma bag. Rarely, peristalsis may expel the stent into the stoma, implying that the stricture may have resolved and stricture status should be re-evaluated on loopography.

Tortuous Ureter

The use of a high-torque, angled-tip catheter with a hydrophilic wire will facilitate navigation of most ureters. Once the wire is in the bladder, it should be exchanged for a stiff wire and a peel-away sheath should be inserted. This will improve the redundancy.

Tight or Rigid Stricture

The stiff end of a hydrophilic wire can be used to forcefully cross an unyielding stricture, but considerable force may be necessary with risk of creating a false passage. Thin stiff wires also have a role. If a subintimal passage is made, then stenting is still feasible once the true lumen has been re-entered distally. The only sure sign that a wire is in the bladder is to exchange it for a catheter and to confirm that the bladder fills with contrast medium. A hydrophilic catheter may be necessary to traverse a rigid stricture. If this fails, a long dilator or a balloon may help. In very resistant strictures, another attempt after 1 week of nephrostomy drainage is often successful.

A Stent Cannot Be Advanced across the Stricture, Even after Dilatation

In such cases, a stiff hydrophilic wire and/or a narrower stent and/or a hydrophilic coated stent should be used. If placement is still not possible, the distal tip of the hydrophilic wire can be snared in the bladder and externalised out of the urethra. This allows a push–pull manoeuvre and the stent can be forced across the unyielding stricture. Retrograde placement of a soft catheter

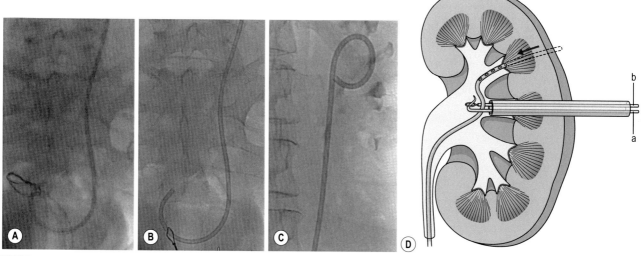

FIGURE 9-16 ■ **Repositioning of a ureteric stent that has been misplaced with the tip in the perinephric space.** A standard transurethral Foley catheter is initially inserted, after which a wire is placed into the bladder. A sheath is then placed in the bladder and bladder distended for ease of snaring. (A) Lower end of stent snared in bladder. (B) Snare loop tightened around stent. (C) Repositioned stent now within collecting system. (D) Line illustration of the antegrade method for repositioning a ureteric stent. Through a new puncture, an angled-tip catheter (a) and snare (b) are advanced to lie on either side of the shaft of the stent, and the tip of the catheter is ensnared. By pulling the catheter and snare together, the stent tip is pulled out of the perinephric space (arrow) and into the collecting system.

across the urethra and ureteric orifice during this manoeuvre protects against tissue laceration.

Improvement in Stent Position

If the stent has been released too soon and the tip is in the renal parenchyma, the simplest method of dealing with the problem is to snare the distal pigtail transurethrally and withdraw the stent (Fig. 9-16A-C). Alternatively, an antegrade approach can be employed, by snaring of the stent shaft (Fig. 9-16D).[42] If the upper pigtail is in the ureter, retraction is straightforward if the threads are still present. If a narrow PUJ makes such retraction difficult, a wire can be manipulated into the ureter and advanced past the upper pigtail, allowing a sheath (or catheter) to be inserted over it until it abuts the stent tip. Simultaneous withdrawal of the stent and sheath/catheter may allow a smooth transition across the PUJ. If there are no threads, repositioning is difficult but can be accomplished by using a snare, or more traumatically with grabbers, through a sheath.

The Thread Loops Will Not Disengage

In this situation a small (3–4Fr) dilator should be advanced over the thread (using a rotatory motion) until it abuts the stent. Pulling the thread will then allow release.

Extra-anatomical Stenting

If the stricture cannot be bypassed with a guidewire, then either a rendezvous technique or a ureteroneocystostomy[43] can be performed. The first is a combined antegrade and retrograde approach with in situ snaring of the wire. The latter can be performed if the

stricture is at the level of the bladder, in which case, under lateral fluoroscopy a curved tip catheter is firmly wedged in the stricture and directed anteromedially towards the bladder. The stiff end of a hydrophilic wire is then used to puncture through the tumour/bladder wall. Both techniques are examples of extraluminal stenting and are of established safety, but the position of the wire within the bladder should be confirmed before a stent is inserted. The final option is true extra-anatomical stenting,[44] by creating a subcutaneous tunnel between the kidney and bladder. A dedicated stent system is available for this technique.

Monitoring Ureteric Stents

Intravenous urography, contrast or radionuclide cystography, renography, supplemented with diuretic renography and Doppler ultrasound measurement of resistive index or ureteric jets can all be used. None are ideal. Plain ultrasound of the collecting system can be confusing, as stent reflux can lead to upper tract distension. However, in routine practice ultrasound correlated with renal biochemistry is simplest, as progressive dilatation is seen with stent dysfunction. For patients requiring long-term stenting, it is prudent to electively change the stent at set intervals (3–6 months) rather than depend on stent patency assessments.

Exchanging or Removing Stents

Stents should be exchanged every 3–6 months. This can be accomplished retrogradely[45,46] or antegradely using a snare. Retrograde exchange is preferable. Under fluoroscopy the bladder pigtail is snared and the stent is retrieved until it just exits the urethra. A full bladder helps retrieval.

A guidewire is inserted through the exiting stent lumen to establish ureteral access. Replacement is then a simple matter, but if difficulty is encountered a peel-away sheath, ureteric dilatation and stiff wire may be helpful, especially in males. Antegrade exchange using a snare can be used, but it is important to have a safety wire in place.

BALLOON DILATATION OF URETERIC STRICTURES

Balloon dilatation of benign ureteric strictures is an alternative to surgical repair. There are many causes of ureteric strictures (Table 9-4).[47] Such strictures can be treated with balloon dilatation. The overall success rate of this procedure is quite variable and ranges between 16 and 83%. Even in cases of technical success, the results are not durable. Balloon dilatation alone has been shown to have a high recurrence rate, but failed balloon dilatation does not prevent a patient from having a surgical procedure.

An interpolar calyx is ideal for ureteric access and a nephrostogram is used to delineate the position and length of the stricture. This may be particularly useful should the patient subsequently require surgical correction. Using an angled-tip catheter and a hydrophilic guidewire, the stenosis can usually be crossed. Either repeated gentle probing or firm direct pressure with the wire tip should be tried, as either technique may succeed, although the former is less traumatic. If the stenosis is very tight, a hydrophilic coated catheter may be required to cross the stricture. A peel-away sheath helps support the catheter and wire during exchange. The hydrophilic guidewire is then exchanged for a stiff guidewire and the stricture dilated using a 6- to 8-mm balloon. High dilatation pressures may be necessary. The pressure is gradually increased until the 'waist' of the balloon disappears. Abolition of the waist with minimal contained extravasation is anecdotally believed to be a 'good' sign. Once the stricture is dilated, a stent is placed as a splint and removed after 4–6 weeks. Ureteric perforation can occur when attempting to cross a tight stricture. When this occurs the procedure should be abandoned if the leak is substantial. External drainage via a PCN should be established. Up to 1 week should be allowed for the perforation to heal before a repeat attempt can be made to cross the stricture.

Treatment of adult-onset pyeloureteric junction obstruction with balloon dilatation has shown to be successful in up to 80% of patients. However, there is a limited role for balloon dilatation in childhood pyelouretic junction obstruction as the results are worse than antegrade and retrograde endopyelotomy or open surgery. In ureteric strictures following renal transplantation, the success rate of high-pressure balloon angioplasty is reported as 16–62%.[34,48,49] Cutting balloon angioplasty has been used for resistant ureteric strictures in the posttransplant ureter, with a primary patency rate of 55% and a secondary patency rate of 78%.[38,39,50] Early treatment of strictures improves the success rate. The best outcome is seen in strictures developing soon after percutaneous nephrolithotomy (PCNL) and ureterolithotomy, early postoperative stenosis and proximal well-circumscribed stenosis. The success rate is lower for dilatations performed at the vesicoureteric junction (VUJ)[39,51] and in ischaemic strictures. Long stenoses (≥3 cm) do not respond as well.

TREATMENT OF URINARY LEAKS AND FISTULAS

Surgical repair of urinary leaks is unsuccessful in up to 12–35% of cases and carries a significant morbidity.[52] Postoperative urine leaks (Fig. 9-17) or leaks secondary to malignant disease or after radiotherapy can all be managed percutaneously. Occasionally ureteric occlusion is performed for severe dysuria, haematuria or to treat total urinary incontinence. Small leaks will usually resolve with external drainage alone. A nephrostomy is inserted and left in place for at least 3 days (Fig. 9-18). If the leak has not resolved, then the nephrostomy should be upsized to a 12–14Fr drain to maximise external drainage. A stent may also be required to splint the ureter.

If simple drainage and splinting is unsuccessful, ureteric occlusion may be necessary. This can be achieved by several different methods and is combined with external drainage. Where the aim is to exclude flow to the bladder, bilateral occlusion may be required. The use of detachable and non-detachable balloons, large-bore occluding catheters, combination of coils and Gelfoam pledgets, plugs, adhesives, intraluminal electrocautery and retroperitoneal clipping have been described.[52] Irrespective of the type of occlusive material used, there is a high rate of dislodgement. Adequate external drainage is critical to the success of the procedure; malfunctioning nephrostomy catheters increase the rate of dislodgement.

SUPRAPUBIC BLADDER CATHERISATION

The need for long-term bladder catheterisation arises mainly in patients with bladder outlet obstruction and neurogenic bladder dysfunction. The procedure is sometimes necessary following bladder or urethral injury or fistula. Studies have demonstrated the superiority of suprapubic catheters over transurethral catheters in long-term bladder drainage[53] with reduced urinary tract infections, less need for recatheterisation, and improved comfort. Image guidance decreases the risk of bowel

TABLE 9-4	Indications for Ureteric Balloon Dilatation
Post-surgical: accidental ureteric ligation, anastomotic stenoses, postrenal transplantation
Inflammatory: postradiation, TB, retroperitoneal fibrosis, calculus
PUJ obstruction
Malignancy

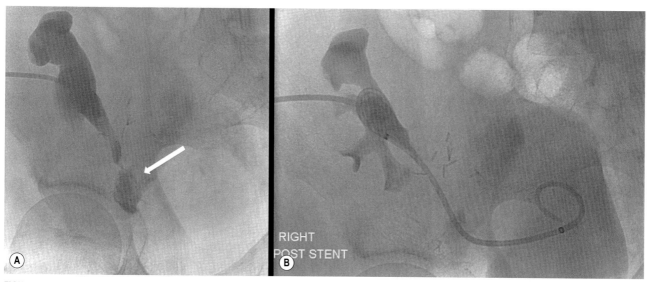

FIGURE 9-17 ■ **Post-surgical urine leak.** (A) Contrast medium injected from catheter in renal pelvis showing extravasation (white arrow) at the site of the transplant anastomosis. (B) Ureteric stent in situ after the site of the leak has been crossed.

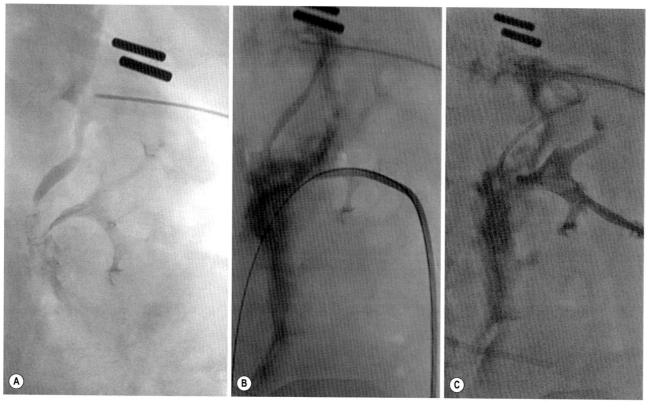

FIGURE 9-18 ■ **PCN for treatment of post-traumatic renal pelvic leak following a gunshot wound.** (A) Fluoroscopic opacification of the collecting system following initial IV contrast medium injection demonstrates a bifid collecting system with contrast medium leak seen from the pelvis. (B) Access via a lower pole calyx into the ureter. (C) Two nephrostomies sited in upper and lower pole to ensure adequate drainage of the bifid collecting system.

injury and is especially recommended when adequate bladder distension cannot be achieved, and in those with previous lower abdominal surgery.[54]

The procedure is performed using sedoanalgesia and prophylactic antibiotics in those likely to have bacterial colonisation of urine. It is important to ensure adequate bladder distension of at least 300 mL, either via an existing urethral catheter or by oral hydration and natural filling. This will displace the bowel loops superolaterally as well as making perforation of the posterior bladder wall by through-and-through puncture less likely. Adequate bladder distension is confirmed using ultrasound. If required, the bladder can be further distended via a 20G Chiba needle inserted into the bladder under ultrasound guidance, which also helps to confirm the absence of any intervening vascular structures or interposed bowel. The catheter should pass through the rectus sheath in the midline, not more than 2 cm above the pubic symphysis or along a safe tract as defined on ultrasound.

Either a Seldinger technique or a trocar (Fig. 9-19) technique can be used. The bladder is punctured under ultrasound guidance. With the trocar technique, once urine is aspirated the catheter is advanced into the bladder. When using the Seldinger technique, urine is aspirated via the puncture needle to confirm intravesical position. A stiff guidewire is inserted into the bladder and serial dilatation of the tract performed, ending with a peel-away sheath of a suitable size to accommodate the catheter. When the catheter is in place and secured by inflating the balloon, final confirmation of position within the bladder can be performed with contrast medium injection under fluoroscopy. CT-guided insertion is indicated in patients with complex pelvic anatomy caused by previous surgery or congenital abnormalities. In a large series of image-guided suprapubic catheter insertion a bowel perforation rate of 0.3% was reported.[53] This compares to a bowel perforation rate of between 2.4 and 2.7% for cystoscopically assisted suprapubic catheter insertion.[55]

MANAGING A NON-DEFLATABLE URINARY CATHETER BALLOON

The balloons of urinary catheters may fail to deflate if the balloon channel becomes obstructed by debris. The balloon can be ruptured by overinflation but this method carries the risks of bladder rupture and retained catheter fragments.[56] Injection of various liquid agents into the balloon can be used to dissolve the balloon, but may induce chemical cystitis. An elegant solution is to reopen the channel by the passage of a hydrophilic or an 0.018-inch stiff guidewire.[57] Alternatively, the sharp end of the guidewire could be used to rupture the balloon, allowing it to deflate. If this fails, the balloon can be punctured under transabdominal ultrasound guidance using a 22G needle, whilst the balloon is fixed by gentle traction per urethra. An alternative is transrectal ultrasound-guided puncture, under antibiotic prophylaxis. Either method may require multiple punctures.

PERCUTANEOUS CYSTOLITHOTRIPSY (PCCL)

Bladder stones are primarily treated by transurethral or open cystolithotripsy. PCCL is indicated when transurethral access is not feasible, e.g. in patients with urethral strictures, following bladder augmentation, and in neurogenic bladders. It is also performed in children as they have a narrow urethra, which makes more difficult the transuretheral removal of fragments. The technique is a hybrid of that described for the insertion of a suprapubic catheter and PCNL. Once guidewire access is obtained

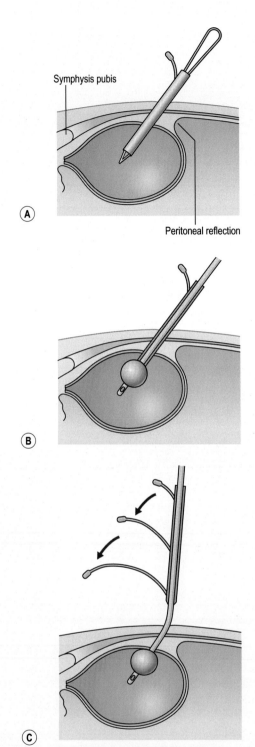

FIGURE 9-19 ■ **Suprapubic catheter insertion.** (A) The suprapubic catheter introducer (trocar and sheath) is advanced into the bladder midline at an angle of approximately 40° from the vertical until urine is seen rising up the trocar. The trocar is then removed from the sheath and the catheter inserted to its midpoint. (B) The catheter balloon is inflated and the sheath is then slid back along the catheter shaft until it is external to the abdomen. (C) The sheath is 'stripped' and removed.

into the bladder, tract dilatation is performed as described for PCNL. A 30Fr rigid sheath is inserted, through which bladder stones are fragmented and removed.

INTERVENTIONAL PROCEDURES IN THE PROSTATE GLAND AND SEMINAL VESICLES

The prostate gland and associated structures, the seminal vesicles and ejaculatory ducts can be accessed easily, as they lie close to the rectum and perineum, and either route is feasible for intervention. Transrectal interventions can be performed as outpatient procedures in the left lateral position, under local anaesthesia. There is a risk of rectal haemorrhage and infection, both of which can be severe. The risk of major complications by the transperineal route is almost negligible but it is painful and requires a general anaesthetic or generous sedo-analgesia. Commonly performed non-vascular interventional procedures in the prostatic bed include biopsy, abscess drainage (prostate or perirectal abscess), seminal vesiculography, prostate brachytherapy and cryotherapy,

and ablation with high-intensity focused ultrasound (HIFU).[58] Balloon dilatation of the prostate gland is ineffective. Insertion of prostatic stents has a high morbidity.

Drainage of Prostate and Perirectal Abscess

Abscess of the prostate may occur after prostatitis, urethral catheterisation or prostate biopsy. Perirectal abscesses are seen after surgery, such as appendectomy. All these can be drained percutaneously. However, abscess secondary to colitis, especially Crohn's disease, should not be drained by this route as a fistula may develop, and are best dealt with via the transabdominal or transgluteal routes. Needle aspiration to dryness is preferred to catheter drainage, as catheter placement can be difficult and is also inconvenient for the patient. The transrectal route is technically easier but may not be tolerated because of pain. Using a prostate biopsy needle guide attached to the transrectal probe, a long 18G needle is directed into the centre of the abscess under US guidance (Fig. 9-20). The needle tip is always very easily seen, and

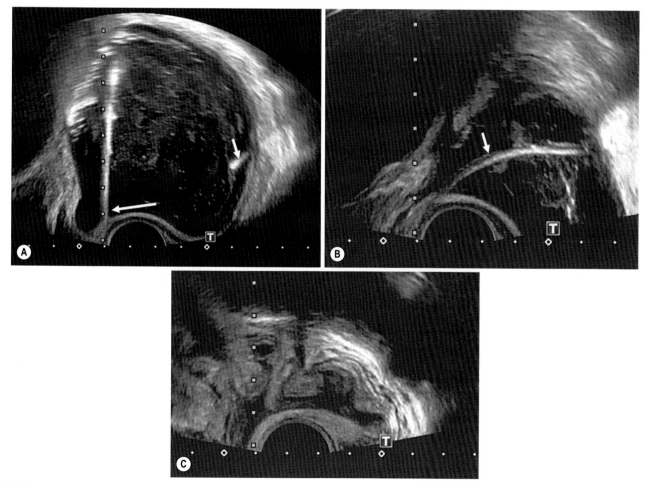

FIGURE 9-20 ■ **Transrectal ultrasound (TRUS)-guided drainage of post-appendectomy pelvic abscess.** (A) A wire (small arrow) has been inserted and looped within the abscess cavity through an 18G long needle (long arrow) inserted into the abscess using the biopsy attachment of the TRUS probe. (B) A catheter (arrow) has been inserted and the abscess is being drained. (C) The abscess is fully drained and the catheter was removed.

once tip position is confirmed, the contents should be completely aspirated. If the pus is thick and difficult to aspirate, a pigtail drainage catheter is inserted into the cavity using the Seldinger technique and removed once the cavity has been thoroughly drained. Loculated collections may require multiple needle aspirations.

Seminal Vesiculography and Cyst Sampling

This is a combined ultrasound–fluoroscopic technique[59] for confirming whether seminal vesicle (SV) dilatation is due to ejaculatory duct obstruction in men with low or absent sperm count. The transperineal route is preferred as the risk of introduced infection is lower, but the transrectal route has been used safely. Initial investigations should have confirmed dilated SVs. By the transrectal route with the patient in left lateral position, the dilated vesicle is punctured using a long 22G needle, and contrast medium is injected with the C arm of the fluoroscopic unit in a horizontal position. If the duct is patent, contrast medium will be seen to flow into the bladder rather than the urethra, as the external sphincter will stop such antegrade flow. Occasionally, aspiration of a prostatic cyst, which is usually a utricle cyst, is required to exclude infection or to sample its content. In this case the transperineal route is preferred to avoid introducing infection.

Prostate Brachytherapy, Cryotherapy and HIFU Prostate Ablation

Detailed description of these techniques is outside the scope of this book, but the guiding principles are similar to those used for other prostatic interventions. Brachytherapy and cryotherapy are carried out under general anaesthesia using the grid template transperineal method. Needles are driven into the grid locations on the predetermined treatment plan, and either radioactive seeds (for brachytherapy) or cooled gases are used to ablate the prostate gland, sparing the urethra and rectum. Both can be used to treat non-metastatic prostate cancer, but only the former is an established technique. HIFU ablation is still under investigation, and uses the transrectal route to ablate the prostate in patients with prostate cancer.

ABLATION OF RENAL CYSTS OR LYMPHOCELES

The clinical indication for either procedure should be soundly established. Very few renal cysts are symptomatic and most lymphoceles are also clinically silent. If necessary, the clinical relevance of either can be established by simple needle aspiration to dryness, to see whether the symptoms improve, before embarking on ablation. Numerous ablation techniques have been tried, but none is universally successfully.[60]

Ablation is performed under combined ultrasound and fluoroscopic guidance. It is important to exclude malignancy using CT or MRI. The cyst is punctured under US guidance, and a 5–6Fr catheter is inserted using the Seldinger technique. The cyst volume is calculated by complete evacuation. The integrity of the cyst and absence of any communication with the renal parenchyma or the collecting system is excluded by filling the cavity with iodinated contrast medium under continuous fluoroscopy. The cavity should be filled to 50% of the cyst capacity (up to a maximum of 100 mL) using > 95% ethanol. The alcohol is left in situ for 1 h, and the patient is asked to change their position by rotating around 90° every 15 min, so the entire cyst wall comes in contact with the alcohol. The alcohol is then completely removed. Some pain may be experienced but is usually not very severe and systemic effects of the alcohol are rare if the 100 mL limit is not exceeded.

Pelvic lymphoceles are seen around renal transplants or after lymphadenectomy. Only a few will require ablation, which can be carried out under US/fluoroscopic or CT guidance, following otherwise similar principles. The diagnosis of a lymphocele can be established by biochemical analysis of the fluid. Lymph contains high triglyceride levels, with serum equivalent levels of creatinine and urea. It is important to ensure cavity integrity with lymphocele as inadvertent peritoneal spill may lead to long-term sequelae. With any cyst ablation, sterile technique is important to reduce the risk of introducing infection.

REFERENCES

1. Sampaio FJ, Zanier JF, Aragão AH, Favorito LA. Intrarenal access: 3-dimensional anatomical study. J Urol 1992;148:1769–73.
2. Sampaio FJ, Aragao AH. Anatomical relationship between the intrarenal arteries and the kidney collecting system. J Urol 1990; 143:679–81.
3. Clark TW, Abraham RJ, Flemming BK. Is routine micropuncture access necessary for percutaneous nephrostomy? A randomized trial. Can Assoc Radiol J 2002;53:87–91.
4. Lewis S, Patel U. Major complications after percutaneous nephrostomy—lessons from a department audit. Clin Radiol 2004; 59:171–9.
5. Mohkmalji H, Braun PM, Martinez PFJ, et al. Percutaneous nephrostomy versus ureteral stents for diversion of hydronephrosis caused by stones: a prospective, randomised clinical trial. J Urol 2001;165:1088–92.
6. Pearle MS, Pierce HL, Miller GL, et al. Optimal method of urgent decompression of the collecting system for obstruction and infection due to ureteral calculi. J Urol 1998;160:1260–4.
7. Wah TM, Weston MJ, Irving HC. Percutaneous nephrostomy insertion: outcome data from a prospective multi-operator study at a UK training centre. Clin Radiol 2004;59:255–61.
8. Farrell TA, Hicks ME. A review of radiologically guided percutaneous nephrostomies in 303 patients. J Vasc Interv Radiol 1997; 8:769–74.
9. Lee WJ, Patel U, Patel S, Pillari GP. Emergency percutaneous nephrostomy: results and complications. J Vasc Interv Radiol 1994;5:135–9.
10. ACR-SIR-SPR practice guideline for the performance of percutaneous nephrostomy. Available at: http://www.acr.org/~/media/ACR/Documents/PGTS/guidelines/Percutaneous_Nephrostomy.pdf (accessed 4 June 2012).
11. Ryan JM, Ryan BM, Smith TP. Antibiotic prophylaxis in interventional radiology. J Vasc Interv Radiol 2004;15:547–56.
12. Barbaric ZL, Hall T, Cochran ST, et al. Percutaneous nephrostomy: placement under CT and fluoroscopy guidance. Am J Roentgenol 1997;169:151–5.
13. Medical Device Alert. 2009 Drainage catheters manufactured by Boston Scientific (MDA/2009/043). Available at: http://www.mhra.gov.uk/Publications/Safetywarnings/MedicalDeviceAlerts/CON051829 (accessed 12 June 2012).

14. Patel U, Hussein F. Percutaneous nephrostomy of non-dilated renal collecting systems with fluoroscopic guidance: technique and results. Radiology 2004;233:226–33.
15. Kobayashi K, Censullo ML, Rossman LL, et al. Interventional radiologic management of renal transplant dysfunction: indications, limitations, and technical considerations. Radiographics 2007;27:1109–30.
16. Barnacle AM, Wilkinson G, Roebuck DJ. Paediatric interventional uroradiology. Cardiovasc Interv Radiol 2011;34:227–40.
17. Khoo L, Anson KM, Patel U. Success and short-term complication rates of percutaneous nephrostomy during pregnancy. J Vasc Interv Radiol 2004;15:1469–73.
18. Vignali C, Lonzi S, Bargellini I, et al. Vascular injuries after percutaneous renal procedures: treatment by transcatheter embolization. Eur Radiol 2004;14:723–9.
19. Horton A, Ratnam L, Madigan J, et al. Nephrostomy—why, how, and what to look out for. Imaging 2008;20:29–37.
20. Patel U, Ghani K, Anson K. Endourology: A Practical Handbook. 1st ed. Taylor and Francis; 2006.
21. Ghani KR, Patel U, Anson K. Computed tomography for percutaneous renal access. In: Preminger G, Smith AD, Badlani G, Kavoussi L, editors. Smiths Textbook of Endourology. 3rd ed. Wiley Blackwell; 2012.
22. Yamaguchi A, Skolarikos A, Buchholz NP, et al. Clinical Research Office of the Endourological Society Percutaneous Nephrolithotomy Study Group. Operating times and bleeding complications in percutaneous nephrolithotomy: a comparison of tract dilation methods in 5,537 patients in the Clinical Research Office of the Endourological Society Percutaneous Nephrolithotomy Global Study. J Endourol 2011;25:933–9.
23. Davidoff R, Bellman GC. Influence of technique of percutaneous tract creation on incidence of renal hemorrhage. J Urol 1997;157:1229–31.
24. Seymour H, Patel U. Ureteric stenting—current status. Semin Intervent Radiol 2000;17:351–66.
25. Argyropoulos AN, Tolley DA. Ureteric stents compromise stone clearance after shockwave lithotripsy for ureteric stones: results of a matched-pair analysis. BJU Int 2009;103:76–80.
26. Lynch MF, Anson KM, Patel U. Current opinion amongst radiologists and urologists in the UK on percutaneous nephrostomy and ureteric stent insertion for acute renal unobstruction: Results of a postal survey. BJU Int 2006;98:1143–4.
27. Joshi HB, Adams S, Obadeyi OO, Rao PN. Nephrostomy tube or 'JJ' ureteric stent in ureteric obstruction: assessment of patient perspectives using quality-of-life survey and utility analysis. Eur Urol 2001;39:695–701.
28. VanSonnenberg E, D'Agostino H, O'Laoide R, et al. Malignant ureteral obstruction: treatment with metal stents—technique, results and observations with percutaneous intraluminal US. Radiology 1994;191:765–8.
29. Lugmayr H, Pauer W. Wallstents for the treatment of extrinsic malignant ureteral obstruction: midterm results. Radiology 1996;198:105–8.
30. Liatsikos EN, Karnabatidis D, Katsanos K, et al. Ureteral metal stents: 10-year experience with malignant ureteral obstruction treatment. J Urol 2009;182:2613–17.
31. Agrawal S, Brown CT, Bellamy EA, Kulkarni R. The thermo-expandable metallic ureteric stent: an 11-year follow-up. BJU Int 2009;103:372–6.
32. Marx M, Bettman MA, Bridge S. The effects of various indwelling ureteral catheter materials on the normal canine ureter. J Urol 1988;139:180–5.
33. Patel U, Kellett MJ. Ureteric drainage and peristalsis after stenting studied using colour Doppler ultrasound. Br J Urol 1996;77:530–5.
34. Hubner WA, Plas EG, Stoller ML. The double J ureteral stent: in vivo and in vitro flow studies. J Urol 1992;148:278–80.
35. Desgrandchamps F, Tuchschmid Y, Cochand-Priollet B, et al. Experimental study of Wallstent self-expandable metal stent in ureteral implantation. J Endourol 1995;9:477–81.
36. Patel U, Abubacker MZ. Ureteral stent placement without post-procedural nephrostomy tube: experience in 41 patients. Radiology 2004;230:435–42.
37. Lu DSK, Papanicolaou N, Girard M, et al. Percutaneous internal ureteral stent placement: review of technical issues and solutions in 50 consecutive cases. Clin Radiol 1994;49:256–61.
38. Atar E, Bachar GN, Eitan M, et al. Peripheral cutting balloon in the management of resistant benign ureteral and biliary strictures: long-term results. Diagn Interv Radiol 2007;13:39–41.
39. Osther PJ, Geertsen U, Nielsen HV. Ureteropelvic junction obstruction and ureteral strictures treated by simple high-pressure balloon dilation. J Endourol 1998;12:429–32.
40. El Faqih SR, Shamsuddin AB, Chakrabarti A, et al. Polyurethane ureteral stent in treatment of stone patients: morbidity related to indwelling times. J Urol 1991;146:1487–91.
41. Pilcher JM, Patel U. Choosing the correct length of ureteric stent: a formula based on the patient's height compared with direct ureteric measurement. Clin Radiol 2002;57:59–62.
42. Lang EK. Percutaneous ureterocystostomy and ureteroneocystostomy. Am J Roentgenol 1998;150:1065–8.
43. Lloyd SN, Tirukonda P, Biyani CS, et al. The detour extra-anatomic stent—a permanent solution for benign and malignant ureteric obstruction. Eur Urol 2007;52:193–8.
44. Patel U, Kellett MJ. The misplaced double J ureteric stent: technique for repositioning using the nitinol 'gooseneck' snare. Clin Radiol 1994;49:333–6.
45. Yedlicka JW, Aizpuru R, Hunter DW, et al. Retrograde replacement of internal double J ureteral stents. Am J Roentgenol 1991;156:1007–9.
46. Cowan NC, Cranston DW. Retrograde radiological retrieval and replacement of double-J ureteric stents. Clin Radiol 1996;51:305–6.
47. Kwak S, Leef JA, Rosenblum JD. Percutaneous balloon dilatation of benign ureteral strictures: Effect of multiple dilatation procedures on long-term patency. Am J Roentgenol 1995;165:95–100.
48. Bachar GN, Mor E, Bartal G, et al. Percutaneous balloon dilatation for the treatment of early and late ureteral strictures after renal transplantation: long-term follow-up. Cardiovasc Intervent Radiol 2004;27:335–8.
49. Fontaine AB, Nijjar A, Rangarji R. Update on the use of percutaneous nephrostomy balloon dilatation for the treatment of renal transplant leak/obstruction. J Vasc Interv Radiol 1997;8:649–53.
50. Cornud F, Chreiten Y, Helenon O, et al. Percutaneous incision of stenotic uroenteric anastomoses with cutting balloon catheter: long-term results. Radiology 2000;214:348–62.
51. DiMarco DS, Le Roy AJ, Thieling S, et al. Long-term results of treatment for ureteroenteric strictures. Urology 2001;58:909–13.
52. Goodwin WE, Scardino PT. Vesicovaginal and ureterovaginal fistulas: a summary of 25 years experience. J Urol 1989;123:370–4.
53. Cronin CG, Prakash P, Gervais DA, et al. Imaging-guided suprapubic bladder tube insertion: experience in the care of 549 patients. Am J Roentgenol 2011;196:182–8.
54. Harrison SCW, Lawrence WT, Morley R, et al. British Association of Urological Surgeons' suprapubic catheter practice guidelines. BJU Int 2011;107:77–85.
55. Ahluwalia RS, Johal N, Kouriefs C, et al. The surgical risk of suprapubic catheter insertion and long-term sequelae. Ann R Coll Surg Engl 2006;88:210–13.
56. Khan SA, Landes F, Paola AS, Ferrarotto L. Emergency management of the nondeflating Foley catheter balloon. Am J Emerg Med 1991;9:260–3.
57. Bui HT, Agarwal D, Clarke A. An easy method of deflating a blocked Foley balloon. ANZ J Surg 2002;72:843.
58. Patel U. The prostate and seminal vesicles. In: Allan P, Baxter GM, Weston MJ, editors. Clinical Ultrasound. 3rd ed. Churchill Livingstone; 2011.
59. Jones TR, Zagoria RJ, Jarow JP. Transrectal US-guided seminal vesiculography. Radiology 1997;205:276–8.
60. Lucey BC, Kuligowska E. Radiologic management of cysts in the abdomen and pelvis. Am J Roentgenol 2006;186:562–73.

CHAPTER 10

VENOUS ACCESS AND INTERVENTIONS

Anthony Watkinson • Richard J. Morse

The placement and maintenance of long-term vascular access catheters accounts for a considerable percentage of the workload of any interventional radiologist, particularly one who works in a large oncology or nephrology unit.

Long-term venous access is usually required for a few, relatively distinct, groups of patients:
- Those requiring access for the instillation of irritant therapeutic agents such as chemotherapy or total parenteral nutrition (TPN), which must be delivered into a large-calibre central vein.
- Those who require access for haemodialysis.
- Patients in whom long-term venous access is required and therefore peripheral venous cannulas are inappropriate, e.g. septic arthritis requiring long courses of antibiotics.

Central access can be gained via either a central or, in certain circumstances, a peripheral vein; the latter is referred to as a peripherally inserted central catheter (PICC).

GENERAL ASSESSMENT OF PATIENTS BEFORE VASCULAR ACCESS PROCEDURES

Before approaching any vascular access case, certain haematological parameters must be checked. As the overwhelming majority of patients referred for access procedures will be elective or semi-elective, there should be time for any clotting abnormalities to be corrected before the commencement of intervention. Central venous access should not be undertaken with a platelet count of $< 50 \times 10^9/L$, and if necessary a platelet transfusion should be arranged after discussion with the local haematology unit. Correction of an international normalised ratio (INR) of > 1.5 should also be performed, ideally with an oral dose of 1–5 mg of phytomenadione (vitamin K_1). The INR measurement should be repeated 24 h later. If there are reasons why a patient cannot wait to have an abnormal INR corrected, then human fresh frozen plasma (FFP) can be administered; however, the prescription and usage of FFP must first also be discussed with the local haematology service.

There is less need to be concerned about abnormalities in clotting parameters when performing PICC lines, but common sense should be exercised. As part of the general pre-procedure, haematological and biochemical work-up, it is also good practice to know the patient's haemoglobin level and glomerular filtration rate (GFR).

Any previous cross-sectional, venographic or ultrasonographic imaging must be reviewed before central access placement. This can alert the practitioner to any unusual anatomical features, the presence of implanted cardiac devices, any previously inserted and now removed long-term vascular access catheters and the presence or absence of venous occlusions.

Informed written consent must be obtained prior to central venous access, ideally in a situation removed in time and place from the interventional suite to allow appropriate consideration of the risks by the patient. The patient should be counselled for the risk of bleeding/haematoma, infection and pneumothorax.

GENERAL PATIENT AND INTERVENTIONAL SUITE PREPARATION FOR CENTRAL VENOUS ACCESS

Strict asepsis must be observed and all staff should wear operating theatre hats and masks. Imaging requirements are a fluoroscopy suite and an ultrasound unit capable of colour Doppler imaging.

The patient should wear a hospital gown which unties at the neck and also an operating theatre hat. It is not essential that they have a peripheral cannula in situ; in many patients peripheral venous access will be very poor and the reason they have been referred for long-term vascular access. The patient should be placed supine on the fluoroscopy table with their head as close to the end of the table as possible. A pillow can be used to support the head and a wedge should also be placed under the knees, for patient comfort but also to help distend the chest and neck veins. Ultrasound examination of the preferred point of access should be undertaken. Usually, the right internal jugular vein (RIJV) is punctured, as it is easily assessed using ultrasound guidance, can be manually compressed in the event of bleeding and provides the most direct route to the superior vena cava/right atrial junction. Ultrasound imaging enables assessment of the venous anatomy and establishes whether the veins are patent and whether they contain thrombus.

The available instruments should include a standard sterile vascular procedure pack and a minor operations surgical set (including scissors, toothed and non-toothed forceps, artery forceps and a needle driver).

INSERTION OF TUNNELLED CENTRAL VENOUS CATHETER

Hickman Line

Once the interventional radiologist and any assistants have scrubbed, the patient's skin should be prepared with an effective skin decontamination agent. Skin preparation should occur from the ipsilateral hairline posteriorly, the angle of the mandible superiorly, the suprasternal notch to the manubriosternal angle anteriorly and across to the lateral border of the ipsilateral pectoralis major laterally. The skin should then be draped; it is the authors' practice to use a standard fenestrated angiographic drape. By placing the top of the fenestration 2–3 cm above the medial aspect of the right clavicle and extending the opening by 2–3 cm inferiorly it is possible to create a well-draped sterile field. The patient's head is covered by the drape; patients are asked to look to their left and the left side of the drape at the head end is elevated on a stand to create a 'tent' under which they stay for the duration of the procedure.

Local anaesthetic is drawn up: 10 mL of 1% lidocaine/1 : 100,000 adrenaline is usually sufficient. The catheter is opened and both lumens are flushed and locked with 5 mL of 0.9% sodium chloride with 1000 IU of heparin. Care should be taken at this point to avoid touching the catheter; if necessary, the non-toothed forceps can be used to handle it.

A sterile ultrasound probe cover is fitted and the RIJV reassessed prior to guided local anaesthetic infiltration of the overlying skin and soft tissues. It is advisable to aim to puncture the vein as close to the clavicle as possible in order to avoid kinking of the catheter. A 5- to 10-mm transverse incision is made and a small pocket created using blunt dissection with the back of the scissors or the needle driver. Ultrasound-guided puncture (in the

transverse plane) can then be performed with a standard 18-gauge one-part needle or with a micropuncture set. It is important to ensure that the tip of the puncture needle is always visible on ultrasound in order to reduce the risk of inadvertent carotid arterial puncture or transgression into the pleural cavity. A 10-mL syringe with 3 mL of 0.9% sodium chloride is fitted to the back of the needle and when RIJV puncture has been performed, aspiration on the syringe is undertaken to confirm correct needle placement. Once the RIJV has been punctured, the left hand holding the needle must remain fixed in position; this is easiest if one or two fingers of the left hand are balanced on the patient's clavicle. The syringe can then be removed immediately followed by the insertion of an 0.035-inch J-wire. A prompt exchange reduces the risk of air aspiration into the vein. The wire is inserted and should run freely. If any difficulty is encountered when advancing the wire, the needle should be turned through 180° before another attempt is made to advance the wire. If this is unsuccessful the wire should be withdrawn and syringe aspiration on the needle should be performed to confirm correct positioning. When the wire has been inserted successfully, fluoroscopic guidance is utilised to confirm its passage through the right side of the heart into the inferior vena cava (IVC). It is not uncommon to encounter difficulty in exiting the right atrium with the wire preferentially passing through the tricuspid valve and into the right ventricle. If simple manoeuvres such as a breath-hold fail to help in exiting the right atrium, a 4 French (4Fr) multipurpose catheter can be used to guide the wire out of the heart.

Once the wire is safely in the IVC, the part outside the patient can be recoiled and fastened to the drape above the patient's right shoulder. Local anaesthetic can then be infiltrated subcutaneously, starting approximately 5–6 cm inferior to the lower border of the right clavicle and continuing superiorly to meet the puncture site. In female patients it is advisable to aim for the catheter to exit as medially as possible to help avoid soft tissues pulling it inferiorly when the patient stands up; this is a less important consideration in thin male patients. Aesthetic considerations may need to be taken into account, especially in female patients who may wish to wear a V-neck style blouse and therefore would want the line exiting more laterally.

An 8- to 10-mm incision is made at the point which the catheter is to exit and a further pocket is made aiming superiorly. The end of the line is attached to the tunnelling device by means of a screw thread at the bottom of the tunneller and the tunneller and line pushed through the subcutaneous tissue to exit at the neck incision site. Two types of tunneller are available, metal or plastic. The metal devices are stiffer and can be bent into a gentle curve. If difficulty is encountered in pushing the tunnelling device through the fascial layers or platysma, a small incision with the scalpel directly onto the device tip will usually free it. The tunneller and catheter are then pulled through the neck incision completely until the cuff of the catheter lies well within the chest wall pocket. Once the catheter is through the tunnel, it should be laid over the patient's chest, aiming to reproduce the path it will follow inside the patient and fluoroscopic screening is utilised to assess where it needs to be cut; its tip should be left near the right atrial/superior vena caval junction— usually 2–3 cm below the carina. The catheter can then be cut using scissors, and the tunneller and the removed section of catheter discarded.

A peel-away sheath one French size greater than the line diameter is inserted over the wire. Then the wire and inner dilator of the sheath are removed and the end of the catheter is advanced into the sheath with the aid of the non-toothed forceps. The patient should lie still, not talk and breathe gently during the line insertion into the peel-away sheath. With a well-hydrated individual the risk of venous air aspiration is very low.

Once the catheter is in place and the peel-away sheath removed, both lumens can be flushed and locked with heparinised sodium chloride solution. Fluoroscopy is used to check the position of the catheter. 3-0 Prolene sutures are used to close the neck incision with a mattress suture and the chest incision with a standard suture subsequently attached to the catheter. Occlusive dressings are applied to the venotomy site in the neck and the catheter exit site on the chest.

Groshong Catheter

The Groshong catheter (Bard Access Systems, UT, USA) has a three-way valve at the tip of the catheter which remains closed at neutral pressure but opens outwards during infusion and inwards during aspiration. This device aims to minimise the maintenance required for a tunnelled central catheter and helps avoid line thrombosis. Many of the principles which apply to the insertion of a Hickman line also apply to the insertion of a Groshong catheter, but there are some important technical differences.

The catheter is always placed via the subclavian vein, at the junction of the outer and middle thirds of the clavicle. The vein is punctured with a Micropuncture (COOK Medical Inc, Bloomington, IN, USA) needle and an 0.018-inch wire introduced into the IVC. After a long peel-away sheath has been inserted over the wire, the inner dilator is removed along with the wire and the catheter inserted. Once the position of the catheter tip is confirmed as satisfactory, the peel-away is removed. It is then that the cuff position is marked on the skin with the line positioned inferomedially across the chest and further local anaesthetic infiltrated and a small incision is made on the chest wall. The tunnelling device is attached to the distal end of the line and inserted through the infraclavicular incision, aiming towards the chest wall incision through which it is brought out. The cuff is left under the skin surface and the hub is then attached and secured before the incisions are closed, again with 3-0 Prolene.

PORT-A-CATH PLACEMENT

Port-a-caths consist of a self-sealing septum encased in a port made of stainless steel, titanium or plastic, attached to a silicone catheter. The port is placed subcutaneously and is accessed via specially designed needles inserted

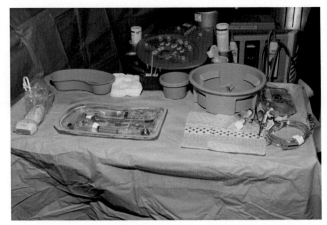

FIGURE 10-1 ■ Trolley laid up before port-a-cath insertion.

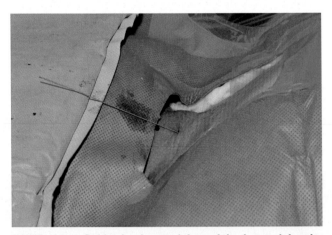

FIGURE 10-2 ■ Guidewire inserted into right internal jugular vein.

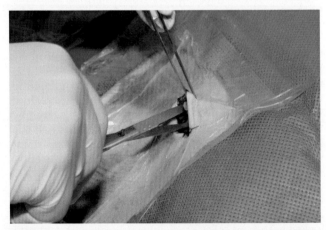

FIGURE 10-3 ■ Subcutaneous pocket formed in anterior chest wall.

into the septum through the skin surface (Figs. 10-1 to 10-8).

The method of insertion of the catheter is generally the same as for other tunnelled devices. It is important to know the type of chemotherapy the patient will receive. The use of bevacizumab (Avastin, Genentech Inc., CA, USA) has been shown to delay wound healing and the manufacturers recommend an interval of 28 days after

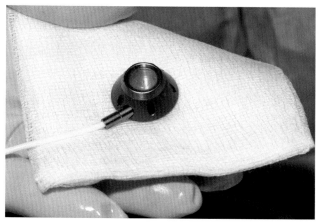

FIGURE 10-4 ■ Port-a-cath hub prior to insertion.

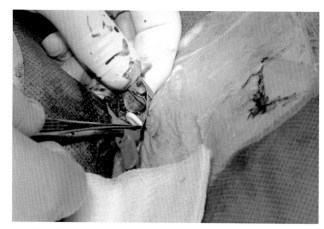

FIGURE 10-7 ■ Catheter inserted into peel-away sheath.

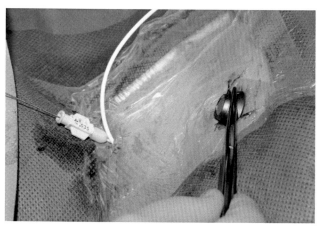

FIGURE 10-5 ■ Catheter has now been tunnelled and the hub is being inserted into the subcutaneous pocket.

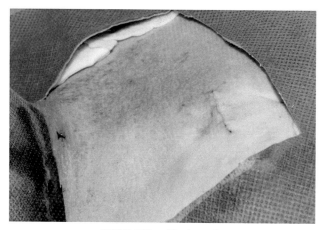

FIGURE 10-8 ■ Final result.

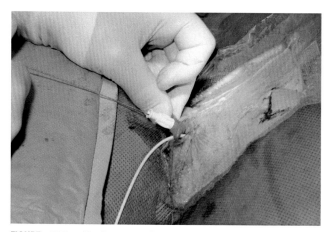

FIGURE 10-6 ■ Peel-away sheath inserted before catheter insertion.

surgery before commencement of the drug. It is also important to try and avoid placement of the port within a potential radiotherapy field as this can also adversely affect wound healing.

An internal jugular venous puncture is made, preferably on the right, and a wire is inserted into the IVC. The site of insertion of the port is generously infiltrated with a local anaesthetic agent, usually 20 mL of 1% lidocaine/1 : 100,000 adrenaline. An incision of 4–5 cm is made in line with the ipsilateral clavicle and a subcutaneous pocket formed. It is very important at this stage to ensure that the subdermal layer is well dissected as this will allow the port to lie correctly within the pocket. The port is also flushed and attached to the catheter by means of a metallic cuff. The port is then sutured to the underlying deep fascial layers by means of three 2-0 Prolene sutures with the septum facing anteriorly. The catheter is measured and cut and inserted through a peel-away sheath in the same fashion as for a Hickman catheter. Two to three 2-0 Vicryl sutures are then used to bring the subcutaneous tissues in apposition over the port before a 3-0 continuous subcuticular Vicryl suture is placed and closed with an Aberdeen knot before dressing. Fluoroscopy is used to check the final position of the catheter.

PERIPHERALLY INSERTED CENTRAL CATHETERS

Initial assessment is made of the venous suitability of the veins of the upper arms using ultrasound and a tourniquet applied high up towards the axilla. The basilic, cephalic or brachial vein can be utilised and assessment should be made for compressibility and the absence of venous thrombosis. Once a suitable site has been identified, preferably just proximal to the antecubital fossa, measurement is taken from the proposed entry site to the ipsilateral mid-clavicular line to the third intercostal space. This measurement corresponds to the desired length of the catheter. The skin is decontaminated and draped appropriately and a sterile ultrasound probe cover-fitted before infiltration of the soft tissues with 3–5 mL of 1% lidocaine under ultrasound control. A tourniquet is used to distend the veins. Using a Micropuncture needle, the vein is punctured and an 0.018-inch wire inserted. The needle is withdrawn and a peel-away sheath inserted. The wire and inner dilator of the sheath are removed and the pre-cut catheter inserted. Asking patients to turn their head to the side of insertion and lowering their chin to their chest helps avoid the catheter turning superiorly into the internal jugular vein. A chest radiograph is then performed to document the position of the catheter tip position before securing the catheter to the skin surface.

CATHETER MAINTENANCE

There is little in the way of maintenance that is usually required to keep a tunnelled central catheter or port-a-cath in good working order. When the catheter is not in use, it is standard practice to flush the lumen(s) with 0.9% sodium chloride before locking a solution of heparin sodium (50 IU/5 mL) into it to help prevent the formation of blood clots. If the catheter is not to be used for a prolonged period, regular flushing and locking of the lumen(s) every 2 weeks maintains patency.

CATHETER REPOSITIONING

It is possible for central venous catheters and port-a-caths to become malpositioned, especially if the line is left short. Malposition may be noted on chest radiography or reported by nursing staff following malfunction. Catheters may enter the contralateral or ipsilateral brachiocephalic or subclavian vein, or the azygos vein.

Repositioning is usually straightforward. Access can be gained via an ultrasound-guided puncture of a femoral vein under standard aseptic conditions. A 5Fr sheath can then be inserted to allow the passage of a guidewire and catheter into the central chest veins. A reverse curve catheter can be hooked over the malpositioned catheter, which is then moved into its correct position. If this technique fails, a snare device inserted via a sheath in the contralateral groin can be used to grasp a wire passed through the reverse curve catheter over the malpositioned catheter and, by gentle withdrawal of the snare whilst grasping the guidewire, the catheter can be pulled back into position.

TUNNELLED DIALYSIS CATHETERS

Whilst the preferred haemodialysis access method is via a surgically formed arteriovenous fistula or graft,[1] there are occasions in which a patient with established renal failure may require a tunnelled catheter for dialysis, e.g. whilst waiting for a surgically formed fistula to mature or if they have exhausted all other potential access options.

The initial patient assessment and preparation are similar to that for tunnelled venous access catheters. It is essential that previous access history is reviewed as a tunnelled dialysis catheter is often the last access option for a patient in whom all other methods have failed. It is not uncommon in this situation to find multiple areas of central venous stenotic disease which may require venoplasty prior to line insertion.

The patient is prepared and positioned as for a tunnelled venous access catheter. The right internal jugular vein is the preferred entry point. The femoral veins, whilst suitable for an urgent non-tunnelled catheter, are unsuitable for a tunnelled dialysis catheter because of the risk of infection but may be used when other venous sites are occluded.

Tunnelled dialysis catheters are available in different lengths to allow for variation in patient body habitus and site of insertion. The technical procedure for insertion of the tunnelled dialysis catheter is similar to that used to insert a Hickman catheter. The main difference is that there is no cutting and measuring of the catheter, as its length is fixed. As a general rule a 28-cm catheter is appropriate from the RIJV and a 32-cm from the LIJV. Prior to insertion of the catheter the two lumens should be gently pulled apart and separated, if appropriate, before attaching them to the tunnelling device. Separation of the catheter tips helps to minimise recirculation of blood and optimises haemodialysis. Inserting a dialysis catheter via the LIJV can be problematic; caution must be utilised when inserting the 16Fr peel-away sheath as rupture of the brachiocephalic vein has been reported. Use of a stiff guidewire can help to minimise the risk of this potentially serious complication.

A variety of alternative access approaches for tunnelled haemodialysis catheters, including the external jugular vein[2] and translumbar,[3–5] transhepatic[6] and transrenal[7] approaches to the IVC, have been described.

DIALYSIS CATHETER MAINTENANCE

Tunnelled dialysis catheters have a high propensity to form a fibrin sheath around the line tips, leading to suboptimal haemodialysis function.

'Stripping' poorly functioning haemodialysis catheters (Figs. 10-9 to 10-11) can deal with this problem. This technique involves snaring the catheter from below, having placed a 6Fr sheath in a femoral vein and stripping away the fibrin from both lumens. It is often necessary to advance a standard J-wire down each lumen in turn and into the IVC in order to grasp this with the snare, as trying to grasp the line itself in the right atrium can be very difficult. This straightforward procedure, which can be performed on an outpatient basis, usually results in

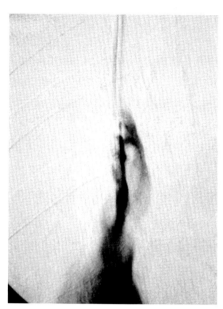

FIGURE 10-9 ■ Linogram demonstrating extensive fibrin sheath formation.

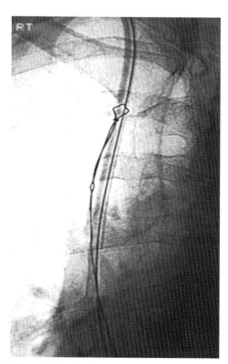

FIGURE 10-10 ■ 'Stripping' the line from below with a snare.

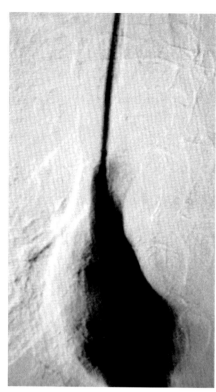

FIGURE 10-11 ■ Post-procedural linogram demonstrates removal of the fibrin sheath.

guidewire. The new tunnelled catheter is inserted through the sheath.

Venoplasty can be performed to disrupt the fibrin sheath immediately prior to catheter exchange; however, this may lead to subsequent central venous stenosis.[10]

REFERENCES

1. National Kidney Foundation KDOQI Guidelines. Updates clinical practice guidelines and recommendations. Am J Kidney Dis 2006;48(Suppl 1):S176–247.
2. Lorenz JM. Unconventional venous access techniques. Semin Intervent Radiol 2006;23(3):279–86.
3. Rajan DK, Croteau DK, Sturza SG, et al. Translumbar placement of inferior vena caval catheters: a solution for challenging haemodialysis access. Radiographics 1998;18:1155–67.
4. Lund GB, Treretola SO, Scheel PJ Jr. Percutaneous translumbar inferior vena cava cannulation for haemodialysis. Am J Kidney Dis 1995;25(5):732–7.
5. Power A, Singh S, Ashby D, et al. Translumbar central venous catheters for long-term haemodialysis. Nephrol Dial Transplant 2010;25:1588–95.
6. Smith TP, Ryan JM, Reddan DN. Transhepatic catheter access for haemodialysis. Radiology 2004;232(1):246–51.
7. Murthy R, Arbabzadeh M, Lund G, et al. Percutaneous transrenal haemodialysis catheter insertion. J Vasc Interv Radiol 2002;13(10): 1043–6.
8. Davies AG, et al. Haemodialysis lines, should we strip? Proceedings of the Cardiovascular and Interventional Radiological Society of Europe Annual Meeting. 2006.
9. Merport M, Murphy TP, Egglin TK, Dubel GJ. Fibrin sheath stripping versus catheter exchange for the treatment of failed tunneled hemodialysis catheters: randomised clinical trial. J Vasc Interv Radiol 2000;11(9):1115–20.
10. Ni N, Mojibian H, Pollak J, Tal M. Association between disruption of fibrin sheaths using percutaneous transluminal angioplasty balloons and late onset of central venous stenosis. Cardiovasc Intervent Radiol 2011;34(1):114–19.

significantly improved dialysis flow rates.[8] The fibrin sheath stripped from the line lodges in small pulmonary arteries but this does not lead to clinical problems.

Alternatively, the catheter can be replaced using an over-the-wire technique.[9] The cuff is dissected out from the skin before a stiff guidewire is inserted through one of the lumens and into the IVC. The catheter is then removed and a peel-away sheath is inserted over the

CHAPTER 11

SPINAL INTERVENTIONS

Konstantinos Katsanos • Tarun Sabharwal

CHAPTER OUTLINE

INTRODUCTION

IMAGE-GUIDED VERTEBRAL BIOPSY

SPINAL INJECTION PROCEDURES

PERCUTANEOUS DISC DECOMPRESSION

PERCUTANEOUS VERTEBRAL AUGMENTATION

ABLATION OF SPINAL TUMOURS

EMBOLISATION OF SPINAL TUMOURS

INTRODUCTION

Spinal interventional procedures are used in the diagnosis and treatment of various spinal pathologies of benign or malignant origin. Procedures described in the present chapter are performed by interventional radiologists, who work within a wider multidisciplinary team of clinical specialists that may include neurosurgeons, orthopedic surgeons and oncologists. Interventional radiologists are appropriately trained to carry out spinal intervention with minimal risks, and can manage any relevant procedure-related complications.

IMAGE-GUIDED VERTEBRAL BIOPSY

Vertebral bone biopsy is a minimally invasive percutaneous procedure with the advantages of low cost, low morbidity, high accuracy and repeatability and it has replaced open surgical biopsy in most cases. Fluoroscopy-guided bone biopsy was first described in the 1970s and image-guided bone biopsy is today a critical part of the management of musculoskeletal lesions, including primary tumours, bone metastases and bone infections. Spinal applications include image-guided biopsy of the vertebrae, the sacrum and the iliac bones. Disc aspiration for the investigation of spondylodiscitis is also widely practiced. Under X-ray guidance a biopsy needle can be used to access and sample small lesions in difficult anatomies, such as the vertebral body or intervertebral discs, without surgical exploration.

Patient Preparation

Before considering an image-guided spinal biopsy all relevant medical history, laboratory tests and relevant imaging findings must be analysed thoroughly and discussed with the multidisciplinary team. The multidisciplinary team usually includes the spinal neurosurgeon, the musculoskeletal radiologist, the responsible oncologist and an experienced cytopathologist. Correlation with plain films and MRI is critical to avoid unnecessary procedures in certain benign lesions with typical imaging appearances ('do not touch lesions'). Well-recognised and accepted indications and contraindications for spinal biopsies are outlined in Table 11-1. In general, spinal biopsy is indicated to identify tumour or infection. If bone metastasis is suspected, biopsy should be undertaken only if the result will influence oncologic management. Spinal biopsy may also be considered for tumour staging, or to compare histological characteristics in patients with synchronous or metachronous metastatic cancer. Primary musculoskeletal tumours require identification, grading and often cytogenetic analysis to determine appropriate treatment strategies and prognosis. Bleeding diathesis is the only absolute contraindication to spinal biopsy as it can cause severe haemorrhage or epidural haematoma that may compromise the spinal cord. Alternative options and the risk–benefit ratio should be considered in all patients with spinal lesions that are difficult to access percutaneously.

Correction of coagulopathy, informed consent and consideration regarding conscious sedation or general anaesthesia constitute key elements of preoperative assessment for all spinal biopsy procedures. Anticoagulants like warfarin and heparin must be stopped prior to the procedure per local institutional policy and a platelet count below 50,000/mL must be corrected with adequate platelet transfusion. Bleeding diathesis with an international normalised ratio (INR) higher than 1.3–1.5 may be reversed with transfusions of fresh frozen plasma or cryoprecipitate as needed. Antiplatelet agents must be stopped in all cases of spinal interventions at least 5 days prior to the procedure to correct platelet dysfunction.

Image Guidance

Image guidance may be real-time plain fluoroscopy based on bony landmarks or computed tomography (CT),

TABLE 11-1 Image-Guided Vertebral Bone Biopsy: Indications and Contraindications

Indications
- Determine the nature of a non-specific solitary bone or soft tissue lesion.
- Confirm or exclude spinal metastases in patients with known primary tumour.
- Determine nature of spinal metastases in patients with unknown primary tumour.
- Exclude metastatic disease or multiple myeloma in patients with vertebral compression fractures.
- Determine causative infectious agent in spondylodiscitis or osteomyelitis.
- Before vertebroplasty or cementoplasty for medicolegal reasons.

Contraindications
- Uncorrectable coagulopathy.
- Uncooperative patient.
- Hypervascular lesion in the cervical or thoracic spine.
- Anatomical location difficult or unsafe to access.
- Risk of infection spreading to the bone.

which offers higher soft tissue resolution, but is not real time. There are several different routes for performing an image-guided spinal biopsy depending on lesion anatomy and size. Typically, patients are placed in a prone or lateral decubitus position. The transpedicular or posterolateral approach is often used for lumbar vertebral body biopsy (Fig. 11-1). The intercostovertebral approach is usually indicated for the thoracic spine and an anterolateral approach with manual displacement of the large vessels is recommended for the cervical spine (Fig. 11-2). Fluoroscopic guidance is the modality of choice for the majority of spinal procedures and may be supplemented by CT for cervical lesions (Fig. 11-3). Biplane fluoroscopy or rotational flat panel angiography with cone beam CT capabilities are emerging modalities for enhanced image guidance during difficult spinal procedures. CT fluoroscopy is readily available in many institutions, but is generally avoided because of the increased radiation exposure. An oropharyngeal approach is indicated for biopsy of C1 or the dens. A posterior oblique CT-guided approach is usually chosen for biopsy of the pedicles and the other posterior spinal elements or the surrounding soft tissues. The access route will also depend on the image-guidance modalities available. Beware that certain musculoskeletal tumour lesions may be eligible for curative surgical resection; thus certain anatomical compartments, not involved by the tumour, must not be breached by the biopsy needle. This is especially true for soft tissue sarcomas and osteosarcomas to limit local recurrence after resection. Nevertheless, the risk of tract seeding

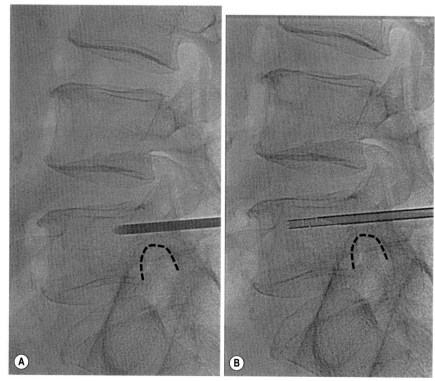

FIGURE 11-1 ■ **Fluoroscopically guided transpedicular biopsy of the L5 vertebral body (lateral projection).** (A) Note the advancement of a beveled 10G needle trocar across the pedicle (black dotted line denotes the superior aspect of the underlying intervertebral foramen). Needle must not breach either the underlying foramen to avoid spinal nerve injury or the medial aspect of the pedicle to avoid epidural haematoma or thecal sac injury. (B) Coaxial insertion of a 12G trephine needle to obtain a bone marrow sample of the cancellous bone of the L5 vertebral body.

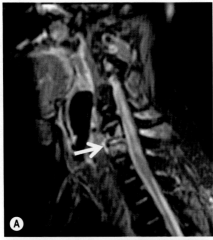

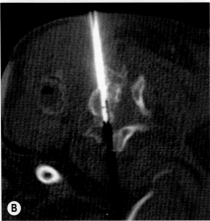

FIGURE 11-2 ■ CT-guided anterolateral biopsy of the C5 vertebral body. (A) Increased signal of the C5–C6 intervertebral disc and the adjacent vertebral bodies (white arrow) in keeping with infectious spondylodiscitis (sagittal STIR image). (B) CT-guided biopsy of the C5 vertebral body using an anterolateral approach and a beveled 10G needle trocar (axial CT image on a lateral decubitus position). A 12G trephine needle has been inserted coaxially for bone sampling. When performing cervical spine biopsies the needle must never breach the transverse foramen to avoid injuring the vertebral artery (dissection or thrombosis), which may induce a vertebrobasilar stroke.

following musculoskeletal fine needle aspiration is very low, estimated at 3–5/100,000 cases.

Performing the Procedure

Routine monitoring of vital signs is necessary during all spinal procedures. Percutaneous vertebral biopsy is a painful procedure because of osseous puncture and conscious sedation is necessary. Sedation is routinely administered using a combination of fentanyl and midazolam according to national and international guidelines. General anaesthesia may be necessary on a case-by-case basis.

In patients with multiple spinal metastatic lesions, the largest and most easily accessible lesion should be chosen. The integrity of the underlying weight-bearing bone must also be considered, although the risk of post-biopsy

iatrogenic vertebral fracture is very low. In patients with painful vertebral pathologic fractures, consideration of palliative cementoplasty following successful histologic analysis is worthwhile to improve quality of life. Bone sampling may be accompanied by sampling of adjacent soft tissues, and percutaneous disc biopsy may include biopsy of the neighbouring subchondral vertebral endplates to increase diagnostic yield. When planning a vertebral biopsy, mixed sclerotic-lytic or contrast-enhancing lesions are preferred as target lesions compared to hypodense or cystic areas that often contain necrotic components. Beware of certain spinal lesions, such as renal cell carcinoma metastases and haemangiomas, which may be highly vascular and can be associated with an increased risk of haemorrhagic complications. Different specimens must be sent for histology, cytopathology and microbiology.

With regard to needle choice, the length of the needle (10–20 cm long) must be appropriate to the depth of the lesion. Spinal bone biopsies require use of 11–15G trephine needles that obtain an adequate core of bone marrow. Spinal trephine needles are inserted through a matching outer cannula that is hammered to penetrate the osseous cortex, as necessary. Routine 16–20G core biopsy cutting needles are used in patients with tumours that have a soft tissue component or extensive osteolysis. Fine needle aspiration with a 20–22G needle (Chiba needle) is usually enough for sampling intervertebral discs and aspiration of collections. Larger bore needles are preferred for percutaneous biopsy of the vertebrae because of their rigidity and ability to be hammered or drilled into the bone. Automated drilling biopsy guns have recently been made available for routine bone marrow biopsy and can be used in patients with bony lesions that have a thick overlying cortex. Depending on the indication, trephine core biopsy for histology may be combined with coaxial fine needle aspiration for cytology and microbiology.

Results

Reported diagnostic accuracy of spinal bone biopsies is above 95%, but there is always a small risk of a non-diagnostic outcome because of insufficient tissue sampling or sampling of necrotic or sclerotic areas. Diagnosis of spinal metastatic tumours is considered generally easier than primary bone tumours, but diagnostic yield also depends on lesion size and accessibility. In general, more than three needle passes are recommended to obtain an adequate volume of tissue and increase biopsy success. Multiple core biopsies are required for diagnosis of lymphoma, whereas fine needle aspiration may suffice for the diagnosis of metastasis and infection. Large core trephine biopsy is indicated for investigation of primary spinal tumours like osteoblastomas. The diagnostic accuracy of percutaneous disc biopsy for the investigation of infectious spondylodiscitis is around 50% and the rate of negative cultures may well exceed 60%, even when paravertebral or intervertebral disc fluid collections are aspirated. The most commonly isolated pathogen in infectious spondylodiscitis is blood-borne *Staphylococcus aureus*, and empirical antibiotic treatment may be initiated even

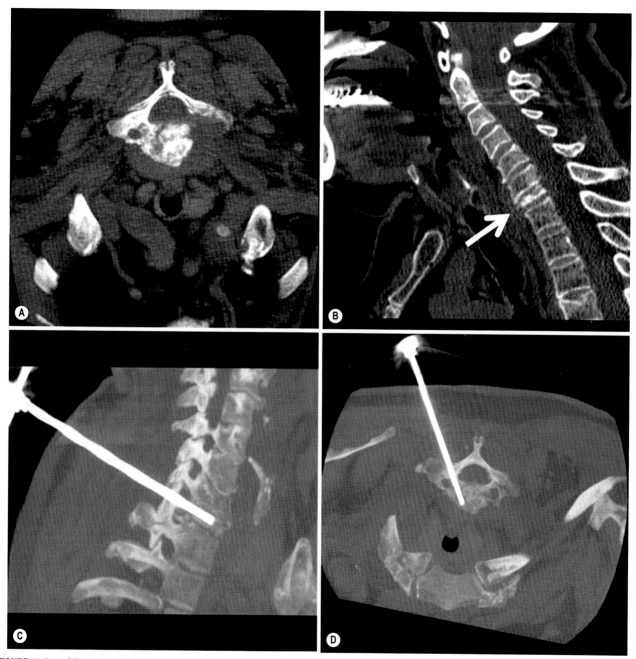

FIGURE 11-3 ▪ **CT-guided transpedicular biopsy of the C7 vertebral body.** (A, B) Collapse and destruction of the C7 vertebral body (white arrow) in a patient with history of metastatic lung adenocarcinoma (A: axial CT image; B: sagittal reformatted CT image). (C, D) CT-guided transpedicular bone biopsy using a beveled 10G needle trocar with coaxial insertion of a 12G trephine needle. Note the oblique needle tract without breach of the spinal canal, the ipsilateral transverse foramen or the over- and underlying intervertebral foramen (C: sagittal CT image; D: axial volume-rendered CT image).

without definite diagnosis. Antibiotics can be stopped 24–48 h prior to tissue sampling to increase diagnostic yield from fluid cultures.

SPINAL INJECTION PROCEDURES

Lumbar Disc Herniation

Lumbosacral radicular pain is defined as pain radiating to one or more lumbar or sacral dermatomes caused by

nerve root compression producing irritation and inflammation. The pathology is also known as sciatica or nerve root pain. Radiculitis (only radicular pain) should be distinguished from radiculopathy that includes objective findings of sensory or motor disturbance. Lumbosacral radicular pain is the commonest form of neuropathic pain with an annual prevalence of 9.9–25% in the general population. Pain usually resolves spontaneously in two-thirds of patients within 12 weeks of onset. However, almost a third of patients continue to suffer from radicular pain after 3 months to 1 year. Before the age of 50 the most frequent cause is disc herniation, while after the age of 50 degenerative spine changes are more prevalent. Radiating pain may be sharp, stabbing, throbbing or burning and diagnosis is based on medical history and medical examination. Dermatomal distribution, pain that increases while bending forward or coughing, and a positive Laségue or crossed Laségue test are the usual clinical findings. Disc herniation most commonly occurs in the L4–L5 (around 30%) and L5–S1 (around 50%) intervertebral segments and the L4, L5 and S1 roots are the ones most commonly affected. MRI may confirm the presence of a disc herniation, but the specificity of the examination is very low because incidental disc herniations are detected in 20–36% of asymptomatic individuals.

Selective segmental nerve blocks, whereby a specific nerve root is anaesthetised via an image-guided transforaminal injection of a small amount of lignocaine, may be helpful in excluding one level if negative, but positive blocks are considered non-specific because of significant overlap between innervation of adjacent segments. Transforaminal blocks may simultaneously block afferent input from the corresponding nerve root, the sinuvertebral nerve that innervates the intervertebral disc anteriorly and the dorsal ramus that innervates the facet joint and the muscles posteriorly at the same level. Therefore, differential diagnosis between true radiculitis, discogenic low back pain and mechanical facetogenic low back pain may be difficult. It is crucial that any red flags (trauma, cancer and infection) are excluded during diagnostic workup of the patient. Watch out for a previous medical history of cancer or unexplained weight loss, structural spinal deformities, symptoms appearing before the age of 20 or after 50 and acute neurological deficits that may require urgent surgical decompression. For example, a patient with acute cauda equina syndrome with saddle anaesthesia, sacral polyradiculopathy and sphincter dysfunction must be referred for emergent surgery.

Indications

Spinal epidural injections with local anaesthetic and corticosteroids are generally indicated in patients with ongoing lumbosacral radicular pain who have failed conservative therapy with non-steroidal anti-inflammatory drugs (NSAIDS), early mobilisation and physiotherapy for at least 6–12 weeks. The primary indication is local compression of a nerve root or exiting spinal nerve by intervertebral disc herniation confirmed by CT or MRI. Spinal injections are also indicated for pain relief in patients with failed back surgery syndrome (FBSS) and degenerative spinal canal stenosis and in elderly patients who are not surgical candidates. The pathophysiology of sciatica combines mechanical nerve compression and the local release of pro-inflammatory mediators such as prostaglandins, nitrous oxide, phospholipase A2 and cyclooxygenase-2. The rationale for epidural corticosteroid injections is based on their potent anti-inflammatory properties. Epidural steroid injections are contraindicated in pregnancy, active peptic ulcers and uncorrectable coagulopathy and caution should be exercised in patients with diabetes and osteoporosis.

Technique

Approaches to epidural peri-radicular injections include (1) the classical interlaminar, (2) the targeted transforaminal and (3) the caudal approach. Transforaminal epidural injection of steroids is reported to provide the best results in patients with segmental radicular symptoms. Compared to the posterior interlaminar approach, the transforaminal approach may achieve more precise delivery at the level of the inflamed root and the drugs may theoretically reach the interface between the disc hernia and the compressed nerve root at the ventral epidural space, more easily. The interlaminar approach may be chosen in posterolateral disc herniations, while the transforaminal approach is usually preferred for foraminal and extraforaminal herniations. However, transforaminal injections can be associated with rare neurological complications, including paraplegia in the lumbar spine and tetraplegia or death in the cervical spine (discussed later). Either fluoroscopy or computed tomography (CT) may be used for image guidance. The latter has the advantage of superb soft tissue contrast resolution, but fluoroscopic guidance is faster and allows for real-time control of needle advancement and drug injection to avoid complications (Fig. 11-4).

When a fluoroscopic-guided interlaminar epidural injection is used, the patient is positioned in the prone position or in the decubitus foetal position based on operator preference. The correct intervertebral segment is identified using fluoroscopic guidance and bone landmarks. Cranial angulation of the tube usually helps to

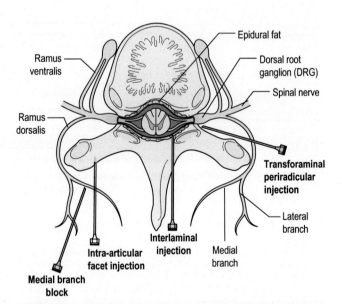

FIGURE 11-4 ■ **Spinal injections.** Schema shows the various different approaches for spinal injections to treat mechanical or radicular cervical and lumbar back pain. Transforaminal and interlaminar approaches are used for the injection of steroids and anaesthetics to the epidural space. Intra-articular injections are used for the injection of steroids into painful degenerated zygapophysial (facet) joints. Medial branch blocks are used for temporary anaesthesia or radiofrequency ablation of the medial branch of the dorsal ramus to achieve long-lasting denervation of the painful facet joints.

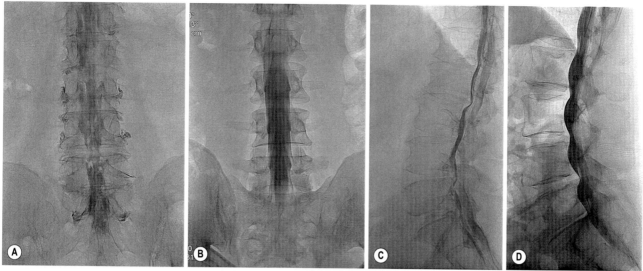

FIGURE 11-5 ■ **Epidurography versus myelography.** (A) Anteroposterior view after injection of iodinated contrast medium into the epidural space (dorsal interlaminal epidurographic approach). (B) Anteroposterior view after injection of iodinated contrast into the subarachnoid space (interlaminal myelographic approach). (C) Lateral projection of epidurography. (D) Lateral projection of myelography. In epidurography and spinal injections the agents are injected into the epidural fat compared to myelography that involves injection of contrast into the cerebrospinal fluid. In epidurography the contrast material outlines the epidural fat and the exiting spinal nerves beyond the intervertebral foramen (AP view), as well as the epidural space in between the thecal sac and the posterior longitudinal ligament (lateral view). In myelography the contrast material outlines the subarachnoid space and opacifies the CSF that surrounds the spinal cord denoting the root sleeves of the nerve roots inside the spinal canal.

adjust for the lordosis of the lumbosacral junction. Typically, a 22G spinal needle (alternatively an 18- to 20G Tuohy needle) is used to enter the interspinous and the flavum ligaments. The latter consists almost entirely of collagen fibres and provides the greater resistance to the needle. Entry to the dorsal epidural space is confirmed with the loss of resistance technique and may be confirmed with the injection of an aliquot of contrast agent. Operators must be familiar with the different imaging features of contrast material patterns between intrathecal (myelography) and epidural (epidurography) injections (Fig. 11-5). The paramedian interlaminal approach with the needle pointing towards the affected side is recommended for more targeted injections (Fig. 11-6). In this case a contralateral oblique projection is used to monitor advancement of the needle and the needle tip enters the epidural space when it crosses the imaginary spinolaminar line (Fig. 11-7).

When a fluoroscopic-guided transforaminal epidural injection is used, the patient is positioned prone and the C-arm is rotated to an ipsilateral oblique projection until the ipsilateral facet column is superimposed midway between the anterior and posterior wall of the vertebral bodies ('scotty dog' projection). The tube may also need to be angled cranially to align the superior and inferior vertebral endplates for the lower lumbar levels. Using tunnel collimation a 22- to 25G needle is advanced into the intervertebral foramen. The needle must slip along the lateral border of the respective facet joint and enter the dorsocranial quadrant of the intervertebral foramen (Figs. 11-8, 11-9). On scotty dog projections the needle target is actually below the junction of the pedicle and the ipsilateral transverse process ('eye of the

scotty dog') and lateral to the inferior articular process of the respective facet joint. The depth of the needle is checked periodically in a lateral projection and elicitation of paresthesia (provoked by puncture of the spinal nerve) is best avoided. Some authors refer to the so-called 'safe triangle' when describing bone landmarks used for transforaminal periradicular nerve injections. On an ipsilateral oblique projection, the triangle is an imaginary triangular area formed cranially by the pedicle and transverse process, laterally by a line connecting the lateral edges of the superior and inferior pedicle and inferomedially by the spinal nerve root, which serves as the tangential base of the triangle. Once the needle tip is in the correct position, contrast medium is injected to outline the nerve sheath of the exiting root and exclude intrathecal, intra-arterial or intravenous injections (Fig. 11-10). After correct opacification of the epidural fat surrounding the spinal nerve, 1 mL of local anaesthetic is injected (bupivacaine 0.5% or lignocaine 1–2%) followed by a dose of steroid. In selective cases the caudal approach through the sacral hiatus may be chosen (Fig. 11-11).

Complications

Spinal epidural injections are generally considered very safe procedures with variable rates of pain relief (50–70%) that depend on a variety of factors (age, duration of symptoms, aetiology, etc). A time interval of at least 2 weeks is recommended between repeat steroid injections and no more than 3–4 injections per annum are allowed. The most frequent complication of a lumbar interlaminal injection is inadvertent puncture of the dura (2.5%)

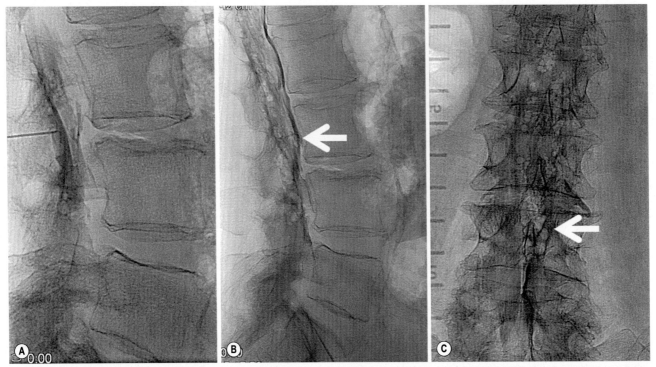

FIGURE 11-6 ■ Interlaminal spinal injection. (A) Interlaminal injection of dilute contrast material with steroids and local anaesthetic at the L3–4 dorsal epidural space in a patient with non-specific mechanical low back pain. (B) Lateral projection. Note spread of the contrast material (and the steroids) to the anterior epidural space (white arrow). (C) Anteroposterior projection after completion of the injection. Note the air bubbles accumulated at the dorsal epidural space because of air injected during application of the loss-of-resistance technique (white arrow).

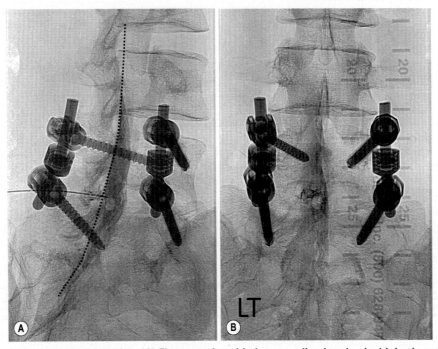

FIGURE 11-7 ■ Paramedian interlaminal injection. (A) Fluoroscopic-guided paramedian interlaminal injection at the L5–S1 level in a young patient with recurrent left-sided radiculopathy 1 year following surgery (failed back surgery syndrome, FBSS). The needle reaches the paramedian dorsal epidural space once the tip of the spinal needle breaches the imaginary spinolaminar line (black dotted line) on the contralateral scotty-dog oblique projection. (B) Anteroposterior view after the injection of the contrast material and steroids confirms selective application of the solution to the affected side.

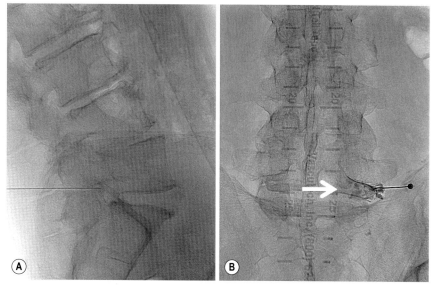

FIGURE 11-8 ■ **Transforaminal periradicular injection.** (A) Fluoroscopic-guided transforaminal periradicular injection of the L5 spinal nerve. Note the location of the tip of the needle at the dorsal aspect of the intervertebral foramen (lateral view). (B) Test injection of contrast material to exclude intravascular needle placement outlines the exiting L5 spinal nerve (white arrow—anteroposterior view).

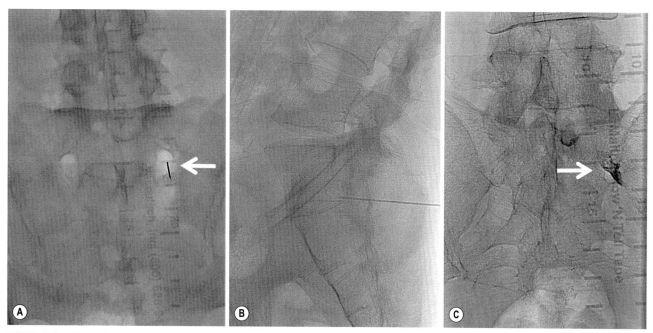

FIGURE 11-9 ■ **Transforaminal periradicular injection.** (A) Fluoroscopic-guided transforaminal periradicular injection of the S1 spinal nerve. The C-arm tube has been rotated cranially to align the dorsal with the ventral sacral foramen. Note the location of the tip of the needle at the superolateral quadrant of the S1 intervertebral foramen (white arrow—lateral view). (B) The needle has been advanced inside the spinal canal (anteroposterior view). (C) Test injection of contrast material to exclude intravascular needle placement outlines the descending S1 spinal nerve (white arrow—anteroposterior view).

which may produce a transient headache. Accidental subarachnoid or subdural punctures may easily be identified with a test injection of contrast agent in the lateral projection to avoid intrathecal injection of the steroid and anaesthetic agents. Radicular pain may also be exacerbated temporarily because of the local effects of the

injection. Other rarely reported complications include arachnoiditis, aseptic or infectious meningitis, epidural abscess and systemic cardiovascular or gastrointestinal side effects from the steroid injection (severe adverse events <0.05%; mild reactions to steroids <5%). Of note, paraplegia is a catastrophic complication that has been

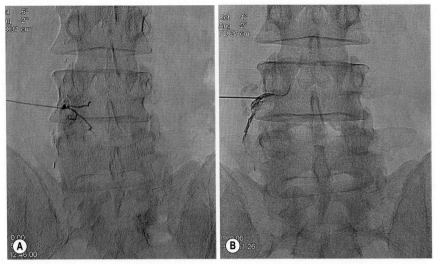

FIGURE 11-10 ■ **Intra-arterial injection.** (A) Test injection of contrast material during an L4 transforaminal injection confirms inadvertent puncture of a radicular arterial branch. Accidental injection of particulate steroids inside a spinal radiculomedullary branch may cause terminal cord ischaemia and result in a catastrophic neurological event (paraplegia). (B) Successful transforaminal periradicular injection after repositioning of the needle under fluoroscopic control. Note how the contrast material now outlines the L4 spinal nerve and diffuses medially to the epidural space.

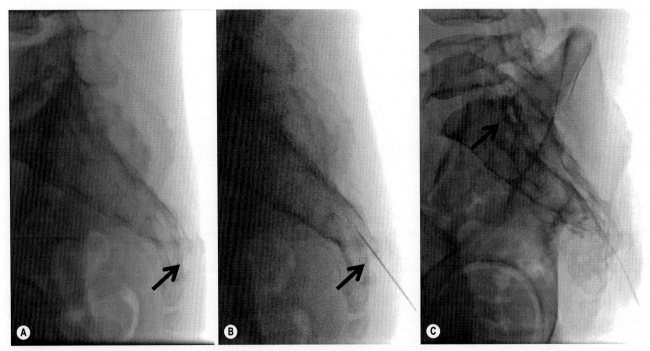

FIGURE 11-11 ■ **Caudal spinal injection (lateral views).** (A) Caudal approach for the injection of agents into the sacral epidural space. The aim is to puncture the superficial dorsal sacrococcygeal ligament (sacrococcygeal membrane) that covers the hiatus (black arrow). (B) The needle follows an oblique ascending course into the sacral epidural space. More injections can be performed at that point (black arrow). (C) Alternatively, a catheter may be advanced up to the L5–S1 level for more selective injection of the steroids (black arrow).

documented in a handful of case reports in association with lumbar transforaminal injections of particulate steroids above the level of L3. The most probable cause is inadvertent intra-arterial injection and embolisation within an unusually low dominant radiculomedullary artery. The largest radicular artery is the arteria radicularis magna (artery of Adamkiewicz), which usually enters the spinal canal on the left side in the lower thoracic level (T9–L1). Accidental injection of particulate steroids into an aberrant radicular branch may then produce terminal

TABLE 11-2 **Steroids**

	Pharmacology	Concentration (mg/mL)	Usual Dose (mg)
Triamcinolone (Kenacort, Bristol-Myers Squibb, New York, NY, USA)	Microparticulate steroid depot	40	40–80
Betamethasone (Celestone, Schering Plough, Kenilworth, NJ, USA)	Microparticulate steroid depot	6	6–12
Dexamethasone (Merck, Whitehouse Station, NJ, USA)	Non-particulate steroid depot	4–10	8–12
Methylprednisolone (Depo-medrol, Pfizer, New York, NY, USA)	Microparticulate steroid depot	40–80	40–80

spinal cord ischaemia with irreversible transverse ischaemic myelitis resulting in paraplegia. Triamcinolone, betamethazone and methylprednisolone have all been found to form aggregations acting as microparticles. Only dexamethasone is considered a particulate-free steroid and is therefore recommended as the drug of choice for all upper lumbar and cervical spinal injections (Table 11-2). No neurologic complications have been reported so far with the use of dexamethasone for spinal injections. Because of the risk of paraplegia, the latest guidelines on spine interventional procedures underline the utility of real-time high-quality fluoroscopy, ideally with digital subtraction angiography, to effectively exclude intra-arterial injections.

Pulsed Radiofrequency Ablation

Epidural corticosteroids are more effective in subacute cases of radiculitis. In chronic cases with established radiculopathy epidural corticosteroids are less effective and they may be combined with pulsed radiofrequency ablation (PRF) of the dorsal root ganglion (DRG) using a routine transforaminal approach. PRF is gaining recognition for effective treatment of persistent neuropathic pain and is applied in combination with corticosteroids. Although its exact mechanism of action remains to be fully elucidated, the rationale of PRF involves modification of transmission of pain signals at the level of the DRG after application of non-thermal pulsed radiofrequency ablation (45 V for 20 ms with a frequency of 2 Hz, for a total of 2–4 min with temperature not exceeding 42°C). No complications or side effects have been reported so far with the use of PRF on the cervical or lumbar DRG.

Adhesiolysis (with hyaluronidase and hypertonic saline) and epiduroscopy are also emerging image-guided techniques for the treatment of persistent or recurrent post-surgery radicular pain, whereas spinal cord neurostimulation is reserved for selected cases with life-disabling pain symptoms.

Facet Joint Syndrome

Axial pain originating from the lumbar zygapophysial joints (facet joint syndrome) is also a common cause of low back pain in the general population. Mechanical pain may arise from any mobile part of the inflamed degenerative facet joints, including the fibrous capsule, the hyaline cartilage and the bone. Painful inflamed facet joints may be associated with spinal canal stenosis because of hypertrophic ligamentum flavum which may also cause sciatica. Advanced age, degenerative disc disease and spondylolisthesis or spondylolysis predispose to facetogenic axial lumbar pain. Diagnosis is always difficult, but paravertebral tenderness on palpation of the facet joints is considered indicative of facetogenic mechanical pain. Intra-articular injection of local anaesthetic with or without steroids or alternatively anaesthetic blocks of the medial branch (medial branch of the dorsal ramus of the spinal nerve that innervates the facet joints) are routinely used for confirmation and treatment of facet joint syndrome (Fig. 11-12). More definite treatment with long-lasting pain relief (6–12 months) may be accomplished with facet denervation using thermal radiofrequency ablation of the medial branch, which is now considered the gold standard treatment of facetogenic pain.

Technique

The technique involves an ipsilateral oblique approach with the patient in the prone position. The needle target is the top of the transverse process, as close as possible to the superior articular process, which is where the medial branch travels. Once the tip of the electrode is in correct position, an RF ablation at 80–90°C for 60 s is performed. Superior and inferior adjacent levels must be treated also because there is significant overlap of zygapophysial joint innervation. Complications are minimal and reported rates of pain relief are well above 60%. Degenerative conditions of the sacroiliac joints may also be responsible for mechanical low back pain radiating to the buttocks and the thighs. In line with facet joint injections, intra-articular steroid injections and thermal radiofrequency denervation are routinely used for pain relief from sacroiliac joint syndrome (Fig. 11-13).

Cervical Spine

Spinal steroid injections and medial branch radiofrequency ablation are equally applicable for the treatment

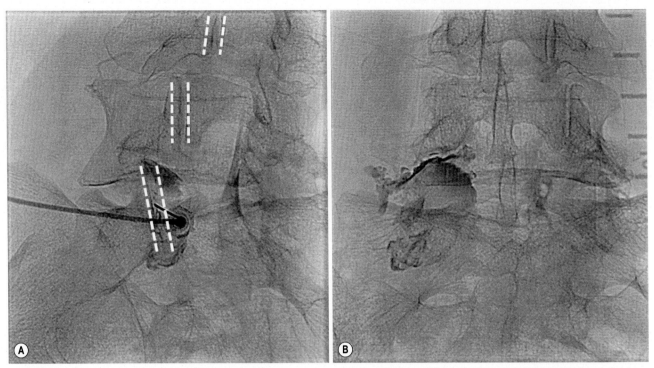

FIGURE 11-12 ■ **Lumbar zygapophysial joint injection.** (A) Intra-articular steroid injection of the L5–S1 facet joint. White dotted tramlines denote the facet joints of the L3–L4, L4–L5 and L5–S1 levels (oblique scotty dog projection). (B) Injection of the steroid–contrast material mixture outlines rupture of the lateral and medial aspects of the facet joint capsule.

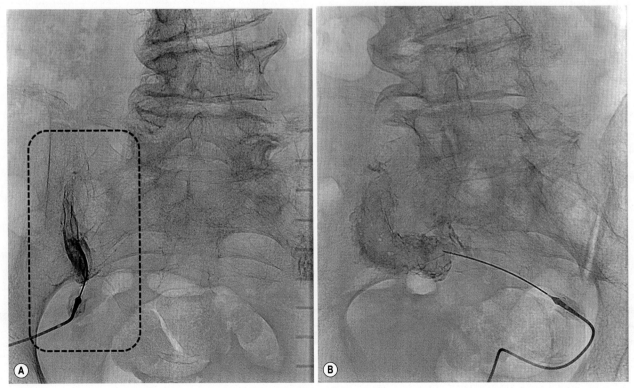

FIGURE 11-13 ■ **Sacroiliac joint injection.** (A) Fluoroscopic-guided injection of the sacroiliac joint for mechanical low back pain radiating to the buttock and the thigh. Point of needle entry should be the caudal aspect of the joint capsule (anteroposterior view). (B) Injection of contrast outlines the ear-shaped configuration of the sacroiliac joint on ipsilateral oblique projection.

of cervical radicular and axial mechanical pain. Cervical radicular pain is defined as electrical or shooting pain perceived in the upper limbs that is caused by compressive irritation of a cervical spinal nerve or its roots. The incidence of cervical radicular pain is approximately 1 person in 1,000. There is a medical history of physical exertion or trauma in 15% of the cases and almost half of the patients report a history of sciatica. The levels of C7 (45–60%) and C6 (20–25%) are affected in the majority of the cases. A detailed neurological examination is necessary to characterise pain distribution, presence of muscle weakness, sensory loss or reflex disturbances. Dermatomal distribution must be correlated with MRI findings of disc prolapse to identify the responsible level. Red flags such as infection, vascular disorders and tumours must be excluded during work-up and imaging may be supplemented by electrophysiological testing in equivocal cases. Interventional treatment of cervical radicular pain includes interlaminal and transforaminal epidural administration of corticosteroids and both approaches can achieve significant relief of pain. In line with the lumbar spine, transforaminal injections offer more accurate administration of the drugs to the affected root. Cervical injections may be performed under fluoroscopic or CT guidance based on the experience and preference of the operator. For cervical transforaminal peri-radicular injections a lateral approach is chosen and the tip of the needle enters the dorsal aspect of the intervertebral foramen posterior to the exiting spinal nerve and in contact with the anterior side of the facet joint, thereby avoiding accidental puncture of the anteriorly located vertebral artery (Fig. 11-14).

The drugs used in the cervical spine are the same as those injected in the lumbar segment, but with a clear preference for particulate-free dexamethasone. Local anaesthetic agents should not be injected in the cervical spine to avoid central nervous system depression and transient phrenic nerve palsy. Steroid injections may also be combined with pulsed radiofrequency ablation of the cervical DRG for enhanced pain relief. Although rare, complications following cervical spinal injections may be catastrophic and deserve special attention. They are divided into spinal cord lesions within the context of anterior spinal artery syndrome and central nervous system side effects involving the brain stem and the cerebellum. The first are attributed to inadvertent injection of a particulate steroid into a radiculomedullary branch feeding the anterior spinal artery and the second are attributed to accidental injection of the anaesthetic and steroid agents into the vertebral artery.

In contrast to the lumbar spine where symptoms of sciatica are more prevalent, facet-related pain is more frequent in the cervical spine. Reportedly, more than 50% of patients presenting with neck pain may suffer from facetogenic pain, usually described as unilateral pain without radiation to the arm, but with limited and painful rotation and retroflexion. Conservative treatment options for cervical facet pain such as physiotherapy, manipulation and mobilisation, although supported by little evidence, are frequently applied before considering interventional treatments. In line with the lumbar spine, interventional pain management techniques, including intra-articular steroid injections, medial branch blocks and radiofrequency ablation denervation are usually offered for the treatment of axial neck pain related to cervical spondylosis and osteoarthritis.

PERCUTANEOUS DISC DECOMPRESSION

The healthy intervertebral disc is avascular and has a complex nerve supply. The sensory innervation of the disc stems from branches of the sympathetic trunk. The dorsal circumference of the annulus fibrosus and posterior longitudinal ligament are innervated by the sinuvertebral nerve, whereas the anterolateral circumference of the annulus fibrosus and the anterior longitudinal ligament are innervated from lateral branches of the communicating ramus and direct branches of the sympathetic trunk. The sinuvertebral nerve stems from the communicating ramus, which in turn interconnects the

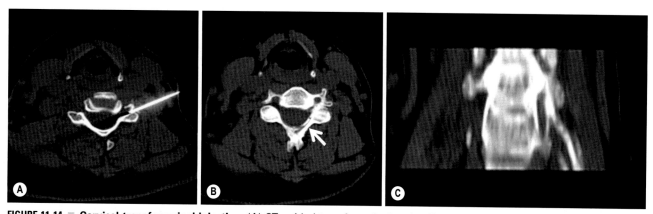

FIGURE 11-14 ■ **Cervical transforaminal injection.** (A) CT-guided transforaminal peri-radicular injection of the left C6 nerve root in a woman with radiculitis. The needle slips posterior to the nerve and in contact with the anterior surface of the facet joint. (B) Note diffusion of the contrast material around the root and into the dorsal epidural space (white arrow—axial image). (C) There is also tracking of the contrast material along the affected spinal nerve (white arrow—reformatted coronal CT image).

sympathetic trunk with the spinal nerves. This extensive nerve plexus has many horizontal and lateral connections resulting in significant overlap in the distribution and projection of painful stimuli originating from adjacent levels and/or structures. Discogenic pain is usually localised medially in the back and may share clinical signs of lumbosacral radicular pain; it is typically provoked by pressure on the spinous processes and exacerbated by coughing, and painful levels are positively correlated with findings of provocation discography.

Disc herniation is defined as local release and herniation of the disc's gelatinous nucleus pulposus because of rupture of the cartilaginous annulus fibrosus. Pain associated with intervertebral disc herniation is a complex process including physical pressure on the adjacent nerve root and local release of proinflammatory cytokines. After failure of 6–12 weeks of conservative treatment, including peri-radicular epidural steroid injections described previously, percutaneous disc decompression is indicated as the next step of treatment. Intervertebral discs constitute a closed hydraulic space. Percutaneous disc decompression aims to reverse spinal nerve compression by removing a small volume of the nucleus pulposus and reducing intradiscal pressure. Techniques of disc decompression (also known as disc nucleotomy) may be chemical (alcohol gel, oxygen–ozone mixture), mechanical (automated discectomy, radiofrequency coblation) or thermal (laser or radiofrequency disc denervation). Percutaneous disc decompression is generally indicated in symptomatic contained disc hernias, but contraindicated in extruded disc hernias and free discal fragments. Red flags should be excluded prior to treatment and acute neurological deficits should be referred for urgent neurosurgery.

Technique

Strict asepsis is required and an approach under fluoroscopic control is used for disc puncture and discectomy. For the lumbar levels the patient is positioned prone and the C-arm tube is rotated first craniocaudally to align with the intervertebral level and second laterally in an oblique 'scotty dog' projection. The needle target lies above the junction of the pedicle and the ipsilateral transverse process ('eye of the scotty dog') and lateral to the superior articular process of the respective facet joint. The needle must slip along the articular process and enter the disc at the lower aspect of the foramen to avoid puncturing the spinal nerve. Intradiscal position of the needle is then confirmed on lateral and anteroposterior projections. For the cervical levels the patient is placed supine and an anterolateral approach is used. Using manual palpation the carotid artery and jugular vein are displaced laterally and the needle is advanced to the intervertebral space travelling between the major vessels laterally and the esophagus medially. Depending on the device used, a needle of appropriate size is used (16–19G) to allow for introduction of the discectomy device from the non-affected side of the disc.

In chemical discolysis (chemonucleolysis), a small dose of an oxygen–ozone mixture or alcohol gel is

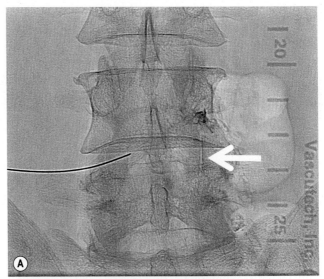

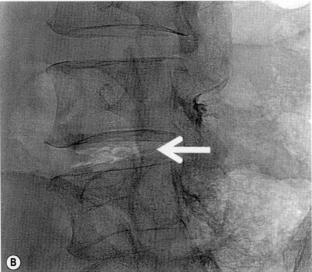

FIGURE 11-15 ■ **Intradiscal ozone injection.** (A) Fluoroscopic-guided injection of the L4–L5 disc (white arrow) with an oxygen–ozone mixture (ozonelysis) for treatment of radiculitis associated with posterolateral disc prolapse (AP view). (B) Note the increased intradiscal radiolucency following injection of the oxygen–ozone mixture into the nucleus pulposus (white arrow—oblique view).

injected inside the disc (Fig. 11-15). The exact mechanisms of ozone action remain unknown, but combined oxidative dehydration of the nucleus pulposus and epidural anti-inflammatory properties are claimed. Chemical nucleotomy aims to dehydrate the nucleus pulposus and decompress the hernia by accelerating disc degeneration. The principle of disc decompression with mechanical devices, laser light or radiofrequency coblation is to reduce intradiscal pressure by vaporising a small amount of the nucleus pulposus and decompress the contained herniation. Mechanical devices may use a variety of automated instruments to extract a small volume of the nucleus pulposus. Thermal energy techniques produce fusion and shrinkage of the peripheral collagen fibres along with denervation of the annulus fibrosus nociceptors responsible for pain. However, there is the risk of thermal damage to the adjacent endplates or the spinal nerves. On the other hand, radiofrequency coblation nucleotomy produces a low-temperature ionic plasma field that disintegrates molecular bonds and cavitates the disc without the risk of heat damage. The coblation electrode debulks the disc by digging multiple channels inside the nucleus pulposus.

Compared to surgical disc decompression, which may cause epidural fibrosis and is associated with a 20–30% risk of FBSS, percutaneous disc decompression with either discectomy or discolysis techniques may achieve 70–90% long-term relief of discogenic and related radicular pain with significant improvement of quality of life. Percutaneous discectomy is also associated with a minimal risk of scar tissue development. Shrinkage of the herniation on CT or MRI is only visible several months following percutaneous disc decompression. The procedure is generally safe and is performed as a day case procedure. Potential complications include infectious discitis, epidural haematoma and vascular or neural injuries (0.25–0.7%).

PERCUTANEOUS VERTEBRAL AUGMENTATION

Percutaneous vertebral augmentation refers to a variety of interventional procedures aimed at stabilising insufficiency or pathologic fractures of the vertebrae and to some extent the pelvis. Vertebral augmentation goes beyond plain cementoplasty, i.e. percutaneous application of cement for bone consolidation, to include interventions that aim to restore the height of the collapsed vertebrae. Procedures like vertebroplasty, kyphoplasty, osteoplasty and sacroplasty are included. Bone packing with cement with or without adjunctive augmentation procedures like kyphoplasty generally aim to treat or prevent pathological fractures and pain in patients with vertebral and pelvic insufficiency fractures or neoplastic osteolytic lesions. Image-guided injection of radiopaque cement is widely used for the stabilisation of painful osteoporotic or malignant vertebral compression fractures and aggressive vertebral haemangiomas. Non-traumatic vertebral compression fractures are defined as reduction in the individual vertebral body height by more than 20% or 4 mm. Vertebral compression fractures produce debilitating back pain with poor quality of life. Most common causes include osteoporosis and bone metastases. Osteoporosis is estimated to afflict more than 10 million people resulting in more than 700,000 vertebral compression fractures per annum in the United States alone. On the other hand, spinal bone metastases, multiple myeloma and lymphoma are the predominant neoplasms associated with spinal pathologic fractures. Well accepted indications for spinal augmentation procedures after failed conservative therapies are outlined in Table 11-3. For osteoporosis the latter is defined as failure to relieve pain even with excessive doses of opiates or inadequate pain management for a period of at least 3 weeks. For metastases, it is defined as unsuccessful pain relief despite

TABLE 11-3   Percutaneous Vertebral Augmentation: Indications and Contraindications

Indications
- Osteoporotic vertebral compression fractures
- Painful osteolytic lesions of the vertebrae (metastases, lymphoma, multiple myeloma)
- Insufficiency fractures of the sacrum and the acetabulum
- Aggressive vertebral haemangiomas and giant cell tumours
- Acute vertebral burst fractures
- Miscellaneous (osteonecrosis, Langerhans cell histiocytosis, vacuum phenomena)

Contraindications
- Spinal cord compression
- Responders to medical therapy
- Uncorrectable coagulopathy
- Osteomyelitis, discitis or active systemic infection
- Allergy to cement or other filler materials
- >5 or diffuse bone metastases
- Lack of neurosurgical support

appropriate oncological treatment and radiotherapy. Patients with aggressive vertebral haemangiomas and giant cell tumours are also candidates for percutaneous vertebroplasty to achieve tumour devascularisation, lesion consolidation and pain relief. In patients with aggressive haemangiomas with anterior epidural spread and/or spinal compression, cementoplasty with adjunctive sclerotherapy may be used as a standalone treatment or as a preoperative treatment.

The ideal candidate for percutaneous vertebroplasty is a patient who presents within 3–6 weeks of a fracture not improving with conservative medical treatment, has mid-line non-radiating back pain that increases with weight bearing and which is exacerbated by manual palpation of the spinous process of the involved vertebra. Preoperative planning for vertebral augmentation involves thorough review of baseline radiographic studies, contrast-enhanced CT and MR imaging in order to identify the level(s) of the fracture, estimate its age, outline the extent of lysis, identify any involvement of the pedicles, evaluate the integrity of the posterior vertebral body wall and exclude epidural or foraminal tumour spread and retropulsed bone fragments, all of which are associated with an increased likelihood of complications. Be extremely careful in case of osteolysis or fracture of the posterior vertebral column, if the tumour extends into the spinal canal, because of a considerably higher risk of complications, including cement leak and further tissue retropulsion. Spinal cord compression with neurologic deficits should be dealt with by operative decompression and posterior spinal stabilisation.

Acute, subacute and non-healing fractures appear hypointense on T1-weighted images and hyperintense on T2-weighted and STIR images. STIR sequences suppress fat and are particularly sensitive in the detection of bone marrow oedema and metabolically active fractures, i.e. acute or chronic non-healing ones. Vertebral haemangiomas are typically hyperintense on both T1- and

T2-weighted images. Of note, an aggressive symptomatic type of haemangiomas with low signal on T1-weighted images and high on T2 has been described. A bone scan is helpful for distinguishing the symptomatic level in case of multiple contiguous fractures and for identifying additional insufficiency fractures of the sacrum and pelvis. Percutaneous vertebral augmentation is not indicated if there is bone sclerosis that suggests successful healing of the fracture of if there is no high signal intensity on STIR sequences.

Vertebroplasty is typically performed with strict asepsis either under local anaesthetic and conscious sedation or under general anaesthesia when larger bore instruments are used, such as those used in kyphoplasty or newer height restoration procedures. Good technique involves, first, proper needle placement and, second, watchful cement injection. Image guidance involves biplane fluoroscopy (Fig. 11-16), but combined guidance with a mobile C-arm placed in front of the CT gantry may be used in lesions difficult to access, such as in osteoplasty

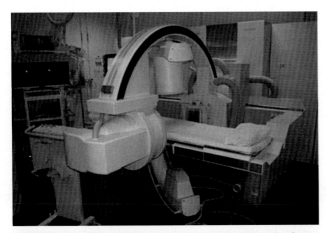

FIGURE 11-16 ■ **Biplane fluoroscopy.** A combination of a C-arm tube and an angiography unit may be placed in an orthogonal configuration for biplane real-time fluoroscopy during vertebroplasty and cementoplasty procedures of the spine.

of pelvic or other extraspinal lesions. Cement injection must always be monitored in real time with high-quality fluoroscopy in the lateral projection. Biplane fluoroscopy allows simultaneous visualisation in two orthogonal planes, but CT guidance is superior in the detection of small cement leaks. Typically, the patient is placed prone and the safest needle pathway is the standard transpedicular approach in the thoracic and lumbar levels with a medial needle trajectory through the pedicle (Fig. 11-17). Alternatively, an intercostovertebral, a parapedicular or a paravertebral pathway may be followed if the vertebral pedicles are not readily visible on frontal X-ray fluoroscopy because of neoplastic infiltration or fracture and collapse. An anterolateral approach by manual lateral displacement of the carotid–jugular complex is typically followed in the cervical spine with the patient in supine position. Note that at least one-third of the vertebral body height is necessary for safe needle insertion and cement injection (Fig. 11-18).

A transpedicular vertebral puncture typically involves the following steps: (1) selection of a large-bore, 10- to 15G, diamond- or bevel-shaped needle, (2) localisation of the relevant pedicle under anteroposterior fluoroscopic projection, (3) local anaesthetic infiltration down to the cortex, (4) needle advancement with a surgical hammer to perforate the cortex at the upper and lateral aspect of the pedicle, (5) avoiding transgression of the medial and inferior border of the pedicle, because the needle might breach the spinal canal or the underlying intervertebral foramen, (6) continuous needle advancement with a 15°–30° angle relative to the midline coronal plane. For unipedicular procedures the needle tip should reach the anterior one-third to one-fourth of the vertebral body, as close as possible to the midline. Kyphoplasty and other vertebral augmentation procedures mandate bipedicular puncture with bilateral needle placement at the lateral aspects of the vertebral body. Such procedures may achieve more symmetrical cement distribution and stabilisation of the vertebral body.

The principle of pain relief with vertebroplasty or kyphoplasty is based on consolidation of the weakened

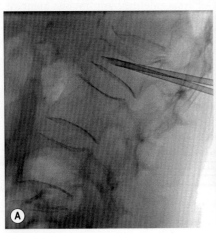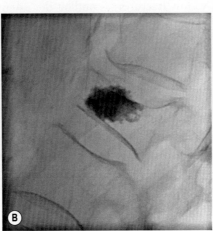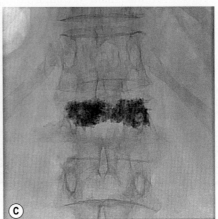

FIGURE 11-17 ■ **Percutaneous vertebroplasty.** (A) Bilateral transpedicular approach for percutaneous vertebroplasty of a painful L1 osteoporotic fracture (lateral projection). (B) There is sufficient cement filling of the anterior and mid-third of the vertebral body (lateral projection). (C) There is optimal cement filling across the midline of the vertebral body (anteroposterior projection).

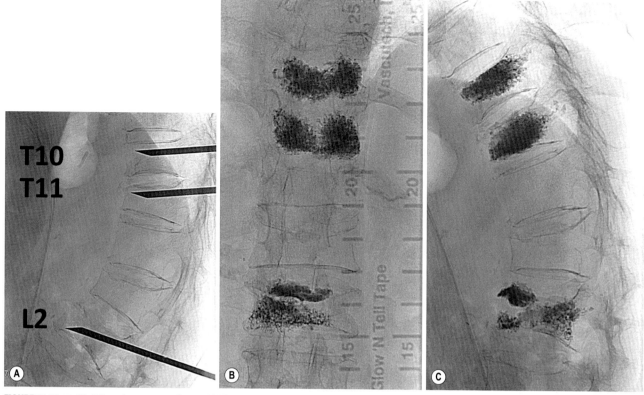

FIGURE 11-18 ■ **Multilevel cementoplasty.** (A) Percutaneous vertebroplasty of three levels in a multiple myeloma patient with several insufficiency fractures of the thoracolumbar spine. Transpedicular approach to the T10, T11 and L2 vertebrae (lateral projection). There is optimal cement filling of all treated vertebrae on the AP view (B) and the lateral view (C). Note the minor cement leak from the anterosuperior aspect of the L2 body towards the disc. Most intradiscal leaks are asymptomatic.

and pathologic cancellous bone. The combined chemical and thermal cytotoxic effects of cement polymerisation also contribute to pain relief. In fact, adequate pain relief may be obtained in metastasis after injection of a volume of only 2 mL of cement. Nowadays, a variety of injectable cements are commercially available. The various cement types are different in terms of chemical synthesis, polymerisation times, biocompatibility, mechanical strength, radiopacity and rheology, and may be indicated for different spinal pathologies. However, polymethylmethacrylate (PMMA) is still the most widely used cement with several decades of experience in orthopedic surgery. Within 1–3 minutes of its recommended preparation, the PMMA increases its viscosity from thin, to thick and pasty. To minimise cement leaks, PMMA must be injected while it remains in this pasty phase. Note that polymerisation of PMMA is an exothermic reaction and cement temperature reaches 80–120°C, which produces local thermocoagulation of tumoural cells, but may also damage healthy neighbouring tissues, like neural roots and the spinal cord itself, in case of extensive leak. Tissue temperatures as high as 70°C have been recorded during PMMA cementoplasty. The suggested endpoint of vertebroplasty is cement packing of the anterior half to two-thirds of the vertebral body with symmetrical cement distribution that extends across the midline to the contralateral side of the vertebra. After completion of the procedure the operator should wait for approximately

30 min for the cement to harden before transferring the patient back to his bed.

The recommended complication threshold for a specialised tertiary centre performing percutaneous vertebroplasty and cementoplasty for pain management is 2% for osteoporotic patients and 10% in malignant patients. Cement leak is the first and most fearsome complication of vertebroplasty, but it is usually asymptomatic. Cement may leak into the epidural veins or the epidural space, inside the neural foramina, towards the disk, the perivertebral venous plexus or into the paravertebral soft tissues. Cement leaks tracking into the arterial system have also been described. Urgent neurosurgical decompression is required in case of cement leak into the spinal canal with cord compression. Cement leaks into the perivertebral venous plexus may continue undetected and produce cement pulmonary embolism that may be potentially fatal. In general, vertebral augmentation procedures are expected to produce satisfactory pain relief with improved mobility and quality of life in approximately 70% of patients with painful bone metastases, 80% of vertebral haemangiomas and 90% of patients with osteoporotic fractures. After vertebroplasty, new compression fractures occur in up to a quarter of patients and almost half of those are located in levels adjacent to the initially treated ones. Kyphoplasty is a modification of vertebroplasty and aims to more effectively restore vertebral height by employing a balloon tamp to create a

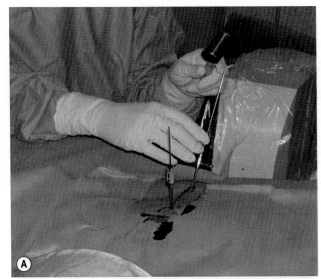

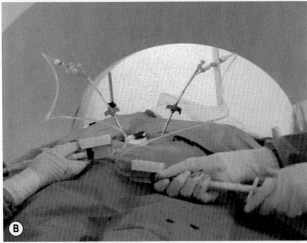

FIGURE 11-19 ■ **Percutaneous kyphoplasty.** (A) Bipedicular advancement of bone trocars under general anaesthesia. (B) Concomitant inflation of bilateral kyphoplasty balloon tamps to try to restore height before cement delivery. (Images courtesy of Professor A. Gangi, Strasburg, France.)

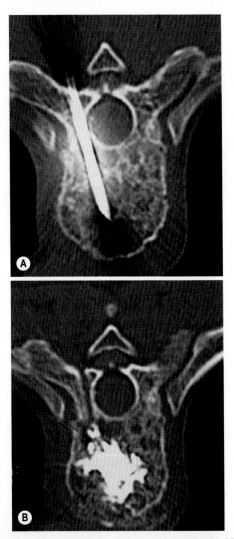

FIGURE 11-20 ■ **Vertebroplasty of haemangioma.** (A) CT-guided vertebroplasty of an aggressive painful haemangioma. Note the transpedicular route of the bone trocar (axial CT images). (B) Final image after successful cement injection. (Images courtesy of Professor A. Gangi, Strasburg, France.)

cavity inside the vertebral body to accommodate the injected cement (Fig. 11-19). The reported mean height restoration after kyphoplasty for compression fractures is around 3–5 mm at the centre of the vertebral body. However, recent data from randomised controlled trials of vertebroplasty or kyphoplasty versus optimal medical therapy have shown that both procedures are significantly better in terms of pain relief and remain most likely equally effective. Osteoplasty refers to radiological cement consolidation of painful insufficiency fractures or malignant osteolyses of the sacrum, the pubic rami, the ischial tuberosities and the acetabulum.

Percutaneous vertebroplasty is also a safe and effective therapy for the treatment of symptomatic vertebral haemangiomas. Its role is limited to pain relief in case of aggressive haemangiomas and in the absence of neurologic deficits (Fig. 11-20). In fact, vertebroplasty was initially described in the late 1980s by Galibert and Deramond for the treatment of a painful aggressive

vertebral haemangioma. Alternatively, vertebroplasty may be used pre-operatively to consolidate the vertebral body and reduce the risk of haemorrhage during subsequent neurosurgical decompression with laminectomy and resection of the epidural extension of the haemangioma.

Latest developments include new mechanical devices for more effective restoration of vertebral height, and the introduction of osteoconductive and osteoinductive cements that may be able to promote more physiological bone healing by being gradually absorbed and substituted by normal osseous minerals. Calcium phospate cements (CPCs) are the most biocompatible and most expensive type of cement commercially available today and are promising because of their osteoconductive properties. CPC consist of calcium phosphate powders dissolved in an aqueous solution. Around room temperature apatite or brushite crystals precipitate from injectable CPC, which in turn stimulate new bone formation. Histological

TABLE 11-4 Cement Fillers

Polymethylmethacrylate (PMMA)	Composite Cements	Calcium Phosphate Cements
Methylmethacrylate polymers	Dimethacrylate resins	Apatite or brushite phosphates
Good radiopacity	Good radiopacity	Low radiopacity
Low cost	Moderate cost	High cost
Exothermic reaction and coagulation (80–120°C)	Abrupt setting at low temperature (<58°C)	Delayed setting at room temperature
Fibrous tissue encapsulation	Surrounding bone mineralisation	Biocompatible and bioresorbable
Recommended for osteoporosis and metastases	Recommended for osteoporosis in younger ages	Recommended for recent burst fractures

examination has shown early bioresorption of CPC after 2 weeks and abundant new bone apposition without inflammation or fibrous encapsulation. Consequently, vertebral augmentation with CPC has been proposed for repair of recent thoracolumbar burst fractures in younger populations (Table 11-4).

ABLATION OF SPINAL TUMOURS

Tumour ablation is defined as the direct application of chemical or physical therapies to a tumour with the aim of achieving complete eradication or substantial destruction. A wide range of radiological locoregional ablative techniques is now available, which induce tumourous cell death primarily through coagulative necrosis or ischaemia. They may be broadly categorised into thermal ablation, cryoablation and transcatheter embolisation. The latter obliterates the vascular supply of the target tumour and can also be combined with targeted chemotherapy.

The main indications for spinal ablation procedures are (1) palliative treatment of painful pre-terminal metastatic bone disease of the spine and pelvis and (2) selected cases of curative treatment of selected benign bone tumours like osteoid osteomas or local control of aggressive vertebral haemangiomas. Typically, thermal ablation is used for pain management in patients with bone metastases and intractable pain that have not responded to radiotherapy and opiates. Up to 85% of patients presenting with breast, prostate and lung cancer have evidence of bone metastases at the time of death. Relief of pain from these deposits is an important aspect of palliative care. Pain from bone metastases is thought to be caused by a combination of periosteal stretching by tumour expansion, cytokine release from tumour cells, osteolysis and fracture fragments that move under compressive loads, and infiltration or compression of nerves or soft tissues. External beam radiation therapy may have variable and transient results. In fact, it can take weeks to take effect and fails to relieve pain in up to 30% of patients.

Spinal tumour ablation can be performed as a day case procedure under conscious sedation and with acceptably low morbidity and mortality. Percutaneous ablation may be repeated for new or recurrent disease and has a low complication rate due to its minimally invasive nature. Pain symptoms must correlate accurately with radiological findings and informed consent must be obtained with realistic patient expectations. Spine ablation procedures

are carried out under CT or X-ray guidance, or a combination thereof. If cement is to be injected, high-quality fluoroscopy is of paramount importance to enhance procedural safety. Lately, real-time open-bore MR guidance systems are available for dedicated state-of-the-art interventional oncology suites. CT guidance is generally adequate for routine procedures because it offers high tissue spatial resolution and may differentiate sensitive adjacent organs and neural structures, at the expense, however, of increased patient exposure to radiation. Conscious sedation (i.e. neuroleptanalgesia) is sufficient for radiofrequency and microwave ablation of lytic lesions, but ablation of osteoid osteomas definitely requires regional or general anaesthesia.

Percutaneous ethanol injection is the simplest and cheapest method of percutaneous tumour ablation. Alcoholisation causes tumour necrosis directly through cellular dehydration and indirectly through vascular thrombosis and tissue ischaemia. Typically, a fine needle (21–22G) is directed into the centre of the target lesion and a mixture of iodinated contrast (25%) and lidocaine 1% (75%) is first injected to assess the extent of tissue diffusion and provide local anaesthesia. Then 5–25 mL of 96% ethanol is instilled into the tumour, provided there is no vascular communication or adjacent vital organ or neural structure communication. Alcoholisation is reserved for ablation and local control of large pelvic tumours or expansile mass lesions, because of the unpredictable diffusion of alcohol which can cause irreversible neurological injury.

Radiofrequency ablation (RFA) was first applied in the early 1990s for the treatment of hepatic tumours and is today the most widely adopted and commonly employed technique for percutaneous ablation of solid organ malignancies. Nowadays, RFA has evolved into a multi-purpose tool for the skeletal system. In general, RFA applicators are available in the form of straight or expandable electrodes that are inserted under guidance into the centre of the target tumour. Then, a high-frequency alternating current (460–500 kHz) is delivered inside the tumour, which causes agitation of the tissue ionic molecules, which in turn produces frictional heat. The applied electrical current exits the body through grounding pads attached usually at the thighs. The thermal effect depends on the electrical conducting properties of the tissues treated. Local tissue temperatures approach 100°C and result in coagulative necrosis of the tumour. Ablation treatment must include a 0.5–1 cm margin of healthy tissue around the target lesion to eradicate any microscopic satellite foci and avoid early local recurrence. Note that the efficacy of RFA may be limited by adjacent high-flow vascular structures, which act as a cooling circuitry (widely known as the heat-sink phenomenon) and increased tissue impedance if tissue vaporisation and/or charring occur. In palliative ablation of bone metastases the principal aim of RF is to ablate the bone–tumour interface, where the pain source arises. Large ablation volumes are generally avoided near the spine and sacrum to minimise the risk of nerve injury. Microwave thermocoagulation is another emerging ablative technology, which depends on the application of an electromagnetic wave (around 900 MHz) through an electrode antenna. Electromagnetic microwaves travelling through tissue produce ultrahigh-frequency agitation of water molecules and production of frictional heat, which results in coagulative necrosis of the tissues. No grounding pads are necessary for the transmission of electromagnetic microwaves. Microwaves are more versatile and efficient than RFA, since they operate independently of any electrical current convection and can achieve higher temperatures and larger ablation zones more quickly than RFA. Microwaves also suffer less from heat-sink phenomena compared to RFA.

Cryotherapy is an alternative technique that freezes lesions to form an 'iceball'. Briefly, miniaturised argon-gas applicators can produce controlled percutaneous tissue freezing under CT or MR imaging (Fig. 11-21). Rapid expansion of argon gas delivered under high pressure inside a sealed cryoprobe reaches −100°C within a few seconds on the basis of the Joule–Thomson effect. Freezing then develops gradually around the cryoprobe to form an ovoid iceball. Cellular necrosis occurs below −20°C via a combination of ice formation and osmosis along tissues causing protein denaturation and rupture of cell membranes. Effective cryoablation involves a freeze–thaw–freeze cycle; i.e. high-pressure argon gas is delivered to achieve a freezing phase followed by a thawing phase with helium gas, and then a second argon gas-freezing phase. Effectiveness of cryoablation may be limited by tissue thawing from nearby high-flow vascular structures (known as the cool-sink phenomenon), which is the opposite of the heat-sink phenomenon occurring during thermoablation. Cryoablation has the added advantages of direct CT or MR visualisation and monitoring of treatment outcome with less peri- and postoperative pain. The iceball is visible in real time under CT or MR. However, cryoablation is a lot more expensive and time-consuming than traditional RFA and MW procedures.

As a general rule, severe pain from bone metastases can be treated with percutaneous ablation when conventional therapies such as opiate analgesia, chemotherapy and radiotherapy are ineffective, too slow acting or cause unacceptable side effects. Significant symptomatic improvement is expected in more than 80% of patients with sustained pain relief for more than 6 months. Ablation of weight-bearing bones must be supplemented with prophylactic cement consolidation if a pathological fracture is anticipated. Proposed criteria to identify bone lesions at a high risk of pathological fracture include cortical destruction >50%, lytic lesion with a diameter >3cm and weight-bearing pain on exertion. For example, cementoplasty of painful expansile osteolytic lesions of the acetabulum may be combined with cryo- or thermocoagulation techniques with the aim of palliative bone consolidation following tumour destruction. PMMA

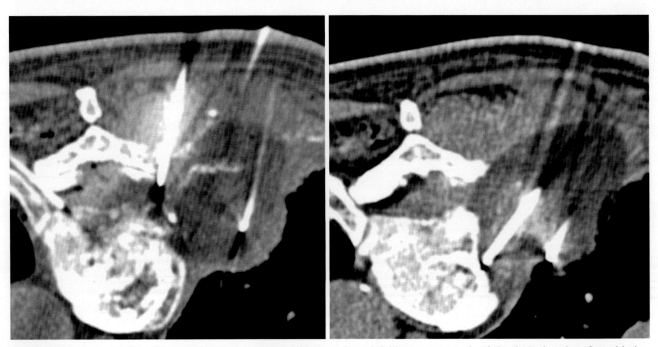

FIGURE 11-21 ■ **Cryoablation.** CT-guided percutaneous cryoablation of a painful bone metastasis of the thoracic spine. Cryoablation allows for real-time monitoring of the treatment effect (hypodense ellipsoid iceball) to avoid neurologic injury. (Image courtesy of Professor A.Gangi, Strasburg, France.)

cementoplasty, which also has inherent antineoplastic properties, may be used either as an individual therapy for painful insufficiency fractures or as adjunctive stabilisation treatment following spine and pelvic ablation therapies. Note that PMMA setting times depend on local tissue temperature. Therefore, higher ambient temperatures, such as after radiofrequency or microwave ablation, will accelerate polymerisation and hardening of the material. In contrast, lower temperatures, such as during subzero cryoablation, will significantly delay cement polymerisation reaction with increased risk of cement leak. Therefore, cement injection may be performed 1 day after ablation to allow for normalisation of tissue temperatures.

Complications

General complications of spinal bone ablation include damage to surrounding structures such as nerve roots with bowel and bladder symptoms, formation of tumour-cutaneous fistulae and pathological fractures or cement leak with the use of adjunctive cementoplasty. Use of appropriate thermosensors and insulation techniques, like carbon dioxide insufflation, may improve safety and efficacy of spinal ablation procedures. During thermal ablation, passive thermocouples, which are available as fine needles, may be inserted alongside the electrodes to monitor temperature rise in sensitive structures, such as at the level of the intervertebral foramina or in the posterolateral epidural space to protect the spinal cord and exiting nerve roots from inadvertent thermal injury. Carbon dioxide can be also very useful for displacement of vital hollow organs and protection of adjacent nerves because of its high insulation coefficient and zero risk of gas embolism.

Osteoid Osteomas

Percutaneous ablation is also considered first-line therapy for eradication of osteoid osteomas. Osteoid osteoma (OO) is a benign skeletal neoplasm of unknown aetiology consisting of both osteoid and woven bone elements that are surrounded by osteoblasts. OO represents 4% of all bone tumours and accounts for 12% of all benign cases. The lesion is usually smaller than 1.5 cm in diameter and may occur in any bone, but it is found in the posterior spinal elements in approximately 6% of patients. Patients complain of dull or aching pain, worse during the night and typically relieved by salicylates. The usual appearance of OOs is of a small sclerotic bone island with a circular radiolucent defect called a nidus. Computed tomography (CT) is the imaging method of choice for precise localisation of the OO nidus and accurate guidance during percutaneous thermal ablation (Fig. 11-22). Intervention is performed under general or spinal anaesthesia, because penetration and ablation of the OO nidus is extremely painful. Regional nerve blocks can be used if the extremities are involved. Typically, the nidus is ablated with a standard non-perfused radiofrequency electrode or with a laser optical fibre that emits near-infrared wavelength laser light (neodymium yttrium

aluminum garnet Nd:YAG). Resolution of pain symptoms is reported after 24–48 h in the majority of the cases with overall clinical success rates of 80–100%. Radiofrequency ablation has also been successfully applied in the eradication of osteoblastomas, chondroblastomas, giant cell tumours, enchondromas and eosinophilic granulomas. Percutaneous ablation for cytoreduction of sacral chordomas and sarcomas, and local control of aggressive desmoid tumours has also been reported.

EMBOLISATION OF SPINAL TUMOURS

Another field of spinal interventional oncology includes arterial embolisation to pre-operatively reduce tumour vascularity or palliate patients who are poor surgical candidates but require symptom relief. The spine is the most common site of bone metastases and primary or secondary spinal tumours may produce pain, mechanical instability, and radiculopathy or compression myelopathy. Transcatheter arterial embolisation of hypervascular spinal tumours can reduce mass effect, relieve cord compression and even improve resectability during neurosurgical reconstruction and stabilisation of the spine. Operators must be skillful in microparticle and microcoil embolisation techniques and be familiar with normal and aberrant cord vascular anatomy to avoid disastrous complications of non-target embolisation. The normal spinal cord is supplied by three longitudinal arteries: one anterior spinal artery that runs anteriorly in the groove of the anterior median fissure and two posterior spinal arteries that run in parallel posterolaterally on the cord itself. Spinal arteries are supplied by terminal branches of the subclavian, vertebral, intercostal, lumbar and internal iliac arteries, the so called segmental or radiculomedullary arteries, the largest of which is the arteria radicularis magna (artery of Adamkiewicz).

Embolisation may be indicated for a variety of hypervascular benign (e.g. haemangioma, aneurysmal bone cyst, osteoblastoma), primary malignant (e.g. chordomas and sarcomas) and secondary malignant spinal tumours (e.g. renal cell carcinoma, thyroid carcinoma and hepatocellular carcinoma) (Fig. 11-23). Pre-operative embolisation is used to reduce tumour size, minimise blood loss during surgery and facilitate radical neurosurgical resection. In patients with unresectable lesions, palliative embolisation of advanced hypervascular spinal tumours may be carried out to relieve pain and improve compressive neurological symptoms. Lately, transcatheter tumour chemoembolisation has been used to combine devascularisation and ischaemia with delivery of regional chemotherapy. In selected occasions, serial arterial embolisation may be offered for curative treatment of certain primary bone tumours such as giant cell tumours and aneurysmal bone cysts.

High-resolution subtraction angiography is critical during spinal embolisation for the identification of the radiculomedullary and spinal arteries. Spinal angiography is performed using routine access from the femoral artery. Non-selective aortograms followed by selective angiograms after catheterisation of the lumbar and intercostal arteries of the affected vertebra and 1–2 adjacent

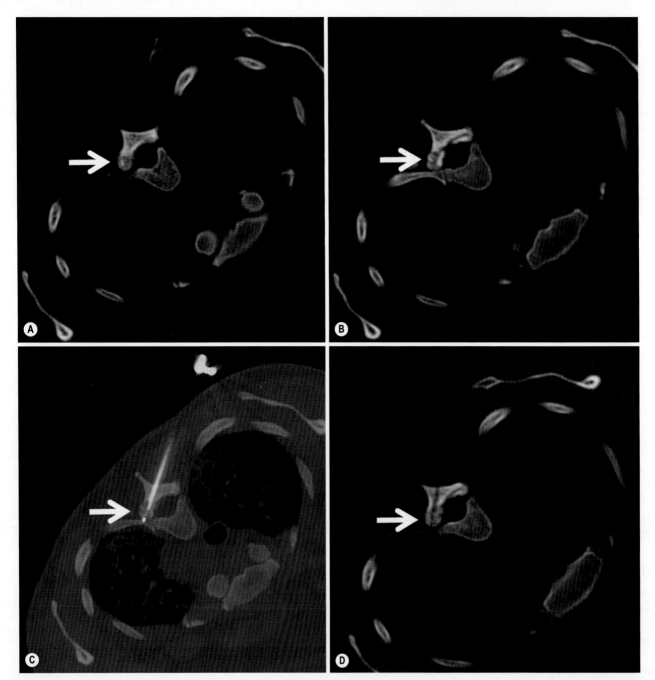

FIGURE 11-22 ■ **Ablation of osteoid osteoma.** (A, B) Painful osteoid osteoma located at the posterior elements of the T4 vertebra. Note the central sclerosis surrounded by a radiolucent area (nidus) (white arrows). (C) CT-guided targeting of the lesion with a beveled trocar to allow for introduction of a non-perfused radiofrequency ablation electrode with a 10-mm active tip (white arrow). (D) Note the needle tract across the lamina after completion of the procedure (white arrow).

segments above and below are obtained. The vertebral, carotid, thyrocervical and costocervical trunks may need to be evaluated in patients with cervical tumours, whereas the iliolumbar and the lateral and medial sacral arteries may provide feeding branches in patients with sacral tumours. Multiple projections may be necessary, but the spinal and radiculomedullary arteries are best identified on an anteroposterior projection. The latter are characterised by a sharp hairpin configuration as they enter the spinal canal and join the spinal arteries. Once the

tumour-feeding branches have been identified and the decision for embolisation has been made, a 3-French microcatheter is advanced co-axially inside the angiographic catheter for superselective embolisation of each feeder without systemic reflux of the embolisation material. Particulate (polyvinylalcohol, PVA, or trisacryl gelatin microspheres), liquid (n-butyl cyanoacrylate, NBA glue) and coils (fibred or non-fibred platinum micro-coils) may be used for terminal tumour devascularisation (Fig. 11-24). Of note, liquid agents may be

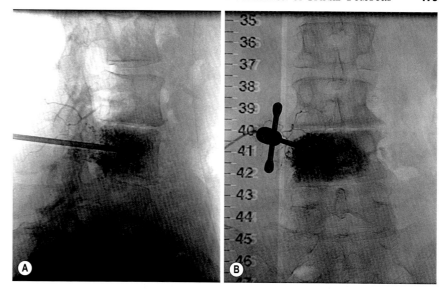

FIGURE 11-23 ■ **Hypervascular tumour.** Transpedicular biopsy of a hypervascular solitary lesion infiltrating the pedicle and most of the L4 vertebral body. Contrast injection through the bone trocar opacifies the extensive tumour neovascularity. Note the retrograde filling of the lumbar arteries at the same level. (A) Lateral and (B) anteroposterior projection.

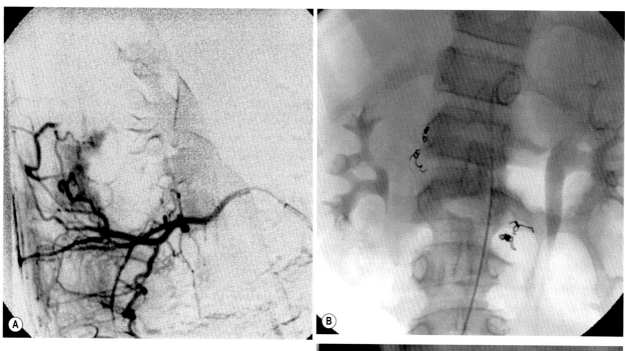

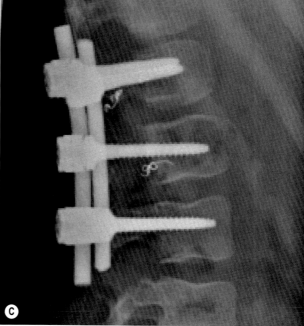

FIGURE 11-24 ■ **Spinal embolisation.** (A) Selective cannulation of the segmental lumbar arteries and angiography in a patient with an aggressive osteoblastoma. Note the hypervascularity of the lesion located at the posterior elements of the lumbar spine. (B) The lesion was embolised with 500 μm PVA microparticles through bilateral lumbar arteries of the same and the overlying level. Micro-coil embolisation was then performed to occlude the major lumbar feeders (anteroposterior view). (C) The patient was operated the following day with minimal blood loss. Note the final outcome after laminectomy and spine fixation of the affected segment. Micro-coils remained in situ (lateral projection).

difficult to control and coils alone are ineffective because they produce proximal occlusion of the segmental branches. However, they are usually used in conjunction with microparticle embolisation to achieve more optimal devascularisation. Coils can also be used to control normal vascular anatomy, i.e. occlude intersegmental anastomoses and prevent non-target embolisation of the cord. Nowadays, 100–500 μm spherical PVA or trisacryl microparticles are preferred because they are controlled and non-absorbable, have homogeneous shape and can penetrate deep into the tumour capillary bed. Microparticle embolisation is performed in each feeder artery under continuous fluoroscopic control applying a slow pulsatile injection until stagnation of flow (near stasis).

A neurologic examination must be performed immediately following successful embolisation to identify potential neurologic deficits. In most cases a mild post-embolisation syndrome characterised by nausea, pain, low-grade fever and elevated inflammatory markers occurs within the first few days because of tissue ischaemia. Neurosurgery should be performed within 1 day of embolisation for reduced intra-operative bleeding, because later tumours are revascularised through collaterals from adjacent levels. In general, the reported success rate of complete tumour embolisation is around 50–80% depending on the morphology of the tumour and the relevant vascular anatomy, and at least a 30–50% reduction in intra-operative blood loss is anticipated. Adequate embolisation of large unresectable spinal tumours has also been shown to provide significant and long-lasting pain relief and improvement of neurologic symptoms. Spinal embolisation is relatively safe, but it carries a low risk of catastrophic spinal cord ischaemia (or stroke when embolisation of cervical tumours is performed) if non-target embolisation of unrecognised radiculomedullary branches occurs. Detailed knowledge of the relevant vascular anatomy and meticulous analysis of subtracted intra-procedural angiograms is vital to avoid complications.

FURTHER READING

1. Katsanos K, Sabharwal T, Adam A. Percutaneous cementoplasty. Semin Intervent Radiol 2010;27(2):137–47.
2. Katsanos K, Ahmad F, Dourado R, et al. Interventional radiology in the elderly. Clin Interv Aging 2009;4:1–15.
3. Sabharwal T, Katsanos K, Buy X, Gangi A. Image-guided ablation therapy of bone tumors. Semin Ultrasound CT MR 2009;30(2):78–90.
4. Kelekis AD, Filippiadis DK, Martin JB, Brountzos E. Standards of practice: quality assurance guidelines for percutaneous treatments of intervertebral discs. Cardiovasc Intervent Radiol 2010;33(5):909–13.
5. Kelekis AD, Somon T, Yilmaz H, et al. Interventional spine procedures. Eur J Radiol 2005;55(3):362–83.
6. Buy X, Gangi A. Percutaneous treatment of intervertebral disc herniation. Semin Intervent Radiol 2010;27(2):148–59.
7. Gangi A, Tsoumakidou G, Buy X, et al. Percutaneous techniques for cervical pain of discal origin. Semin Musculoskelet Radiol 2011;15(2):172–80.
8. Gangi A, Dietemann JL, Ide C, et al. Percutaneous laser disk decompression under CT and fluoroscopic guidance: indications, technique, and clinical experience. Radiographics 1996;16(1):89–96.
9. Rybak LD, Gangi A, Buy X, et al. Thermal ablation of spinal osteoid osteomas close to neural elements: technical considerations. Am J Roentgenol 2010;195(4):W293–8.
10. Gangi A, Tsoumakidou G, Buy X, Quoix E. Quality improvement guidelines for bone tumour management. Cardiovasc Intervent Radiol 2010;33(4):706–13.
11. McGraw JK, Cardella J, Barr JD, et al; SIR Standards of Practice Committee. Society of Interventional Radiology quality improvement guidelines for percutaneous vertebroplasty. J Vasc Interv Radiol 2003;14(7):827–31.
12. Ozkan E, Gupta S. Embolization of spinal tumors: vascular anatomy, indications, and technique. Tech Vasc Interv Radiol 2011;14(3):129–40.
13. Owen RJ. Embolization of musculoskeletal bone tumors. Semin Intervent Radiol 2010;27(2):111–23.
14. Van Zundert J, Huntoon M, Patijn J, et al. Cervical radicular pain. Pain Pract 2010;10(1):1–17.
15. van Boxem K, van Eerd M, Brinkhuizen T, et al. Radiofrequency and pulsed radiofrequency treatment of chronic pain syndromes: the available evidence. Pain Pract 2008;8(5):385–93.
16. van Eerd M, Patijn J, Lataster A, et al. Cervical facet pain. Pain Pract 2010;10(2):113–23.
17. Welch BT, Welch TJ. Percutaneous ablation of benign bone tumors. Tech Vasc Interv Radiol 2011;14(3):118–23.
18. Peh WC, Munk PL, Rashid F, Gilula LA. Percutaneous vertebral augmentation: vertebroplasty, kyphoplasty and skyphoplasty. Radiol Clin North Am 2008;46(3):611–35, vii.
19. Van Boxem K, Cheng J, Patijn J, et al. Lumbosacral radicular pain. Pain Pract 2010;10(4):339–58.
20. van Kleef M, Vanelderen P, Cohen SP, et al. Pain originating from the lumbar facet joints. Pain Pract 2010;10(5):459–69.
21. Benyamin RM, Manchikanti L, Parr AT, et al. The effectiveness of lumbar interlaminar epidural injections in managing chronic low back and lower extremity pain. Pain Physician 2012;15(4):E363–404.
22. Kallewaard JW, Terheggen MA, Groen GJ, et al. Discogenic low back pain. Pain Pract 2010;10(6):560–79.

SUBJECT INDEX

Page numbers followed by '*f*' indicate figures, '*t*' indicate tables, and '*b*' indicate boxes.

Printed in the United States
By Bookmasters